HAND
SPLINTING
ORTHOTIC INTERVENTION

Principles of Design and Fabrication 2nd Edition

JUDITH WILTON

VIVID
PUBLISHING

Copyright © 2013 Judith C. Wilton

ISBN: 978-1-925086-15-7

Published by Vivid Publishing
A division of the Fontaine Publishing Group
P.O. Box 948 Fremantle
Western Australia 6959
www.vividpublishing.com.au

National Library of Australia Cataloguing-in-Publication entry
Author: Wilton, Judith, author.
Title: Hand splinting / orthotic intervention : principles of design and fabrication / Judith Wilton.
Edition: 2nd edition - International
ISBN: 9781925086157 (paperback)
Subjects: Hand--Wounds and injuries--Treatment.
             Splints (Surgery)
Dewey Number: 617.575044

To order further copies or to contact the author, please visit
www.vividpublishing.com.au/judithwilton for further information.

CONTENTS

CHAPTER 2: BIOMECHANICAL PRINCIPLES OF DESIGN, FABRICATION AND APPLICATION

CHAPTER 3: MATERIALS AND METHODS

CHAPTER 7: THE THUMB

CHAPTER 8: ORTHOTIC INTERVENTION AND CASTING IN THE PRESENCE OF NEUROLOGICAL DYSFUNCTION

ABOUT THE AUTHOR

JUDITH WILTON   MSc, PGradDipHthSc, BAppSc(OT) has worked in upper limb rehabilitation as a clincal practitioner and acaedemic since graduating as an occupational therapist over 35 years ago. She currently works in hand therapy private practice, and consults to numerous organisations providing services to clients with neurological disabilities.

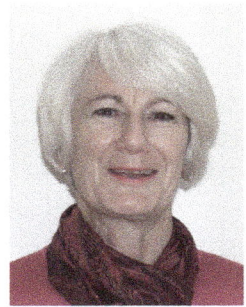

Judith was a member of faculty of Curtin University's School of Occupational Therapy for over 20 years teaching undergraduate and post graduate courses. She established the first Australian university based postgraduate hand and upper limb rehabilitation programme for occupational therapists and physiotherapists. She has published numerous journal articles and presented many courses and workshops on hand therapy and orthotic fabricaton across Australia and internationally.

Judith is an active member of Australian Hand Therapy Association (AHTA) holding numerous executive committee positions including national president. She is responsible for the development and continued presentation of courses on Hand and Upper Limb Orthotic Fabrication conducted by AHTA across Australia. She was awarded life membership of AHTA in 2002.

ACKNOWLEDGEMENTS

I would like to express my thanks to: Simon Garbellini, Helen Fitzgerald and Joelene Colliton who contributed to sections of the text, the therapists who contributed photographs, and the many students and colleagues whose questions and ideas stimulated and challenged my splinting/orthotic practice. I also acknowledge the significant contribution of Terri Dival to the first edition. To Jason Swiney, Vivid Publishing, my grateful appreciation for his patience and expertise in making this book a reality. And finally to my unsung hero David Turner, who faithfully supported and sustained my motivation throughout the writing of this book, my sincere thanks.

CONTRIBUTORS

Joelene Colliton BSc OT, BBA - *Chapter 6*.
Hand Works Occupational Therapy, Perth Western Australia

Helen Fitzgerald BSc OT - *Chapter 3*.
Sir Charles Gairdner Hospital, InHand Occupational Therapy, Perth Western Australia

Simon Garbellini MHlthServMgt, BSc OT - *Chapter 8*. Princess Margaret Hospital for Children, Perth Western Australia

Photographic contributions:
Terri Dival MSc BAppSc(OT)
Helen Fitzgerald BSc OT
Michael Fitzgerald BA, BSc OT
Celeste Glasgow PhD, MSc, BOccThy(hon)
Cathy Merry MHlthSc, BAppSc (PT), CHT
Ceri Pulhman BSc OT
Maryanne Simpson BAppSc (OT)
Stuart Wilson BSc OT

PREFACE

Hand therapy is increasingly recognized as a specialization within the practice of occupational therapy and physiotherapy. *Hand Splinting / Orthotic Intervention: Principles of Design and Fabrication* is intended to be a very practical book for therapists and students who do not have extensive knowledge or experience in this domain of practice. The interchangeable terms splinting/ orthotic intervention; splints, orthoses, and braces refer to therapy practices and devices primarily used in the management of trauma, diseases affecting musculoskeletal systems, principally arthritis, and central nervous system dysfunction. The standardized international terms 'orthosis' and 'orthotic fabrication' have been adopted throughout this edition of the text.

This second edition continues the same format as the first with extensively revised content in all chapters reflecting latest research, theories, practice, techniques, and products. The first section contains three chapters of theoretical and technical information essential to prescription, design and manufacture of upper limb orthosis. Chapter 1 focuses on clinical reasoning to assist the therapist to determine the role of orthotic intervention in optimizing hand function for a given patient or client. The functions of an orthosis – to immobilize, mobilize, restrict or transmit torque– are discussed in relation to healing and disease processes, and the requirements for occupational performance. Chapter 2 addresses the biomechanical principles that pertain to the design of an orthosis, while Chapter 3 provides more technical information about materials, equipment and resources used to manufacture an orthosis.

The second section contains four chapters that address regional orthoses in the elbow and forearm, the wrist and hand, the fingers and the thumb for the conditions of trauma and arthritis. Each of these chapters highlight anatomical features pertinent to orthotic intervention, reference current literature, and describe technical procedures. Orthoses are described according to their function with one or two orthoses identified for more detailed information as to their design and fabrication procedure. It is the desire of the authors that the basic pattern-making and fabrication skills will form the building blocks for competency in design and manufacture of more complex orthoses. It is recommended that these chapters are not read in isolation from the first section.

The third section addresses orthotic intervention and casting in the presence of central nervous system dysfunction. The need for a specific chapter arises in part from the complexity of issues associated with this population and the fact that orthotic intervention is not the usual domain of the neurological therapist.

Whilst many diagnostic specific orthoses are described in the literature, it is not the intention of this book to address orthosis design and fabrication from this premise. Therefore, there are no 'orthotic intervention protocols'. Many excellent resources exist which address the therapeutic processes, including orthotic prescription, involved in the management of specific diagnoses.

In this text, the focus is directed to the orthosis product, however, fabrication of a quality orthosis is only a small part of the total process. Orthotic intervention is a therapeutic modality that can achieve some very specific therapeutic goals in partnership with the patient. Unlike many other aspects of therapy, the evidence of intervention is worn by the client outside the therapy environment. Therefore, the quality of intervention, the competence of the therapist, and his or her skills in prescription, design and fabrication can be judged by the patient, the family, the medical team and others. Confident application of thermoplastic materials to injured or painful hands to fabricate effective orthoses comes with practice.

Judith Wilton

1

ORTHOTIC/SPLINT PRESCRIPTION: CLINICAL REASONING ISSUES

INTRODUCTION

Rehabilitation of the hand is one of the significant challenges for therapists working with persons with disease or trauma affecting the upper limb. Hands, and hand function, are such a vital and demonstrative part of one's body and personality that impairment or disability has serious implications for emotional well-being and performance of occupational tasks. Restoration of, or maximizing potential for, optimum hand function is a common objective of therapy intervention. Orthotic or splinting intervention is an integral part of this therapy. It is but one of many tools used and should not be considered as a separate entity in hand therapy practice.

Clinical reasoning is the thinking and decision-making process associated with clinical practice. The theoretical information that must be synthesized prior to making a decision about the use of an orthosis as an integral part of a therapy regime is extensive.

1

It includes:

1. Knowledge of pathology, anatomy and kinesiology so that the problem presented by the client can be identified.
2. Knowledge of the procedures and practice of therapeutic intervention of which orthotic fabrication is but one modality.
3. Knowledge of the purposes, functions and principles of orthotic design and fabrication.
4. Technical skills and knowledge of orthotic fabrication procedures.

The development of clinical expertise requires knowledge and skill to be used in practice where the unique characteristics of the patient influence decisions made by the therapist. Splinting/orthotic intervention is an integral part of hand therapy practice that may include modalities that address physiological, psychological, functional and vocational domains. A focus to "physiological" components of hand function such as range of motion (ROM), strength, sensibility and coordination will not meet the needs of a patient unless they are used in therapy in the context of the current and future occupational performance demands of the patient. In addition the culture in which the practice occurs will also determine the course of intervention. Factors such as health policy, medical hierarchy, and economics have to be considered.

The focus of this chapter is to provide information that will facilitate clinical reasoning and assist a therapist to determine the role of an orthosis in achieving objectives to optimize hand function for a given patient or client. Issues pertinent to problem identification are addressed prior to identifying the purposes and functions of various types of hand orthoses/splints. The last section focuses upon the patient and their characteristics, which will impact upon the prescribed treatment.

NOMENCLATURE

Various orthoses, braces and splints have been used for many centuries evolving with the emergence of diseases, and changes in medical practice, technology and education. This has resulted in orthosis/splint nomenclature that is extensive, creative and not always helpful to the novice therapist. Orthoses/splints have been labelled by the diagnosis that they address (e.g. Mallet Splint, De Quervain's Splint), others are named after the practitioner who first described the fabrication (e.g. Grainger Orthosis [16], Collello[14]), while others have their own stories to tell (cockup splint, aeroplane splint).

'Orthosis', 'splint' and 'brace' are interchangeable terms used to describe an external device applied to support a body part. Numerous definitions are available however all focus on immobilization, support or restriction of a specific part of the body by the application of an external device made of rigid or flexible materials.

The International Organization for Standardization (ISO) published a 'Prosthetics and Orthotics Vocabulary' in 1998 identifying terms for external limb orthoses.[35] Orthosis is the **true term** for a brace, splint or appliance that is designed and fitted to the body to achieve specific goals related to movement, pain management and functional independence. The term 'splint' applied to upper limb devices has been largely the domain of occupational and physiotherapy practice. Traditionally it was used to describe devices made of low temperature thermoplastic materials used to resolve pain, deformity and or contracture and to facilitate movement and function. The term orthosis is used by Orthotists to describe the devices they fabricate, which are made from high temperature thermoplastic materials primarily for persons with more permanent disabilities. However, the distinction between the professional practice and fabrication materials is now irrelevant with an international definition that resolves around the purpose of the device.

In response to widely variable 'splint' terminology and usage, adoption of the term 'orthosis' by the ISO, major government departments, health insurance providers, hand therapy associations are adopting common nomenclature to describe the majority of hand orthoses fabricated by members. The nomenclature systems adopt some of the basic elements of the ASHT Expanded Splint Classification System.[20] The vast majority of orthoses are articular as they impact upon joint motion, with a separate category for non-articular orthoses. Familiar examples of nonarticular orthoses are the 'tennis elbow

brace' and some fracture braces. The four primary objectives of articular orthoses are immobilization, mobilization, restriction, or transmission of torque. Detailed descriptions of these objectives follow later in this chapter. The final element relates to the extent of the orthosis, whether it is finger, hand, or wrist and hand based. Refer to Appendix.

ASSESSMENT FOR ORTHOTIC INTERVENTION

Whilst many patients are referred to therapy 'for an orthosis/splint', the therapist should acknowledge that the patient has been referred for 'therapy' that in the opinion of the referring doctor, or surgeon, should include the application of an orthosis. As with any other form of therapeutic intervention an evaluation is required. The process and instruments selected by the therapist are determined by the patient, the diagnosis, and the information required.

In the acute phases of injury or disease the therapist is concerned with the anatomy and physiology of tissues involved in the pathology. Knowledge of the mechanism of injury, the surgical intervention, and duration from onset of pathology, will assist in determining the degree of tissue integrity, the response of tissues to the injury, surgery, or disease process, and the stage of the healing process. Function of the hand is evaluated at the level of impairment with determination of joint motion, muscle strength, sensory status, level of amputation, and severity of pain experienced. Good communication between the referring doctor and the therapist will ensure all relevant information is gleaned prior to commencing intervention. This is essential for the formulation of a treatment plan, including the choice of media and modalities. Orthotic intervention is one therapeutic modality that can achieve some very specific goals, but it is rarely used in isolation.

In less acute stages of injury or disease, or in the case of long term disability, the focus of assessment changes from the various tissues of the upper limb, to the accomplishment of tasks undertaken by the patient using the affected limb. While the instruments that quantify or describe hand function at the level of disability are valuable, of equal importance is a discussion with the patient identifying their specific occupational performance priorities and limitations. Disability of the upper limb cannot be assessed with one instrument as the demands that a person places on the hand and arm may vary from fine co-ordination and dexterity to considerable power and endurance. Many instruments are described in the literature to assess occupational performance in activities of daily living (ADL) and work capacity. Input from both patient and therapist must guide clinical decisions in relation to orthotic intervention. Whilst the primary goal of hand rehabilitation is to optimize the patient's ability to function in their environment, it is essential that the assessment is undertaken to ascertain that the orthosis prescribed facilitates and does not hinder this objective. Thus reassessment is necessary following use of the orthosis in usual occupational tasks.

Irrespective of the level of hand function assessed, instruments provide information to identify the need for patient treatment, to evaluate progress of dysfunction or outcome of intervention, to compare the patient's hand function status to the norm, and as a basis of professional communication and accountability. However the quality of the information gathered is determined by the reliability, validity and sensitivity of evaluation instruments used.

On completion of evaluation, the therapist will have identified a number of issues to be addressed. The next stage in the therapeutic process involves prioritizing these and identifying the most appropriate therapeutic interventions to address each one. Orthotic intervention may be the media of choice. One orthosis may address several problems, or in some instances several orthoses may be designed and fabricated. As the patient progresses in rehabilitation, obviously the problems will change along with the objectives and types of orthotic intervention.

The process of assessment, which identifies a potential role for orthoses in achieving the therapeutic objective, must ascertain that the patient's expectations and understanding of the purpose of the orthosis correlate with those of the therapist. This incorporates an understanding of the wearing schedule, application procedures, potential limitations, restrictions and discomfort associated with wear, possible precautions and contraindications. Precautions in the use of orthoses as a therapeutic intervention pertain to the integrity and sensibility of the skin and the viability of the peripheral vascular system, irrespective of the diagnosis.

THE PURPOSE OF ORTHOTIC INTERVENTION

Orthotic intervention may be used to:
1. Immobilize, stabilize or protect tissues in the acute phases of wound healing post injury, surgery, or exacerbation of disease.
2. Immobilize, stabilize or protect tissues when their integrity has been compromised by chronic disease.
3. Protect tissues that are at risk of deformity and contracture subsequent to paralysis or altered muscle tone.
4. Optimize functional use of the upper limb.
5. Substitute for paralysed musculature.
6. Correct deformity.

FUNCTIONS OF AN ORTHOSIS

Identifying that the client requires an orthosis as an integral part of the treatment process, presupposes a knowledge of the purpose and functions of an orthosis. Immobilization, mobilization, restriction and torque transmission are identified as the key functions an orthosis can perform on a body part. Prescription of an orthosis, or orthoses, with one or more of these functions will fulfil the medical requirements for tissue management and the objectives of the patient for recovery of optimal function. This section will consider the key issues pertaining to selection of orthosis function to resolve identified problems in the upper limb. Descriptions of individual orthoses that fulfil these functions are discussed in later chapters.

ORTHOTIC INTERVENTION TO IMMOBILIZE TISSUES

When using orthoses to stop joint motion, and thus immobilize tissues, there is a distinction between those that immobilize tissues to facilitate wound healing and those that allow the tissues to rest in optimal positions to limit pain or support paralysed musculature. The differences pertain to the position of immobilization, and to the duration and frequency of orthosis application.

IMMOBILIZATION FOR REST

The normal resting position adopted by the hand is determined by the bony architecture, capsular length, and the length and resting tone of the intrinsic and extrinsic muscles of the wrist and hand. The wrist is generally positioned between 10°-20° extension with minimal ulnar deviation, the metacarpophalangeal (MCP) joints in 20°- 40° flexion, and the interphalangeal (IP) joints 0°-15°flexion.

The thumb is slightly abducted at the carpo-metacarpal (CMC) joint, and in a few degrees of flexion at the MCP and IP joints. Orthoses designed to rest tissues should adopt a similar position for immobilization (Figure 1). Following injury, or exacerbation of disease, the hand assumes a posture determined by the impact of pathology on the normal tension within the wrist and hand muscula-ture, the degree of swelling in the wrist and hand, and the integrity of the bony, capsular and ligamentous structures. The tendency is for wrist flexion and ulnar deviation, MCP joint extension, proximal interphalangeal (PIP) joint flexion greater than 45°, and slight distal interphalangeal (DIP) joint flexion. The thumb is slightly abducted and extended to a position just lateral to the index finger. This position flattens the normal longitudinal and transverse arches found in the hand, in addition to altering the arches of the thumb. In the presence of paralysis, adoption of this posture will result in significant compromise of function should contracture result and then re-innervation occur or reconstructive surgery be attempted. Regaining motion secondary to contracture associated with this position is most difficult in abduction of the thumb, flexion of the MCP joints, extension of the PIP joints, and flexion of the DIP joints.

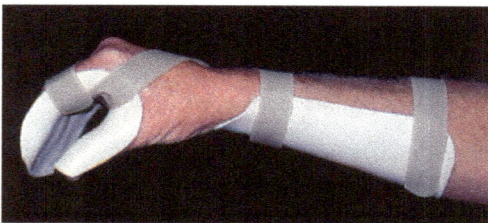

Figure 1: Immobilization of the wrist and hand in a position of rest.

The positions of immobilization of the hand, achieved by orthotic intervention aim to maintain normal anatomical relationships. Deformity is commonly seen following joint and tissue destruction associated with arthritic diseases. Altered biomechanics of the muscles entrench certain positions that may lead to contracture of tissues. Gentle correction of a deformity, whilst immobi-lized in a resting orthosis, can provide pain relief and prevent permanent shortening of tissues. Orthoses that immobilize the hand in the presence of paralysis, or diseases with permanent deformity, are worn for extended periods of time, and thus should position the hand to minimize possible complications associated with loss of length and flexibility of capsular structures and muscle tendon units. Further discussion on immobilization of specific parts of the hand is found in subse-quent chapters.

IMMOBILIZATION TO FACILITATE THE WOUND HEALING PROCESS

Knowledge of the responses of tissue to injury and the physiology of the subsequent wound healing process is the basis for clinical decision making in hand and upper limb re-habilitation. It is also the basis for orthotic design and application. Wound repair, as characterized by the three phases of inflam-mation, fibroplasia, and remodelling, is well described in the literature.[67] The major issue with application to orthotic design and fabri-cation is that of wound strength.

Surgical repair to restore the association of structures can provide stability through various pins, plates, screws and external fixation devices in the case of bone, and strength from suture materials in the case of connective tissues and skin. Immobilization, by casts and orthoses, is a common method used to provide external strength or stability until the tissues have regained sufficient strength to withstand the normal stresses associated with their function. Where immobilization is required post injury or surgery, the position required, along with the duration of immobilization, is determined by the specific pathology of the tissues involved. Thus good communication with the surgeon is necessary.

In the presence of acute inflammation, whether from trauma, surgery or infection, the immediate vascular and cellular response is designed to destroy bacteria and clear the tissue space of dead and dying cells so that repair processes can begin. The wound is predominantly cellular with little inherent strength, owing to lysis of collagen within and at the margins of the wound. The increase in tensile strength that takes place during the fibroplastic phase, beginning 2-5 days post injury, corresponds to increasing amounts of collagen in the wound. This phase consists of fibroplastic proliferation and capillary growth as a result of endothelial cell migration and proliferation. During this period, immobilization helps prevent collagen fibre and capillary disruption, and facilitates the increase in tensile strength of the wound.[57]

Collagen content increases rapidly for approximately three weeks at which time it reaches a plateau as a result of balancing rates of collagen degradation and synthesis. At this time the wound is a single unit with newly synthesized collagen tissue invading all aspects of the wound. Whilst this has advantages for re-establishing integrity and strength, it has serious implications to the free gliding of mobile structures. This 'one wound' concept as described by Peacock[57] results in adhesions between skin and tendon, and tendon and bone that have the potential to severely limit motion. Re-establishment of a gliding function requires motion and stress to be applied to the tissues, so that randomly orientated collagen fibrils uniting all injured structures during the early phase of the healing, become orientated to a structure resembling the pre-injury state. Orthotic intervention is thus combined with other movement modalities designed to gain differential glide between tissue structures. A progressive increase in tensile strength of the wound continues for up to a year.

Wound contraction is an important aspect of the fibroplastic phase designed to close a wound in which there has been loss of tissue. This results from a centripetal force generated by interaction between fibroblasts and the matrix to advance the edges toward the centre of the wound.[32,57] Manipulation of wound contraction remains primarily mechanical via surgery or the use of orthoses or casts to maintain tissues in a lengthened position. Where there is sufficient tissue mobility contraction is not a problem, however deformity may occur if the wound crosses a concave

Table 1

Joint	Resting position	Safe Position (in relation to capsular structures)	Functional Range[#]
Wrist	10°-20° extension	Neutral-10° extension	15°-40° extension
Finger MCP	20°-30° flexion	Greater than 45° flexion	15°-70° flexion
Finger PIP	Slight flexion	0°-10° flexion	0°-60° flexion
Finger DIP	0°-20° flexion	0°-10° flexion	20°-40° flexion
Thumb	Slightly extended & abducted at CMC with slight flexion of MCP & IP	Abduction extension and rotation at CMC, extension of MCP & IP	Abduction and opposition at CMC with slight flexion of MCP & IP

[#] Angle of immobilization will be determined by the patient's requirements in performance of occupational tasks.

or joint surface. A possible end result of the process of contraction is a deficit in passive ROM, flexibility and or differential glide of tissues. Scar contracture is a result of the contractile process occurring in a healed wound and often results in an undesirable fixed rigid scar causing deformity. Where wound contraction is a significant risk, as in the case of burns, the position in which the hand is immobilized in the orthosis becomes critical. The 'position of safe immobilization' a term coined by Boscheinen-Morrin et al.[8] considers the relative length of capsular structures of the MCP, PIP and DIP joints in addition to the ultimate functional demands of the hand requiring length and extensibility of the dorsal skin of the hand.

Orthotic intervention to minimize the complications associated with wound contraction is quite specific to the location of the wound and the tissues involved. When instigating a therapy programme that addresses this issue it is important that all tissues are considered. For example, it might be ideal to maintain the hand in an extended position to maintain full length of palmar skin following palmar burns and skin grafting, however this position will compromise the length of capsular structures of the MCP joints. Thus the clinical decision-making of the therapist demands synthesis of pathology and anatomy to plan an orthotic programme that addresses the unique requirements of the tissues for an optimum healing environment, without compromise of the ultimate functional result. As the strength of the wound increases, the need for continued immobilization declines. The duration of immobilization of injured tissues is directly related to their inherent strength and function. For example skin grafts are immobilized for three to five days whilst bone fractures are immobilized up to six weeks. The maturation or remodelling phase may last for many months. Tensile strength progressively increases with approximately half of normal tensile strength regained by 6 weeks ultimately achieving 80% of the tensile strength that was present initially.[32,63] At this stage the objective of orthotic intervention may change from immobilization to mobilization.

IMMOBILIZATION TO FACILITATE FUNCTION

Orthoses that immobilize joints whilst facilitating functional use of the hand generally address the thumb and/or wrist. Rarely are fingers immobilized. Immobilization of an unstable or painful joint in the position of function commonly used by the patient can increase the potential for involvement of the hand and upper limb in self-care, vocational or avocational activities. The position of immobilization should be determined in consultation with the patient as dominant and non-dominant hands often have different functional requirements. Table 1 provides a summary of positions for immobilization of the wrist and hand.

CONSEQUENCES OF PROLONGED IMMOBILIZATION

The dilemma commonly faced by therapists and surgeons is to protect injured structures long enough to allow them to repair, yet allow motion early enough to avoid the complications of immobilization and / or scarring. Restriction in the ROM of a joint is fundamental to the development of contracture. This restriction may arise from pain, joint destruction or incongruity, wound contraction, immobilization imposed by a cast or orthosis, neurological disorders affecting muscle function, or indeed a combination of several factors.

The effects of immobilization on tissues are well documented.[1,2,18] Akeson et al.[1] summarizes the changes in synovial joints as:

- Proliferation of fibro fatty connective tissue within the joint space that adheres to the cartilage surfaces.
- Formation of adhesions between the folds of the synovial lining.
- Atrophy of the cartilage.
- Disorganisation of the cellular and fibrillar arrangement of the ligaments and their attachment to the bone.
- Generalized osteoporosis of cancellous and cortical bone.

The response of skeletal muscle to immobilization is atrophy with a significant decrease in the rate of protein synthesis, and adaptation to immobilized position with changes in the number and length of sarcomeres.[64,68]

It is not uncommon for the patient to immobilize the injured part and in severe cases, the whole upper limb. When pain is combined with fear complete immobilization of the limb results.

Immobilization of tissues in any orthosis carries some significant responsibilities for the therapist. The benefits of joint rest in terms of pain relief, decreased inflammation, or increasing potential healing must be weighed against the possible adverse functional deficits that may arise secondary to disuse, atrophy and contracture. While immobilization is deemed to be essential to promote optimal tissue healing and length, therapists should make every effort to limit the extent, involving only those joints necessary, as well as duration through appropriate patient education. Figure 2 illustrates the consequences of poor orthotic intervention to rest a hand with pain associated with complex regional pain syndrome.

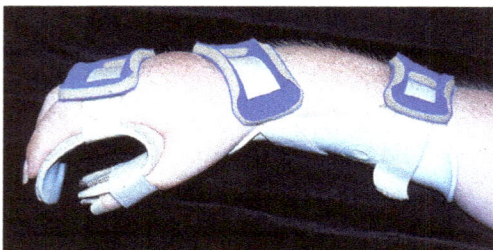

Figure 2: Joint contracture in the position of immobilization and chronic oedema are the consequences of poor orthosis design.

ORTHOTIC INTERVENTION TO MOBILIZE TISSUES

Mobilization orthoses essentially fall into two categories:

1. Those designed to remodel tissue according to it's functional requirements of length and extensibility and address **passive** ROM deficits, which may or may not be associated with active motion deficits, and

2. Those that substitute for weak, paralysed or spastic musculature and address deficits in **active** motion.

The principles underlying the application of the mobilizing force differ in each instance. Traditionally mobilizing splints/orthoses were described as serial static, static progressive or dynamic.[21] All three types of mobilizing orthoses are used to address deficits in passive ROM, with only dynamic designs used to address deficits in active motion.

TYPES OF MOBILIZING ORTHOSES
Serial Static Orthoses (and Casts)

Serial static orthoses are moulded in one position at the end range of the elastic limit of tissues (Figure 3). A period of time is allowed for tissues to respond to the position prior to the orthosis being remoulded, or cast replaced, in the new lengthened position. The therapist has full control of the end range position and therefore the amount of force applied to contracted tissues. Serial orthoses, in the same way as casts, maximize the time tissues are maintained at end range as they are generally worn for periods between 10 and 24 hours per day. The therapist must undertake incremental adjustments at intervals appropriate to tissue response. Serial orthoses and casts are used to address deficits in ROM where a lower force applied for a longer period of time may be preferred, such as persistent joint swelling or where muscle spasticity remains a potential driving force for contracture irrespective of tissue extensibility.

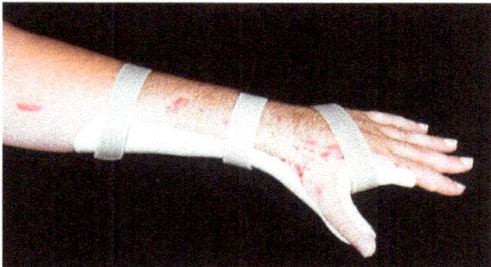

Figure 3: Regaining length and extensibility in the thumb index web, and in wrist extension, is the purpose of this orthosis worn by a patient with severe fractures of the distal radius and ulna.

Static Progressive Orthoses

These orthoses have a static base and the mobilizing component consisting of an outrigger and non-dynamic traction components such as Velcro®, hinges, screws, or turnbuckles (Figure 4). The tissues are positioned at end range of their elastic limit for a period of time. As the viscoelastic components of the tissues respond to the force joint position changes, so the patient must adjust the traction or hinge. Education is critical to encourage vigilance as infrequent adjustments of the traction tension may result in force becoming too low. Similarly limitations are required for the 'over enthusiastic' patient who wants to rush the mobilizing process by adjusting

traction frequently without allowing sufficient time for tissue response. In this type of orthosis active muscle contraction against the mobilizing force is not possible, thereby maximizing time spent at the predetermined joint range.

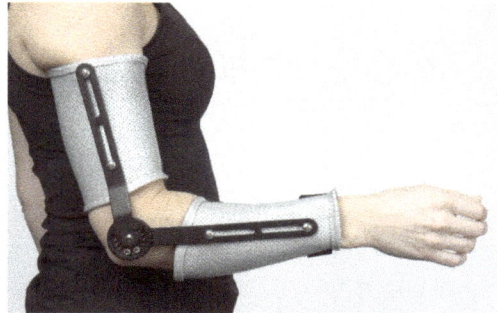

Figure 4: A hinge at the elbow allows the range of elbow motion to be progressively increased as tissues respond to mobilizing force. (Courtesy Michael Fitzgerald)

Static and serial progressive mobilization orthoses eliminate motion of the targeted joints while applying their corrective forces to increase ROM. However, unnecessary prolonged rigid immobilization should be avoided to promote optimal nutrition of tissues and decrease risk of articular surface damage by compression of the involved joint/s.[62]

Dynamic Orthoses

Dynamic orthoses create a mobilizing force on a segment, resulting in passive or passive assisted motion of a joint or successive joints.[20] Orthoses have a static base to secure them to the limb, with the mobilizing component an outrigger and elastic bands, or springs or mechanical devices to create the force (Figure 5).

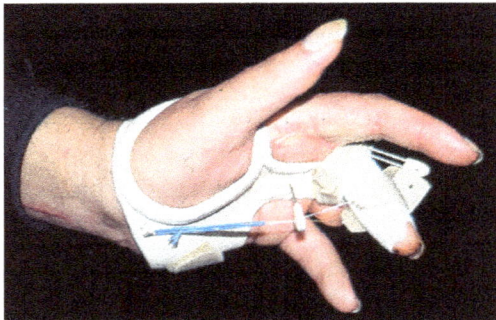

Figure 5: Mobilizing orthosis with elastic traction applied to the finger proximal phalanx in the directions of flexion and extension.

In dynamic orthoses designed to address joint contracture and increase passive ROM there is interplay of forces. The elastic force initiates movement that slows down, and eventually stops by reduction in kinetic energy and or an increase in tissue resistance. The size of the force applied is measured (refer to chapter 3) to ensure that the skin and subcutaneous tissues can tolerate the pressure[65] and the contracted tissues tolerate the torque while not causing trauma to the tissues with associated inflammatory response. The therapist sets the tension in the elastic traction system that continues to apply force when the tissues reach their maximum length. Viscous changes in tissues are generally greatest in the first hour or so then slow throughout the duration of application. Adjustments to traction are not required within a daily period of wear that makes this an ideal mobilizing system when worn during sleep.

Traction tension should be set and measured by the therapist at each treatment session, with patients educated how to make minor adjustments to the dynamic component should it stretch or break between therapy sessions. Active movement against the traction is possible, thereby minimizing risks of sustained tissue compression. However the patient needs to understand that any active movement diminishes time tissues are held at end range.

In some post surgical joint replacement and tendon repair protocols, dynamic orthoses passively assist joint motion through a predetermined range. Active motion is encouraged in the direction opposite the mobilizing force, therefore the dynamic force applied must be sufficient to take joint/s through the range and overcome the resistance of targeted tissues and gravity. The quantity of force applied is determined by the patient's capacity to work with and against the traction to move through the desired ROM and is often greater than predetermined pressure and torque measures used to address passive motion deficits. Dynamic orthoses that facilitate active motion are generally worn during waking hours.

PRINCIPLES OF APPLICATION OF MOBILIZING ORTHOSES TO ADDRESS DEFICITS IN JOINT RANGE OF MOTION

Therapists experienced in the practice of upper limb rehabilitation know from practice that splinting/orthotic intervention is the most efficient method available for improving joint ROM.[5,6,13,20,44,62] Michlovitz et al.[50] in a systematic review of therapeutic interventions used for improving joint ROM reported positive effects of mobilizing orthoses in the management of joint contracture. More recent studies by Glasgow et al.[27,28,29,31] have increased the evidence underpinning use of mobilizing orthoses in the management of joint contracture.

While theory and research findings suggest a high level of evidence for use of mobilizing orthoses in the management of joint contracture, there is little evidence to guide therapist's selection in the type of mobilizing orthoses.[30] Few studies have compared the effectiveness of differing types of mobilization orthoses. Lindenhovius and colleagues[42] identified no differences in contracture resolution following traumatic elbow injuries in persons treated with dynamic orthoses worn 6 to 12 hours a day and those treated with static progressive orthoses worn twice daily for 30 minutes. Similarly Li-Tsang et al[41] found no difference in resolution of extension deficits in finger proximal interphalangeal joints of persons with rheumatoid arthritis following intervention with dynamic or serial static orthoses. However patients in the group wearing dynamic orthoses had better flexion range at the conclusion of six weeks of intervention. Further research is required to determine the most efficient orthosis to administer the ideal 'dose of stress' in terms of amount of force and torque for different upper limb joints and the duration of orthotic wear in hours per day or number of days and weeks. Numerous 'expert opinions' are published in the literature, however until clear evidence exists it is necessary for therapists to base their clinical decisions upon an understanding of the nature of tissue stiffness and contracture and its response to stress.

Nature of Contracture

Many factors contribute to loss of tissue extensibility and joint ROM with few joint and tissue contractures being equal. Diagnosis, specifically the type of tissue injury and potential for healing, the number of tissues involved, and the time since injury strongly influence the nature and potential severity of contracture. Glasgow et al.[28] in a study of 56 MCP and PIP joint contractures found diagnosis was a strong predictor of improvement in active ROM following mobilizing orthotic intervention. Joints with extra-articular fractures made greater progress than intra-articular fractures. In the same study she also found that the shorter the time since injury to mobilizing orthotic intervention, the greater the gains in active ROM.

Tissue Response To Stress

Mobilizing orthoses are used to correct deformity through application of gentle forces, resulting in an increase in passive range of joint motion. In order to safely apply stress, to resolve joint contracture, an understanding of viscous and elastic changes in the extracellular matrix in response to stress is required. Brand and Thompson[10] and Brody[11] describe four phases in the lengthening response of tissues. The initial phase, where fluid in the extracellular matrix moves from the area under tension allowing collagen fibres room to unfold, is followed by gradual alignment of internal elements with the primary stresses. Stiffening of tissue elements occurs when all elements are aligned with the stress. Further incremental increase in stress results in smaller and smaller amounts of lengthening until ultimate failure is caused by internal disruption of the tissue (Figure 6). The focus of mobilizing orthoses is to apply stress in phases two and three.

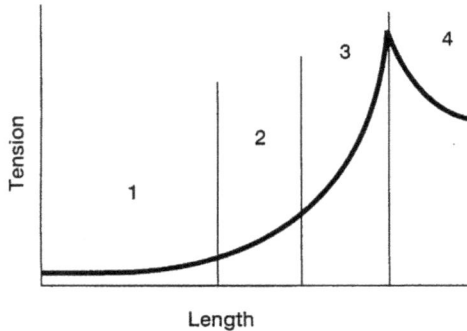

Figure 6: Soft tissue response to applied tension. Phase 1 unfolding, 2 alignment, 3 stiffening and 4 failure.

When the force used stretches tissues beyond their normal elastic limit, microscopic tears of fibres and cells may cause an inflammatory reaction. This inflammation may cause fibrinogen to be laid down resulting in an even greater limitation in motion. Where failure or disruption of tissues has not occurred, their response to unloading will be determined by the nature of the tissue, the proportion of elastic verses inelastic components, and the length of time the force was applied. Recovery of shape and dimension on removal of the force is described as elastic deformation, whilst retention of length and shape is due to the viscous nature of tissues demonstrating plastic deformation.

When safe forces are applied to tissues, either statically or cyclically, they demonstrate a transient lengthening depending upon viscoelastic properties of the tissues. Brand and Thompson[11] note that elongation of tissue accompanied by stretch will shorten again once the force is relaxed. The lengthening that occurs within 24-48 hours is mechanical creep or response to the stretch. Biological creep is the lengthening that occurs in material held under constant load over time. Generation of new tissue or growth occurs over weeks and is associated with the normal turnover of tissue. Thus remodelling in tissues held in a lengthened position, for a period of hours or days, ultimately depends on the ability of the cells to sense and transduce the mechanical force into biological action and grow.[3] Orthoses are an efficient therapy to hold tissues in a lengthened position over the days and weeks required for growth to occur.

Proponents of stretching and orthotic protocols that use the principles of high load of short duration stretch techniques, via bidirectional static progressive orthoses, describe their effectiveness in producing tissue elongation through stress relaxation.[7,45,46,46,66] They propose that short daily periods of orthotic wear-one to three 30-minute treatment sessions per day-are more efficient than using dynamic orthoses to achieve permanent tissue elongation. The mechanism by which tissues gain range in these protocols is not well understood nor underpinned by empirical evidence, but it is thought that stretching the tissue in this way may break some of the bonds between irregularly arranged collagen bundles, which may increase the length of the tissue without causing damage. Protocols like this need careful monitoring to ensure internal disruption of the tissue does not occur.

Diminished stress to tissues associated with loss of capacity to put joints and associated tissues through a full active ROM will contribute to sustaining contracture of traumatic origin. It may also potentiate contracture in diseases such as arthritis and in the presence of neurological dysfunction. The orthotic intervention is not used for a short period with the goal of resolution of contracture, but becomes a longer intervention designed to sustain current range and function with minimization of progression over time.

Measurement of Joint Stiffness

Numerous measures are used to determine severity of stiffness. Historically 'end feel' and Torque Angle Curves (TAC) have been used to determine the type of mobilizing intervention, however recent research has questioned the foundation of these recommendations.

1. Active ROM and Passive ROM

Goniometric measurement of active motion records the patient's 'own effort'. Passive motion requires application of a force to move tissues to end range within the limits of pain. Reliable measures are required.

2. End Feel

Joints that were rated as "springy" are those that when held at the end of available PROM demonstrated further increase in ROM with therapist application of increased manual stretch. In contrast, joints with a "non-springy" hard end feel were those that demonstrated minimal improvement in PROM on therapist application of manual stretch.[13] The expert recommendations that relate type of mobilizing orthosis to the end

feel - dynamic traction be used for joints with springy end feel[12,13,23,25] and non elastic traction for more fixed hard end feel[13,23,25,62] - are not supported by more recent research data.[27, 31, 42, 58] Research findings suggest end feel has minimal relation to speed of resolution of contracture, or to outcome of differing orthotic interventions.

3. Torque Angle Curve

Measurement of torque ROM has been used to determine the mechanical quality of tissues that limit joint motion. This measurement has traditionally been recommended prior to determining the appropriate orthotic intervention for stiff joints.[6,10,23,24,62] Torque ROM (TROM) is a reliable method of measuring a joint with a standard goniometer whilst a known force is used to position the joint.[10,30] Starting at the joint's resting position, higher and higher torque is applied until the joint's end range is reached.[24] A gentle curve is suggested as characteristic of compliant tissues with a 'soft end feel' whilst a steep curve is characteristic of non-compliant tissues with dense parallel collagen fibres and thus a 'hard end feel' to joint motion (Figure 7).

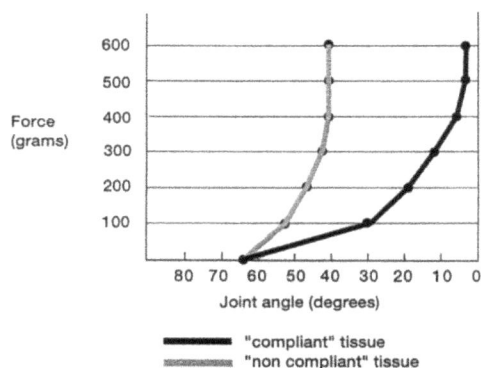

Figure 7: Graph of torque angle measurements for two interphalangeal finger joints.

It has been suggested gentle curves have a good prognosis with dynamic orthoses, while steep curves require static or static progressive orthoses, and very steep curves are more likely to require surgery to resolve the contracture.[12,13,24,25,62,69] However, studies of finger joints by Prosser[58] and Glasgow et al.,[31] found no direct association between torque angle curve and ultimate resolution of contracture following treatment with various types of mobilizing orthoses.

4. Modified Weeks and Wray Test (1973)

This test determines the amount of 'creep' shown in response to an identified sustained force over a period of time. Initially described in 1973 and modified by Flowers[24] it uses a standard passive ROM measure recorded on the unstressed stiff joint prior to application of a thermal modality that allows movement for 20 minutes. This is followed by tolerable pressure applied by the patient at end range of joint motion for 10 minutes. A second passive ROM (preconditioned) is recorded with the difference between the two recordings determining the amount of tissue stiffness. The smaller the change, the greater the stiffness.

Glasgow and colleagues[28] use active ROM, instead of passive ROM, due to greater reliability of the active measure. In a study of 56 stiff finger joints, they found the Modified Weeks Test was a superior measure in predicting improvement in active ROM over TAC and 'end feel', and recommend it should be used in treatment planning.

Intensity And Timing Of Force Application – Dose of Stress

Factors critical in the resolution of deficits in joint ROM are the time of initial application and the intensity and duration of force applied. When deficits in ROM exist, an orthotic programme will minimize long-term deformity. This is achieved by gently influencing the laying down of collagen fibres during the fibroplasia and early remodelling phases of wound healing. The timing of the initial application of stress is crucial as stress applied too early post injury may prolong the inflammatory response, with greater caution required where tissues have not stabilized and fluctuation in oedema still occurs. Similarly stress applied some months post injury may be too late to be effective in resolving contracture in mature scar tissue. Poorer progress has been shown when orthotic intervention has commenced after two to three months post injury.

The total stress used to modify contracture is a product of the force, tension or compression, and the time, duration and frequency it is applied to the tissues. McClure et al.[44] and Flowers et al.[22,26] suggests that therapists consider total stress applied to the tissues as a 'dose' of treatment. An insufficient dose of stress will have no therapeutic effect, while an excessive dose may produce complications such as pain and inflammation.

Brand and Hollister[10] encourage the use of a gentle force for a prolonged period of time to effect permanent changes in length of tissues. While the principle of low load prolonged stress is accepted as the premise of mobilizing orthotic intervention, the quantity of force required to mobilize a deficit in ROM remains unclear. Commonly recommended forces of 100-300 gms for small hand joints[10,20] are based upon the skin and the subcutaneous tissue tolerance to pressure and not the rotational effect of the stress on the actual contracted tissues. Rotational effect or torque is the product of the stress and the distance from the axis on which the stress is applied. Adjusting the force and the distance it is applied from the axis of the joint allows the torque stress to the contracted tissues to be modified, particularly in larger joints.

Kottke et al.[37] investigated the association between time and intensity of force application in addressing chronic joint contractures. They found that prolonged stretching at moderate tension produced significantly greater restoration of motion, within the limits of pain and without evidence of tissue tearing, than did intense stretching of short duration. Kolumban[36] suggested eight to eleven hours per day over an extended time.

Flowers and Michlovitz[23] introduced the term 'total end range time' (TERT) to focus attention on the summation of all the time the joint is held at end range to stimulate growth of tissue. Results from a 24-hour per day casting intervention for PIP flexion contractures by Flowers and LaStayo[22] showed subjects who experienced a TERT of six days showed twice the improvement in PROM than those in the 3-day group. It is worth noting that measurement was recorded

immediately after cast removal with the differences between the two groups being less than 10 degrees.

The directly proportional relationship between increase in passive ROM and TERT identified by Flowers and LaStayo[22] in their *casting* study is not evident in subsequent studies with *mobilizing orthoses,* used for daily intervention periods of greater than 6 hours per day with the observation period extending to many weeks. Prosser[58] observed between 65%-90% of the improvement in PIP joint ROM was achieved within the first two weeks of wearing a dynamic orthosis for between six and fourteen hours per day. The balance of improvement occurred over a period of three to five months.

Glasgow et al.[31] explored the importance of the daily end range time (ERT) in the efficacy of low force mobilizing orthoses for finger joint contracture resolution. They found a daily ERT of greater than 6 hours per day facilitated contracture resolution at a faster rate than a daily ERT of less than 6 hours a day, over four weeks of intervention. However daily ERT beyond 12 hours per day did not result in a statistically significant improvement in active ROM, passive ROM, or torque ROM compared with daily ERT between 6 to 12 hours per day.[27] Many participants assigned to the longer duration of orthosis wear found it difficult to reach their target for more than 12 hours per day suggesting that it may be impractical to expect patients to comply with a daily ERT beyond 12–14 hours.

Further research by Glasgow et al.[27] investigated the long-term relationship between the number of weeks of treatment using a dynamic orthosis and progress with contracture resolution in 48 stiff PIP joints. They found a statistical association between orthosis wearing time and resolution of contracture. While the TERT accrued each week was strongly associated with contracture resolution differences were noted between joint flexion and extension deficits. In the flexion deficit group, with daily ERT of orthosis wear of 6.2 hours, AROM and TROM increased in a linear fashion with minimal improvement in AROM observed after 12 weeks. In the extension deficit group, with daily ERT of orthosis wear of 10.8 hours, slowing of progress with TROM extension was observed after four weeks with continuing slow improvement in both AROM and TROM, during the 17 weeks of treatment. The PIP joint extension deficits were stiffer on average than flexion deficits and appeared to recover more slowly, despite averaging greater daily ERT.

When choosing the time to apply mobilizing orthoses the therapist must consider the client's requirements for functional hand use, the application of therapeutic modalities other than orthoses, and in some cases the number of orthoses incorporated into the programme. While longer daily orthotic use is considered desirable Glasgow et al.[29] found many patients were unable to find sufficient time in the day to wear mobilizing orthoses for longer than 12 hours. Sleep affords the hand an extended period of rest each day and is often an ideal time to apply orthoses. Without the demands for functional use, orthoses can be worn for extended periods of uninterrupted time. Prior to application at night it is important to ensure there are no problems from extended wear during waking hours. It is also important to ensure components such as traction, cannot be inadvertently altered by bedding or poor positioning.

Cessation of orthotic intervention is appropriate when the deficit in passive ROM is resolved and can be maintained by active motion. If a contracture has not resolved, but gains in passive ROM have plateaued, increases to dose variables should be trialled – daily ERT and or intensity of force applied. If changes result in no further gains, gradual weaning from the orthosis is appropriate to ensure passive ROM is not lost. The exception is where active ROM does not sustain passive gains. Intermittent periods of wear may continue, generally at night so that function is not impaired, until stabilization of the wound healing process has occurred; or muscles have regained strength to move through full ROM. Remodelling of tissue can occur for many months and discarding orthoses prior to maturation of the scar tissue is unwise. In some cases this may mean orthoses are worn for several hours per day for many months.

It is accepted the duration of treatment using mobilizing orthoses is a key factor influencing contracture resolution. With few empirical guidelines as to the 'dose of treatment' applied via mobilizing orthoses in terms of intensity of force, and the frequency and duration of application to different upper limb joints, therapists are encouraged to monitor patient responses so adjustments can be made to ensure effectiveness of intervention.

Precautions To Application Of Mobilizing Orthoses

Exacerbation of pain and swelling may be indicators of problems arising from application of mobilizing orthoses. Some discomfort is not uncommon when the mobilizing force is first removed from the tissues, however persistence of pain and discomfort, directly attributable to the orthosis, for periods longer than 10 minutes is indicative that the dose of stress was too great. In this situation manipulation of the force should be considered, adjusting both traction tension and daily ERT. The type of force application via traction, dynamic verses static, may also be a consideration.

ORTHOSES TO RESTRICT MOVEMENT OF TISSUES

Restriction orthoses are those that limit a specific aspect of joint ROM. Restriction of joint motion is used to provide an optimum environment for wound healing and to facilitate functional use of the limb.

RESTRICTION OF TISSUES TO FACILITATE HEALING

Tissues in the hand glide in relation to each other to permit intricate complex movements essential to function. Injury to one structure or system in the hand is rare. Therefore the interrelationship between intrinsic and extrinsic structures requiring different excursion will be affected if complete immobilization of the hand is undertaken in order to allow one or several structures to heal. Maintenance of gliding will only happen if controlled motion is allowed minimizing the possibility of one wound resulting in one scar. Studies have shown that early motion increases the tensile strength in repaired tendons[63] and speeds repair of cartilage.[59] Orthoses used following tendon repairs fall into this category. Finger or thumb movement is restricted in one ROM so that undue stress is not placed on the tendon repairs. Secondary joints, such as the wrist, are commonly immobilized.

RESTRICTION OF TISSUES TO FACILITATE FUNCTION

Problems associated with rigidity, compromise of some aspects of hand function, and the discomfort from orthoses made of thermoplastic materials, have lead to increased availability of a wide range of 'soft' orthoses. Custom made and prefabricated orthoses in elastic, neoprene or leather materials provide tissue constraint and support. Complete immobilization of joints and tissues is not possible due to the nature of materials but restricting the motion of the joint to prevent instability or pain at extremes of movement will increase functional potential. Comfort from softer fabrication materials that allow some 'give' often leads to greater acceptance by patients with more chronic conditions.

TORQUE TRANSMISSION ORTHOSES

ORTHOSES TO ADDRESS PARALYSIS

In the presence of paralysis, without joint contracture, orthoses can redirect active motion of non-paralysed muscles to effect motion in target joints. The unique coupling of the wrist and finger musculature in the tenodesis action allows a therapist to design orthoses to facilitate grip and pinch function. The action of the wrist musculature can be harnessed to approximate the fingers to the thumb for pinch, or to extend the fingers for reach. Similarly in ulnar nerve palsy if MCP joint extension is restricted the extensor digitorum communis (EDC) tendons can affect PIP and DIP extension and flexor digitorum profundus (FDP) and flexor digitorum superficialis (FDS) can flex the fingers towards the palm for effective reach and grasp. These orthoses are effective for specific movements with wearing schedules determined by the patient's functional activities. In the presence of paralysis, orthoses are worn until recovery of function occurs by either reinnervation or tendon transfer.

ORTHOSES DESIGNED TO FACILITATE 'EXERCISE'

By restricting movement of proximal or distal joints exercise orthoses adopt this principle of transferring torque along the kinetic chain of extrinsic finger muscles. Torque transmission orthoses can also transfer motion in a transverse direction in the fingers. Movement of an adjacent normal finger, or buddy, can be harnessed to transfer movement to a problematic MCP or PIP joint if the orthosis effectively connects them.

ORTHOTIC INTERVENTION TO FACILITATE FUNCTION

Many orthoses manufactured to specifically facilitate functional use of the hand may be classified within the categories of immobilization, mobilization, restriction or torque transmission. However, there is a group of orthoses designed to facilitate a particular functional task that do not. Orthoses designed to hold a pen, pencil or an eating utensil, to allow control in driving a car, or to isolate a digit to facilitate computer access are commonly used in the presence of permanent paralysis or dysfunction.

PATIENT ISSUES PERTINENT TO ORTHOTIC DESIGN AND FABRICATION

In the majority of therapeutic interventions used to address musculoskeletal dysfunction the therapist has direct control of the procedure. However in orthotic intervention the patient or their carer has the control. If orthotic intervention is to achieve its objectives the patient must wear the orthosis. Consideration of factors unique to the patient, their attitudes, lifestyle and living and working environment, will increase the potential for an optimal outcome. Interactive reasoning, based upon face-to-face communication between the therapist and the patient, will directly influence many aspects of orthosis design. Failure to consider the unique aspects of the patient, and their lifestyle, may jeopardise the success of the very best orthosis.

PATIENT RESPONSIBILITY IN ORTHOTIC INTERVENTION

Immediately following an acute injury, decisions regarding the orthotic design, the fabrication material, and the wearing regime are generally made by the therapist or surgeon, with minimal contribution from the patient. In many instances no choice is offered as the patient is either too sick, or has no experience or foundation upon which to make any decisions about orthotic intervention. The nature of the injury determines the orthosis requirements and wearing regime. The positive effects of the orthosis in facilitating tissue healing are outweighed by the negative impacts such as movement limitations or restricted function. In the acute phases of intervention it is accepted that orthoses may compromise functional performance, with the goal that the result of the intervention will be a better outcome in the future. Communication with the patient is essential to explain the process.

In the presence of lifetime disability however, the patient will have more extensive experience with hand dysfunction and often orthoses, so may identify specific orthotic requirements to facilitate a functional goal.

The patient contributes information on their unique characteristics related to physical, psychological and cognitive attributes, occupational demands and culture. The therapist provides a clear explanation as to the purpose for orthotic intervention, the reasons and rationale for the design, the wearing regime and precautions, the limitations and impact of wearing an orthosis, and the consequences of not wearing an orthosis. McKee and Rivard[47,48] describe this as a partnership between therapist and patient to optimize orthotic intervention outcomes that are important and achievable within the context of the patient's lifestyle. In paediatric settings the family should be included, with both child and family preferences considered in the selection and use of orthotic devices and adaptations. Family members need to understand the underlying mechanisms and potential benefits of the orthosis, so as to ensure that they incorporate its use as a routine part of daily activities. Any negative consequences of use of the devices (e.g. self-image, sleep disturbances, discomfort) need to be "solved" by the treatment team, in partnership with the child and family. Prior to the patient making a decision that orthotic fabrication should proceed it is also imperative that the therapist addresses any disparity between the patients expectations of the orthosis with the capacity of the orthosis to meet those objectives.

A systematic review on adherence to prescribed upper limb orthosis wear identified high rates (75%) in acute conditions[55] with lower rates (between 25% to 65%) for chronic conditions[4]. The literature suggests adherence to orthotic intervention is greater when:

- The benefits of the intervention are immediately obvious. [15,33,34,41,52,53,56,60]
- The therapist provides education to the patient on the benefits and limitations of the orthosis and expected wearing regime.[15,19,38,54]
- The therapist affirms their belief in the positive benefits of orthotic intervention for the patient.[17,19,20,38,40,54]
- The orthosis is comfortable and aesthetically acceptable.[4,18,38,48,52]
- The orthosis makes a difference in a person's life enabling them to pursue valued occupations.[39,48,52,56]
- The family supports the intervention.[55,61]
- Therapists give examples of how other patients have successfully adapted functional activities without compromising the orthotic regimen.[54]

For those patients who are very young, very sick, who have altered levels of consciousness or an intellectual impairment, or who are unable to communicate their response to intervention, the therapist must assume the responsibility for safe application of orthoses. The therapist must involve parents, relatives, or those responsible for the patient's care in decisions regarding orthotic intervention. Education of carers and implementation of strategies that monitor intervention are essential to minimize risk of injury.

Compliance to orthotic intervention has long been considered in terms of obedience, and motivation with the non-compliant patient considered uncooperative. Comfort,

cosmesis, convenience and, thus, usability, are key factors[48,53] to the success of orthotic intervention which is dependent upon the patient wearing the orthosis. Thus it is important that the therapist creates opportunity for review and feedback, and investigates and addresses any reasons for non-adherence to a wearing protocol. Effective communication is essential in this regard.

AGE

Age is also a strong determinant of the type and design of orthosis intervention.

Children

For very young children the challenge is to maximize the effects of orthotic intervention within the context of the child's intelligence and tolerance to therapy. Issues of co-operation during orthosis fabrication can be addressed by establishing the parent's and child's confidence in the process, by having a non threatening environment where tools and the heating pan are not in direct view of the child, by allowing the child to play with the fabrication material and perhaps make an orthosis for a favourite toy (Figure 8) or a parent prior to fabrication. It is important to mould the orthosis right on the first attempt as distressing the child will not facilitate a positive attitude to the orthosis, orthosis wearing, or returning to therapy. Burns, from heated thermoplastic materials and hot water, are a very real risk when fabricating orthoses for very young children. Ideally thermoplastic materials should have a low activation temperature, a quick set up time and a memory, or the ability to be remoulded several times to accommodate for growth.

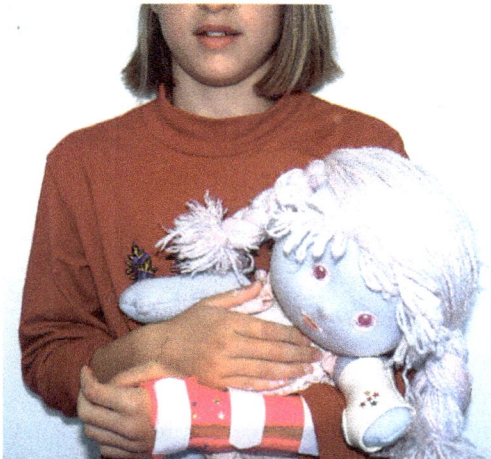

Figure 8: A wrist immobilization orthosis for both child and doll. Decorative features were later added by the child's mother.

Design features specific to children often require:

1. *Inclusion Of More Proximal Joints To Anchor The Orthosis.*

Orthoses need to be more extensive where they are required to protect structures post operatively to eliminate risks of further injury during play. Incorporation of the elbow to anchor an orthosis to the arm is not uncommon. Risks associated with immobilization of uninvolved joints and structures are minimal in this age group.

2. *Use Of Circumferential Designs To Gain Strength And Ensure Good Pressure Dispersion Over Very Fragile Skin.*

Circumferential orthosis designs made of lighter thinner materials (1.6 mm width) use contour to gain strength, disperse pressure and eliminate any risks of straps being applied too tightly. Baby and toddler skin, with its subcutaneous fat, does not tolerate straps well. All straps should be wide and

contour to the area applied. Fabrication of a 'tough' orthosis that is not too heavy or cumbersome, yet able to protect structures during play, will alleviate some of the fears of parents and reduce restrictions necessary for children during orthosis wear.

3. *An Effective Means To Secure The Orthosis To The Limb*

Laced ties and buttons combined with Velcro® may be necessary to impede ingenious and inquisitive little people removing orthoses during unsupervised periods of wear. An orthosis may also be held in place by self-adhesive bandage such as Coban, or a crepe bandage secured by tape. A sock or stocking cover will also provide some degree of protection against the orthosis injuring another body part following spontaneous arm movements.

4. *Incorporation Of Features That Facilitate Compliance To Wearing.*

Special features applicable to the child's age and interests may be incorporated into the orthosis. The use of coloured thermoplastic materials, trims in sporting team colours, decorative transfers or disguises in the form of gloves or puppets, should assist adherence to the wearing regime. However, it is important that features applied to increase compliance do not detract from the use of functional hand orthoses.

Parents and carers of children have a unique role in ensuring adherence to an orthotic wearing schedule; therefore they should contribute to the decision-making processes associated with design and fabrication.

Adolescents

Compliance to orthotic intervention is a major consideration when addressing deformity and dysfunction in the hand of adolescent clients with permanent conditions such as rheumatoid arthritis or cerebral palsy. In this age group body image is particularly important and therefore any form of orthotic intervention must also fit into this schema. Logical reasoning by the therapist based upon long-term gains will not necessarily win out over short-term acceptance within a peer group.

Maintaining hand function and skill for activities with high motivation or interest, particularly those associated with computer technology and games, can provide a persuasive rationale for orthotic intervention.

The first step in the fabrication process is for the patient to make an informed decision that the proposed benefits of an orthosis outweigh the potential feelings of discomfort, inconvenience and self-consciousness. The second step is for the therapist to ensure the aesthetic appearance is acceptable to the patient. The final step is to determine a wearing schedule that is sensitive to the patient's lifestyle whilst still achieving the specific requirements of the intervention.

Elderly

Issues pertaining to orthotic intervention for the elderly are centred on fragility of the skin and it's ability to tolerate stress. With little subcutaneous fat and a slowed healing response, consideration must be given to meeting the objectives for orthotic intervention whilst being fully aware of the risks of loss in function or injury from an orthosis. Where toughness of skin is not maintained by normal functional use of the hand, it becomes very soft and vulnerable to breakdown. In a fisted hand, the lack of airflow around the fingers and thumb maintains a warm moist environment that increases the risks of bacterial and fungal infection. Choice of materials is critical. Perforated thermoplastic materials and washable lining materials are recommended.

Cognitive status is also a critical issue. Orthoses with simple designs, including strapping, and clear written instructions, to assist both the patient and their carer, are often required to accommodate diminished memory and a confused state of mind. Acceptance of change is often difficult for the elderly person so gradual introduction to an orthotic wearing schedule may be necessary in non-acute situations. Modified straps and closures for orthoses may also be necessary for those persons with dementia.

It is recommended that the focus of assessment for orthotic intervention go beyond the hand and upper limb, as many elderly patients have a complex medical history. Whilst the medical problem may not be the focus of orthotic intervention it may have a direct impact upon the design and fabrication. Common examples are diabetes where design features may change in the presence of compromised peripheral circulation and sensibility, or rheumatoid arthritis where immobilization of one joint may place un-acceptable demands on other upper limb joints.[49]

ENVIRONMENT AND LIFESTYLE FACTORS

Consideration of the environment in which the orthosis will be worn will identify those persons who will assume responsibility for application of the orthosis. In an acute setting such as a burns unit it may be the nursing staff, in a school setting it may be a teacher's aide, but in the majority of cases it will be the orthosis wearer. Experience suggests that persons who contribute to the decision making process, who are well informed as to the purpose of orthotic intervention and who are convinced that the therapist believes the orthosis will achieve its objectives, are more likely to be compliant and incorporate it into their usual daily activities. Attitudinal and motivational factors impact upon adherence to orthotic regimes, with experience a powerful influence, particularly for patients with a chronic disability.

For those patients who independently manage their own orthotic programme, the possible functional impact of wearing an orthosis on self-care, mobility, vocational and avocational activities should be discussed. Design should maximize independent appli-cation and accommodate lifestyle demands. Tolerance to moisture and various chemicals, flexibility, friction to accommodate grip on tools and walking aids in the hand are just some of the factors that impact upon choice of fabrication materials.

Musicians and athletes form a unique category of patients due to their motivation to return to their vocation early in the phase of healing. This often demands creative orthotic designs to address both the therapeutic objectives and the performance requirements of the instrument or sport (Figure 9).

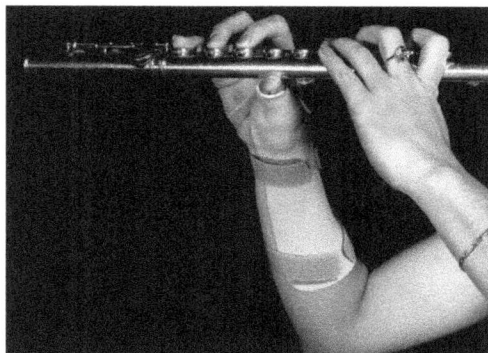

Figure 9

GEOGRAPHICAL AND CLIMATIC FACTORS

The geographical location of the client's home and work will influence the availability for follow-up, and indicate the climatic condi-tions under which the orthosis will be worn. Many of the orthotic protocols, which address deficits in ROM, require regular attendance at therapy for modification to the position of the orthosis, the angle of the outrigger, and the force of mobilizing traction. If distance prohibits regular attendance, the design must accommodate change without loosing effectiveness. Alternatively education of the patient as to how to modify the orthosis com-ponents to accommodate change is possible in selected cases. In environments where care and maintenance of the orthosis may be less than ideal, for example isolated areas such as mining camps, off shore drilling rigs or fishing trawlers, simple orthoses may be a better choice than complex orthoses, due to lessor risks of complications of broken or modified components.

Climate will influence the type of thermoplastic and lining materials selected. Comfort is a major factor in adherence to orthotic protocols; therefore, the need to use perforated thermoplastic materials where heat and humidity are a major issue will dictate the design options. The use of orthosis 'socks' which can be changed and washed regularly will assist in minimizing adverse skin reactions. In the presence of extreme cold, methods to maintain warmth in the hand in the orthosis should be considered.

AESTHETIC FACTORS

Aesthetic considerations are an important issue for a majority of clients. Consider the person you are making the orthosis for; their appearance and care associated with their grooming will give some indication as to their expectations of an orthosis. Essentially the orthosis becomes like an item of clothing. Therefore care should be taken to ensure smooth surfaces and edges on both the thermoplastic materials and the Velcro® with the colours of thermoplastic material, the straps, the finger loops, and lining materials, integrated for an acceptable cosmetic product. An important question for all therapists to answer is *'Would I be prepared to wear in public the orthosis I have just made for my patient?'*

Obviously some designs are 'eye catching' with their function dictating their structure, however the quality of the finished product provides evidence of the skill and craftsmanship in the design and manufacture.

Some light coloured thermoplastic materials do soil with continued use that can impact patient acceptance and wear. Thermoplastic material manufacturers do not recommend cleaning products however a paste of 50:50 glycerine and talcum powder applied to the *orthosis*, left for several minutes, then rinsed off with cool water has been found to be effective.

COST FACTORS

Cost of therapeutic and orthotic intervention is a real consideration for all consumers. Whilst one would wish to provide the best options, cost may dictate the use of less costly materials for orthotic intervention, the use of materials that have a memory and can be remoulded several times, or the use of designs that accommodate several objectives in the one orthosis. Cost should not compromise design or the objectives of the intervention. Prefabricated or commercially made-to-measure orthoses may be perceived to be more expensive, however in some instances the cost savings in reduced consultation time may warrant their use.

The cost of an orthosis that fails to meet its objective is extremely high. Both thermoplastic materials and therapist time are expensive, however the cost incurred by the patient should not be disregarded. When confronted with a problem requiring a complex orthosis beyond the expertise of the primary therapist referral to, or consultation with an experienced therapist competent in orthotic fabrication can be a cost effective solution to the problem.

PATIENT EDUCATION

Education of the patient and carers has been shown to increase participation in therapeutic intervention. Verbal instructions given at the time of fabrication are often forgotten. The event can be quite stressful with the patient coping with a lot of new experiences and a lot of information. Written instructions provide a permanent reminder and allow reference at a later date.

Written instructions should name and state the purpose of the orthosis and include:
1. A wearing schedule for both day and night.
2. Problems or complications that may arise from wearing an orthosis.
3. Precautions when wearing the orthosis.
4. How to care for, clean and maintain the orthosis.
5. How to contact the therapist should problems arise.
6. A date of review appointment.

It is very important to review the provision of an orthosis to determine the effectiveness of the intervention. It will allow the patient and therapist to address and clarify any concerns such as discomfort or pressure, application or wearing issues and maintenance. Review will also determine if the orthosis is being used for its intended purpose and is meeting the clinical objectives.

ORTHOSIS WEARING REGIMES

Wearing regimes are as variable as diagnoses and clients. In determining an initial or ongoing regime the following factors should be considered:
1. The pathology of the effected tissues and acuity of problem.
2. The goal of the orthosis, and on re-evaluation its effectiveness in achieving this goal.
3. The patient's lifestyle with specific focus on self-care, vocational and avocational demands of the involved hand.
4. The number of orthoses in the programme and other therapeutic objectives for active motion and functional performance.

The bottom line to successful intervention is the fact that the patient must participate in the orthotic intervention and wear the orthosis if it is to achieve its objectives. Therefore realistic expectations must be set in conjunction with the patient.

CONCLUSION

Information presented in this chapter underpins clinical reasoning in relation to prescription of orthoses to address dysfunction in the upper limb. Appropriate orthotic intervention is dependent upon a sound knowledge of the functions of an orthosis and the purposes it can achieve. Accurate assessment and determination of the objectives for intervention are the first stages in successful design and fabrication. Whilst the function of the orthosis may be immobilization, mobilization, or restriction of specific joints, the objective may vary widely according to the diagnosis, time from onset of the condition, and the unique qualities of the patient and their requirements for function in his or her upper limb.

Orthotic fabrication for the hand and upper limb presents a constant challenge to the therapist as the unique characteristics of the patient combine with their pathology to determine orthosis requirements. Sensitivity to the patients' needs, their attitudes and lifestyle, and their living and working environment will maximize participation in the therapy interventions and will thus increase the potential for an optimal outcome.

References

1. Akeson WH, Amiel D, Abel M et al. Effects of immobilization on joints. Clinical Orthopaedics and Related Research. 1987;219: 28–37.

2. Akeson WH, Amiel D, Woo S. Immobility effects on synovial joints: The pathomechanics of joint contracture. Bioheology. 1980;17: 95–110.

3. Arem AJ, Madden JW. Effects of stress on healing wounds: intermittent noncyclical tension. Journal of Surgical Research. 1976;20: 275–286.

4. Belcon MC, Haynes RB, Tugwell P. Critical review of compliance studies in rheumatoid arthritis. Arthritis and Rheumatism. 1984;27: 1227–1233.

5. Bell-Krotoski JA. Biomechanics, splinting and tissue remodelling. In: Fess EE, Gettle KS, Philips CA, Janson JR editors. Hand and Upper Limb Splinting Principles and Methods. St Louis:Elsvier Mosby; 2005. p. 103–112.

6. Bell-Krotoski JA. Tissue remodelling and contracture correction using serial plaster casting and orthotic positioning. In Skirven TM, Osterman AL Fedorczyk JM, Amadio P, editors. Rehabilitation of the Hand and Upper Extremity. 6th ed: Philadelphia:Elsvier Mosby; 2011. p. 1599–1609.

7. Bonutti PM, Windau JE, Ables BA, Miller BG. Static progressive stretch to reestablish elbow range of motion. Clinical Orthopaedics Related Research. 1994;303: 128–134.

8. Boscheinen-Morrin J, Davey V, Conolly WB. The Hand Fundamentals of Therapy. 2nd ed. Oxford: Butterworth Heinemann; 1992.

9. Brand P. Thompson DE. Clinical Mechanics. In: Brand PW and Hollister A editors. Clinical Mechanics of the Hand. 2nd ed. St Louis:CV Mosby; 1992. p. 92–128.

10. Brand PW, Hollister A editors. Clinical Mechanics of the Hand. 2nd ed: St Louis:CV Mosby; 1992.

11. Brody GS. The biomechanical properties of tissue. In: Rudolf R. Problems in Aesthetic Surgery. St Louis:CV Mosby; 1986. p. 49–64.

12. Callahan AD, McEntee P. Splinting proximal interphalangeal joint flexion contractures: a new design. American Journal of Occupational Therapy. 1986;40: 408–13.

13. Colditz JC. Therapists' management of the stiff hand. In: Hunter JM, Makin EJ and Callahan AD, editors. Rehabilitation of the Hand: Surgery and Therapy. St

Louis:Mosby 2002 p. 1021–1049.

14. Collelo-Abraham K. Dynamic pronation-supination splint. In: Hunter JM, Schneider LH, Makin EJ, Callahan AD, editors. Rehabilitation of the Hand: Surgery and Therapy, 3rd ed: St Louis:Mosby; 1990 p. 1134–1139.

15. Copley J, Turpin M, Brosnan J, Nelson A. Understanding and negotiating: Reasoning processes used by an occupational therapist to individualize intervention decisions for people with upper limb hypertonicity. Disability and Rehabilitation. 2007; 1–13.

16. Crotchetiere W, Granger CV, Ireland J. The 'Granger' orthosis for radial nerve palsy. Orthotics and Prothetics. 1975;27: 27–31.

17. De Boer IG, Peeters AJ, Ronday HK, et al. The usage of functional wrist orthoses in patients with rheumatoid arthritis. Disability and Rehabilitation. 2008;30(4): 286–295.

18. Donatelli R, Owens-Burkhart H. Effects of immobilization on the extensibility of periarticular connective tissue. Journal of Orthopaedic and Sports Physical Therapy. 1981;3: 67–72

19. Feinberg J. Effect of the arthritis health professional on compliance with use of resting hand splints by patients with rheumatoid arthritis. Arthritis Care and Research. 1992;5: 17–23.

20. Fess EE, Gettle KS, Philips CA, Janson JR. Hand and Upper Extremity splinting: Principles and Methods. 3rd ed St Louis: Mosby; 2005.

21. Fess EE, Philips CA. Hand Splinting Principles and Methods, 2nd ed, St Louis: CV Mosby; 1987.

22. Flowers KR, LaStayo P. Effect of total end range time on improving passive range of motion. Journal of Hand Therapy. 1994;7: 150–7. Reprinted in January 2012.

23. Flowers KR, Michlovitz SL. Assessment and management of loss of motion in orthopaedic dysfunction. Post Graduate Advances in Physical Therapy II-VIII. 1988. American Physical Therapy Association.

24. Flowers KR, Pheasant SD. The use of torque angle curves in the assessment of digital joint stiffness. Journal

of Hand Therapy. 1988;1: 69–74.

25. Flowers KR. A proposed decision hierarchy for splinting the stiff joint, with an emphasis on force application parameters. Journal of Hand Therapy. 2002;15: 158–62.

26. Flowers KR. Reflections on mobilizing the stiff hand. Journal of Hand Therapy. 2010;23: 402–403.

27. Glasgow C, Fleming J, Tooth LR, Hockey RL. The Long-term relationship between duration of treatment and contracture resolution using dynamic orthotic devices for the stiff proximal interphalangeal joint: a prospective cohort study. Journal of Hand Therapy. 2012;25(1): 38–46.

28. Glasgow C, Fleming J, Tooth LR, Peters S. Dynamic splinting for the stiff hand after trauma: predictors of contracture resolution. Journal of Hand Therapy. 2011;24(3): 195–205.

29. Glasgow C, Fleming J, Tooth LR, Peters S. Randomized controlled trial of daily total end range time (TERT) for Capner splinting of the stiff proximal interphalangeal joint. American Journal of Occupational Therapy. 2012;66: 243–248

30. Glasgow C, Tooth LR, Fleming J. Mobilizing the stiff hand: Combining theory and evidence to improve clinical outcomes. Journal of Hand Therapy. 2010;23: 392–401.

31. Glasgow C, Wilton J, Tooth L. Optimal daily end range time for contracture resolution in hand splinting. Journal of Hand Therapy. 2003;16(3): 207–18.

32. Goldberg SR, Diegelmann RF. Wound healing primer. Surgical Clinics North America. 2010;90(6): 1133–46.

33. Groth GN, Wulf MB. Compliance with hand rehabilitation: Health beliefs and strategies. Journal of Hand Therapy. 1995;8: 18–22.

34. Hicks JE. Compliance: A major factor in the successful treatment of rheumatoid disease. Comprehensive Therapy. 1985;11: 31–37.

35. International Standard ISO 8549-1 Prosthetics and Orthotics Vocabulary Part 1. 1st edition 1989. Interna-

tional Organization for Standardization. Switzerland.

36. Kolumban SL. The role of static and dynamic splints, physiotherapy techniques and time in straightening contracted interphalangeal joints. Leprosy in India. 1969;40: 323–8.

37. Kottke FJ, Pauley DL, Ptak RA. The rationale for prolonged stretching for correction of shortening of connective tissue. Archives of Physical Medicine and Rehabilitation. 1966;47: 345–352.

38. Kuipers K, Rassafiani M, Ashburner J, et al. Do clients with acquired brain injury use the splints prescribed by occupational therapists? A descriptive study. NeuroRehabilitation. 2009;24(4): 365–75.

39. Langlois S, Pederson L, MacKinnon JR. The effects of splinting on the spastic hemiplegic hand: Report of a feasibility study. Canadian Journal of Occupational Therapy. 1991;58: 17–25.

40. Law M, Cadman D, Rosenbaum P, et al. Neurodevelopmental therapy and upper-extremity inhibitive casting for children with cerebral palsy. Developmental Medicine and Child Neurology. 1991;33: 379–387.

41. Li-Tsang CP, Kim Hung L, Mak AFT. The effect of corrective splinting on flexion contracture of rheumatoid fingers. Journal of Hand Therapy. 2002;15(2): 185–91. Lindenhovius AL, Doornberg JN, Brouwer KM, et al. Prospective randomized controlled trial of dynamic versus static progressive elbow splinting for posttraumatic elbow stiffness. Journal Bone Joint Surgery. 2012;94A: 694–700.

42. May-Lisowski TL, King PM. Effect of wearing a static wrist orthosis on shoulder movement during feeding. American Journal of Occupational Therapy. 2008;62: 438–45.

43. McClune PW, Blackburn LG, Dusold C. The use of splints in the treatment of joint stiffness. Biologic rational and an algorithm for making clinical decisions. Physical Therapy. 1994;74:1101–1107.

44. McGrath MS, Ulrich SD, Bonutti PM, et al. Evaluation of static progressive stretch for the treatment of wrist stiffness. Journal of Hand Surgery. 2008;33A:1498–1504.

45. McGrath MS, Ulrich SD, Bonutti PM, et al. Static progressive splinting for restoration of rotational motion of the forearm. Journal of Hand Therapy. 2009;22: 3–9.

46. McKee P, Rivard A. Biopsychosocial Approach to Orthotic Intervention. Journal of Hand Therapy. 2011;24: 155–63.

47. McKee P, Rivard A. Orthoses as enablers of occupation: Client-centred splinting for better outcomes. Canadian Journal of Occupational Therapy. 2004;71: 306–14.

48. Mell A, Childress B, Hughes R. The effect of wearing a wrist splint on shoulder kinematics during object manipulation. Archives of Physical Medicine and Rehabilitation. 2005;86: 1661–1664.

49. Michlovitz SL, Harris B, Watkins MP. Therapy interventions for improving joint range of motion: a systematic review. Journal of Hand Therapy. 2004;17:118–30.

50. Minami A. Ligament stability of the MCP joint: a biomechanical study. Journal of Hand Surgery. 1985;10A: 255–260.

51. Nicholas JJ, Gruen H, Weiner G, Crawshaw C, et al. Splinting in rheumatoid arthritis: I. Factors affecting patient compliance. Archives of Physical Medicine and Rehabilitation. 1982;63: 92–94.

52. O'Brien L. Adherence to therapeutic splint wear in adults with acute upper limb injuries: a systematic review. Journal of Hand Therapy. 2010;15:3–12.

53. O'Brien L. The evidence on ways to improve patient's adherence in hand therapy. Journal of Hand Therapy. 2012;25: 247–250

54. Oakes TW, Ward JR, Gray RM, et al. Family expectations and arthritis patient compliance to hand resting splint regimen. Journal of Chronic Diseases. 1970;22: 757–764.

55. Paternostro-Sluga T, Keilani M, Posch M, Fialka-Moser V. Factors that influence the duration of splint wear in peripheral nerve lesions. American Journal Physical Medicine Rehabilitation. 2003;82(2): 86–95.

56. Peacock EE. Some biochemical and biophysical aspects of joint stiffness: Role of collagen synthesis as opposed to altered molecular bonding. Annals of Surgery. 1983;164: 1–12.

57. Prosser R. Splinting in the management of proximal interphalangeal joint flexion contracture. Journal of Hand Therapy. 1996;9(4): 378–86.

58. Salter RB, Simonds DF, Malcolm BW, et al. The biological effects of continuous passive motion on the healing of full thickness deficits in articular cartilage: An experimental investigation in the rabbit. Journal of Bone Joint Surgery. 1980;62A: 1232–1251.

59. Sandford F, Barlow N, Lewis J. A study to examine patient adherence to wearing 24-hour forearm thermoplastic splints after tendon repairs. Journal of Hand Therapy. 2008;21(1): 44–52.

60. Schroder N, Crabtree MJ. Lyall-Watson S. The effectiveness of splinting as perceived by the parents of children with idiopathic arthritis. British Journal of Occupational Therapy. 2002;65: 75–80.

61. Schultz-Johnson K. Static progressive splinting. Journal of Hand Therapy. 2002;15(2): 163–78.

62. Strickland JW. The scientific basis for advances in flexor tendon surgery. Journal of Hand Therapy. 2005;18:94–110.

63. Tabary JC, Tabary C, Tardiue C, et al. Physiological and structural changes in the cat's soleus muscle due to immobilization at different lengths by plaster casts. Journal of Physiology. 1972;224: 231–244.

64. Thompson DE. Dynamic properties of soft tissues and their interface with materials. Journal of Hand Therapy. 1995;8(2): 85–90.

65. Ulrich SD, Bonutti PM, Seyler TM, et al. Restoring range of motion via stress relaxation and static progressive stretch in posttraumatic elbow contractures. Journal of Shoulder and Elbow Surgery. 2010;19: 196–201.

66. Van Der Heyde R, Evans RB. Wound classification and management. In Skirven TM, Osterman AL, Fedorczyk JM, Amadio P. editors. Rehabilitation of the Hand and Upper Extremity. 6th ed. St Philadelphia: Elsevier Mosby; 2011. p. 219.

67. Williams PE, Goldspink G. Changes in sarcomere length and physiological properties in immobilized muscle. Journal of Anatomy. 1978;127: 459–468.

68. Wong JMW. Management of stiff hand: an occupational therapy perspective. Journal of Hand Surgery. 2002;7(2):261–9.

2

BIOMECHANICAL PRINCIPLES OF DESIGN, FABRICATION AND APPLICATION

INTRODUCTION

The science underpinning successful orthotic and splinting intervention is based on engineering principles. Therefore, an understanding of biomechanical principles is essential to successful design and fabrication of any orthosis/splint applied to the upper limb. Biomechanics is the unique marriage of physiology and physics that provides sound principles and a simple explanation to successful application of orthoses. This chapter presents explanations of essential biomechanical principles and their application to orthotic design and fabrication.

Mechanically orthoses can be considered one of two systems – levers that apply three reciprocal forces to affect joint motion in a linear design, or coaptation circuits that apply two opposing forces in the same plane in a circumferential design. The major biomechanical principles to consider are minimization of pressure, advantageous application of forces, and the use of mechanical characteristics of materials. In each section, the concept and

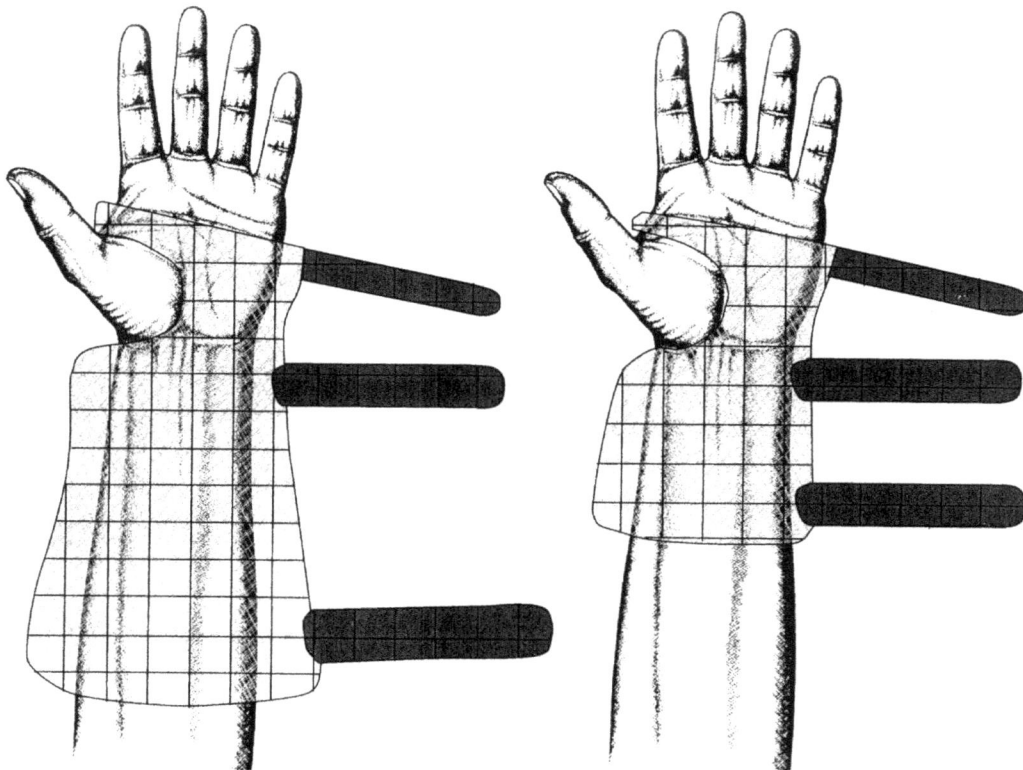

Figure 1: Area of Force Application. Increase the area of force application to decrease the pressure exerted on the tissues of the forearm. The orthosis on the left will produce less pressure than the orthosis on the right.

its relevance are introduced. Biomechanical analysis explains the theory behind the principle. Clinical implications address those considerations the therapist must think about when applying the principle to the patient and his or her pathology. Clinical applications gives readers a summarized list of rules for the principle that shows how to utilize the information when treating a patient.

The dominant action of all orthoses is to apply force to the limb with the intent to position, to move or to prevent movement. Force may be considered as compression (push) or tension (pull). Compression is an issue with all types of orthoses, whilst tension is a critical issue in those orthoses that use mobilizing traction to achieve their effect.

MINIMIZATION OF PRESSURE

One of the prime functions of the hand is to apply force to objects in the performance of self-care, vocational and avocational tasks. Tissues are designed to withstand certain amounts of tension and compression and, indeed, the lack of such forces can result in an alteration in histology of bone, cartilage and connective tissues. High force is commonly transmitted through the skin on the volar surface of the hand and often tissues respond by forming a callous. The dorsal surface of the hand rarely has to withstand much force. The skin is thinner with minimal subcutaneous tissue to disperse the force. Skin over muscle tolerates greater locally applied loads and deformations because the pressure within the tissue is lower than when similar loads and deformation are applied to skin over bone.[16] In the application of force to the hand by an orthosis, compression forces, and therefore pressure, becomes an issue. This is further complicated by the fact that most upper limb orthotic interventions are secondary to trauma with compromised and potentially sensitive tissues. Whilst the focus is on the tolerance of skin tissues to external pressure, vascular tissues must also be considered to avoid compromising arterial and venous supply. Some areas, such as the volar forearm, are better able to tolerate pressure than others.

Compression forces may be applied in many directions to the skin. Those applied perpendicularly (generally referred to as *pressure*) are better tolerated than those applied tangentially (at an angle) across the surface of the skin with a rotational effect on the tissue. These directional forces cause what is commonly termed *shear stress*.

When pressure is applied to the skin a series of events can be observed. There is blanching of the skin due to compression of the microvasculature and occlusion of the venous return.[19] A change in the contour of the surface also occurs depending upon the type, consistency and mechanical properties of subcutaneous tissues. Scar tissue can be rigid and noncompliant compared to normal tissue. Thus when pressure is applied in presence of either an internal or external scar variations in deformation and concentration of stresses need to be considered and managed.[9] Low stress to the skin of short duration is a normal part of living. However, prolonged low stress to the skin results in displacement of the fluids in the tissues and may eventually change capillary flow and ultimately result in ischaemia. Discomfort and pain can also result from sustained or repetitive pressure. On release of pressure, an area of hyperaemia (redness due to capillary blood flow) may exist. Discomfort and hyperaemia are signs of pressure being greater than tissue tolerance.[19] Hyperaemia lasting longer than 15 minutes is evidence of inflammation from pressure.

Repeated pressure has a cumulative effect that may cause a progressive inflammatory change, finally resulting in tissue damage. Brand[4] demonstrated that tissues that responded to stress with minor inflammatory changes one day required less stress for less time the next day, prior to the same response occurring.

BIOMECHANICAL ANALYSIS

Pressure is defined as force per unit area of application, i.e.

Pressure = $\dfrac{\text{Total force}}{\text{Area of force application}}$

Therefore, the larger the area over which a predetermined amount of force is applied the smaller the pressure. One hundred grams of force applied to an area of 1 cm^2 equals 100 gm/cm pressure. The same force applied to an area 2 cm^2 equals 50g/cm pressure. Therefore, when designing an orthosis consider the length and width of the orthosis and its components so that pressure is distributed over a large area (Figure 1 - overleaf). Narrow components of orthoses, including straps, generally apply higher pressure. Following the contours of the hand will ensure an even pressure distribution between convex areas at high risk (commonly bony prominences) and the periphery of low pressure on concave surfaces (Figure 2).

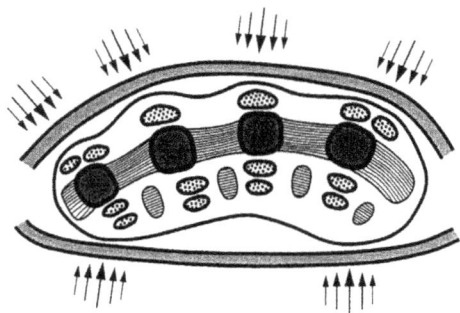

Figure 2: Cross Section Through Hand at Proximal Palmar Crease. The arrows denote areas of potential pressure if the contour of the orthosis does not equal the contour of the hand.

Shear stress occurs when there are large changes in applied stress, particularly at the interface of the hard thermoplastic material edges and the soft underlying and adjacent tissues. Joint movement, changes in muscle bulk associated with muscle contraction or migration of the orthosis with movement can also cause shear stress. To minimize shear, the edges of the orthosis are rolled to ensure a more gradual change in pressure.

Similarly, straps or slings which are not angled to contour to the forearm, hand or finger, can cause shear stress when one edge of the strap or sling lifts away with the sheer stress localised to the other. The same thing occurs if slings used in mobilizing orthoses no longer pull at 90° (Figure 11).

CLINICAL IMPLICATIONS

Pressure is more critical in those areas of the hand that have minimal subcutaneous tissue (fat or muscle) to disperse the pressure. Particular care is necessary in the dorsum of the hand, the heads of the metacarpals, the radial styloid and the ulnar head to ensure even application of pressure. Identify the potential pressure areas on your own hand. Look closely at your patient's hand and assess skin condition, scar pliability, soft tissue extensibility, and joint alignment - all factors that may alter hand shape and contour.

The therapist must consider the patient's pathology, as conditions that increase fragility of the skin increase the risk of pressure from an orthosis and thus the potential to cause

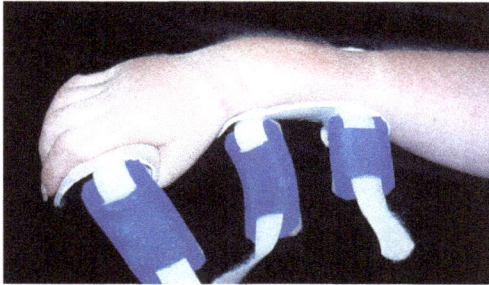

Figure 3: Circulatory Compromise from Strap Pressure. Inattention to presence of pitting oedema has resulted in very obvious circulatory impairment in this patient with Chronic Regional Pain Syndrome. Distribution of pressure over the entire surface by uniform circumferential bandaging would have avoided this complication.

an injury. Pressure can also compromise vascularity, lymphatic drainage (Figure 3), and sensibility.

CLINICAL APPLICATION
1. Assess Tissue Tolerance To Pressure And Shear Stress

Considering all orthoses apply pressure, determine the body part's ability to tolerate stress. Repeated stress resulting in minor inflammation decreases on subsequent application in normal tissues and, therefore, is of greater concern in the presence of denervation, circulatory disorders and oedema, fragile skin (as in the case of the elderly or very young), scar tissue, those persons on steroid therapy or with wounds, grafts or flaps.

It is necessary to ensure no pressure problems exist after an hour of orthosis wear prior to extended wear. Similarly, application of a low force on mobilizing traction, which is subsequently increased with tissue tolerance, is preferable to tissue injury from too great a force.

2. Reduce Pressure - Increase Application Area

Design orthoses, including straps, wider and longer to apply less pressure. In situations where anatomy dictates narrow components, acknowledge that pressure may be problematic.

3. Reduce Pressure - Provide Maximum Contour

Contouring to all skin surfaces increases the area of orthosis contact and, therefore, increases the area of application of force. All orthosis components should contour both convex and concave surfaces of the hand to ensure continuous uniform pressure.

4. Reduce Pressure - Protect Areas Of Risk

Padding is not a solution to a pressure problem. Padding that does not bottom out may mimic subcutaneous tissue, and dissipate and absorb some compression force. However, in areas of high risk, such as bony prominences and scar tissue, padding concentrates and therefore, worsens the risk of pressure. Adding padding over bony prominences only increases the compression by decreasing the space between the tissue and the orthosis. The solution is to pad out the bony prominence prior to orthotic fabrication with a small piece of exercise putty moulded over the prominence. If padding is to be used when there are no areas of risk, it is essential that the padding is incorporated into the design and fabrication, and not added as an afterthought to solve a problem of pressure.

Cutting holes in orthoses is not a solution to a pressure problem. This has the potential to create greater pressure around the edges of the cut out or allow extrusion of soft tissue into the cut out area.

The stabilization of fractures often involves the surgical introduction of external fixation or internal fixation in the form of wires, pins, screws and plates. Care is required to avoid pressure between these components and the orthosis, particularly if part of the orthosis must be cut out to accommodate them. Patients need to be educated to monitor the areas carefully to avoid pressure on both the device and underlying soft tissues as post-operative oedema subsides.

5. Reduce Shear Stress - Avoid Large Sudden Changes In Pressure

Rolling the edges to ensure a more gradual change in pressure reduces the shear effect caused by a sudden change in the pressure gradient at the edge of the orthosis. Sheer stress at the edges of straps and slings is avoided by ensuring contour to the limb or digit. Applying straps at an angle may be necessary to achieve good contour.

ADVANTAGEOUS APPLICATION OF FORCES

An orthosis may be considered a series of related systems of force application. These force systems are easiest to analyse, apply and remember if described by their intended purpose. This must not be confused with the key functions of immobilization, mobilization or restriction that an orthosis performs on a body part (as described in Chapter 1).

The types of forces applied by orthoses to the limb are:

- Stabilizing forces are those forces that are applied to stabilize and secure the orthosis on the limb.
- Manipulatory forces produce a counter-force to oppose gravity, tissue tension or muscle action in order to position, prevent movement or restrict movement.
- Mobilizing forces are dynamic forces that produce movement and allow movement.

The method of application needs to make the best use of the available force. Inherent in this concept is the notion that the most efficient use of force means using the least energy possible to effect change. The use of minimal force reflects the principles of pressure minimization to protect tissue integrity.

1. STABILIZING FORCES

A well-designed stabilizing system prevents migration or rotation of the orthosis on the limb, avoids zones of pressure concentration by the proximal orthosis component and maximizes transmission of force by the orthosis to the targeted tissues. Stabilizing forces provide the base from which manipulatory and mobilizing forces can effectively be created. They must balance and counteract the forces produced internally by the limb and externally by the distal orthosis components to produce a system in equilibrium.

2. MANIPULATORY FORCES

The manipulatory forces are those static forces that direct, control or regulate internal and external forces to produce the desired outcome position. In orthoses that traverse more than one joint, the system must account for movement and position at one joint influencing movement and position of another.

3. MOBILIZING FORCES

Mobilizing forces require a system to generate force (e.g. the traction system), a method of applying or directing this force to the limb (e.g. the outrigger or hinge) and a method of attachment of these to the stabilizing orthosis base.

BIOMECHANICAL ANALYSIS

An understanding of some principles of biomechanics is required at this point. In an effort to create more accessible information, this section will look at the definitions and principles in isolation, remembering in reality the principles are interlinked. The following sections (Clinical Implications and Clinical Applications) will integrate the information.

Newton's Laws

Newton's third law states that to every action there is always opposed an equal reaction. This is the law of interaction, whereby the mutual actions of two bodies upon each other are always equal and directed to the diametrical parts. Thus, where a body part, a lever or an orthosis imparts a force to another, the target will impart an equal force back.

Newton's second law states that acceleration of a body part is equal to the force applied to it. Movement initiated by the orthosis slows down and eventually comes to a stop by a decrease in kinetic energy or by an increase in resistance. This principle has particular application for mobilizing orthoses using traction devices to gain joint motion.

Leverage

A lever is a rigid structure that pivots at a fixed point designed to effect movement. It serves to impart pressure or motion from a force applied at one point to a resisting force at another point. It is a tool used to effect movement. In all types of levers there is one or more manipulatory force, one or more resistive force, and an axis around which these two sets of forces are applied. The lever itself consists of a fulcrum or axis (the pivot point), a force arm (that part between the axis and the applied force) and a resistance arm (that part between the axis and the resistance). In orthotic fabrication, the axis is generally the joint the orthosis is designed to influence. The resistance is the part of the limb to which manipulatory (or mobilizing forces) are directed, and the force is the stabilizing or manipulatory force created by the orthosis.

For simplicity levers are classified depending on the configuration of the force, axis and resistance, but it should be remembered this is purely arbitrary. It is only intended to make analysis of force and mechanical advantage less complicated and should not be the source of pedantic analysis. In any lever, there must be clockwise and counter-clockwise forces around the axis. The same action often can variously be described as a first, second or third class lever, depending on what point is chosen as the axis (Figure 4). The essential element is that all forces and their associated distances are considered in the analysis.

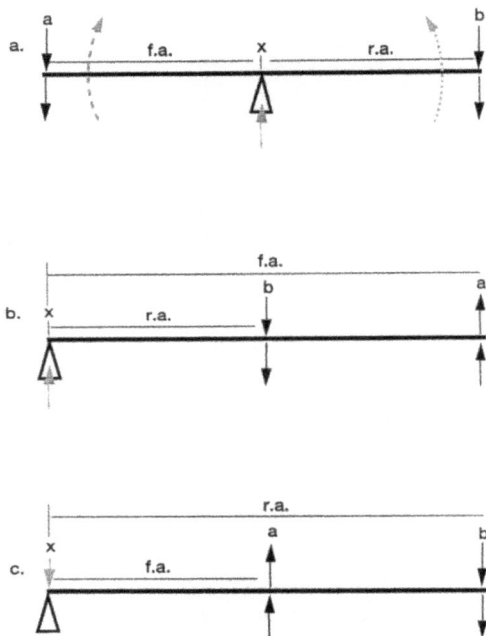

Figure 4: Levers. Illustrations of orthoses acting as levers where x = axis; f = force; r = resistance; f.a. = force arm; r.a. = resistance arm. Solid arrows denote direction of force application; broken arrows denote potential direction of movement. (a) The first class lever has the axis situated between the force and the resistance. (b) The second class lever has the resistance between the axis and the force. (c) The third class lever has the force applied between the resistance and the axis.

In a well-fabricated immobilization orthosis, the forces will always be directed perpendicularly to the longitudinal axis of the body part to be influenced. Resolution of forces is addressed in Advantageous Application of Mobilizing Forces.

The designation of a force does not indicate whether it 'pushes' or 'pulls' at the lever. It is the quantity, point of application and the direction of application that is important.

Systems in Equilibrium

In any leverage situation, the system is said to be in equilibrium when the sum of the clockwise rotational forces equals and balances the sum of the counter-clockwise rotational forces and there is no resultant movement about the axis. These forces are calculated by the equation:

Force x force arm = resistance x resistance arm

$$f \times f.a. = r \times r.a.$$

i.e. force torque = resistance torque

Forces can be applied at any angle to a lever. The force refers to the rotary or perpendicular component of the applied force (refer to Resolution of Forces). The length quantity (f.a. and r.a.) is the distance between the axis and the point of application of force. Where there is force or resistance applied over the whole length of the force or resistance arm, which is usual in immobilization orthoses, the centre of gravity of the lever arm is the point designated to measure length. If the rotary effects are equal, the lever will not move. If one is greater than the other, there will be resultant movement about the axis.

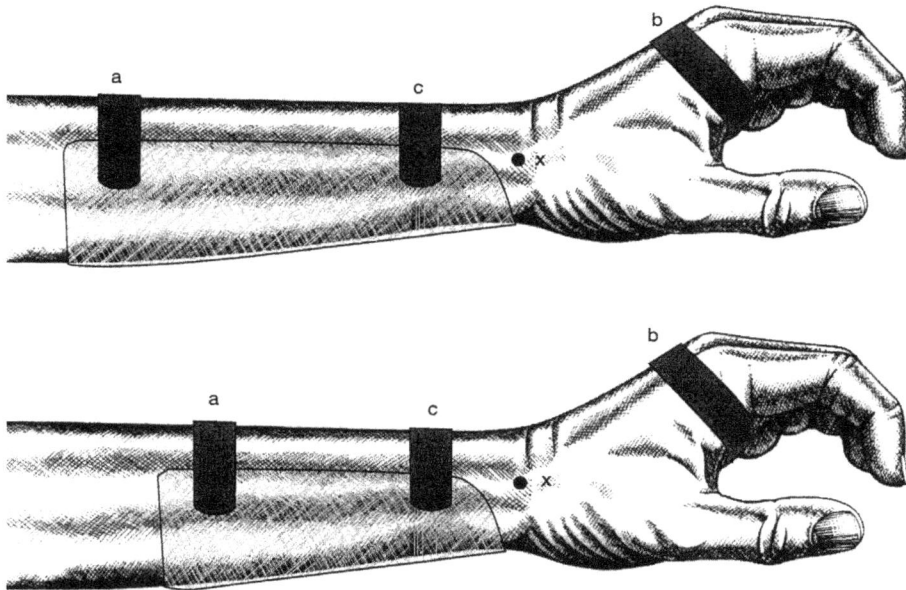

Figure 5: Mechanical Advantage. x = joint axis; a, b, c = positions of force application. Increasing length of the proximal component of a wrist orthosis increases the mechanical advantage.

Mechanical Advantage

Mechanical advantage = $\dfrac{\text{force arm}}{\text{resistance arm}}$

The function of a lever is to produce more efficient work. The intent is to create a mechanical advantage to effect the desired output. The longer the force arm then the greater the mechanical advantage. A long resistance arm signifies mechanical disadvantage (Figures 5 and 6).

Direction of Force Application

Many orthoses applied in the clinical setting utilize three points of pressure arranged in a linear pattern to control or effect joint motion.[8,9,20] The middle force is generally directed opposite to the proximal and distal forces. Generally, one force is directed

to targeted tissues to maintain a position or to increase joint range (Figure 7). The balance of forces is used to control other joints, so that the force is not dissipated by unwanted motion of the more mobile joints or migration of the orthosis with associated shear forces. Orthoses that impact multiple joints may require a series of three-point systems to affect desired action at each joint. Circumferential orthoses use circumferential forces directed inward to a central point and so have no opposing middle force.

In order for the application of force to result in a desired motion or maintenance of position, a reactive force must be applied to ensure the potential work is directed to the target joint axis. Without these reactive forces, unwanted movement will occur, such as motion at joints proximal or distal to the

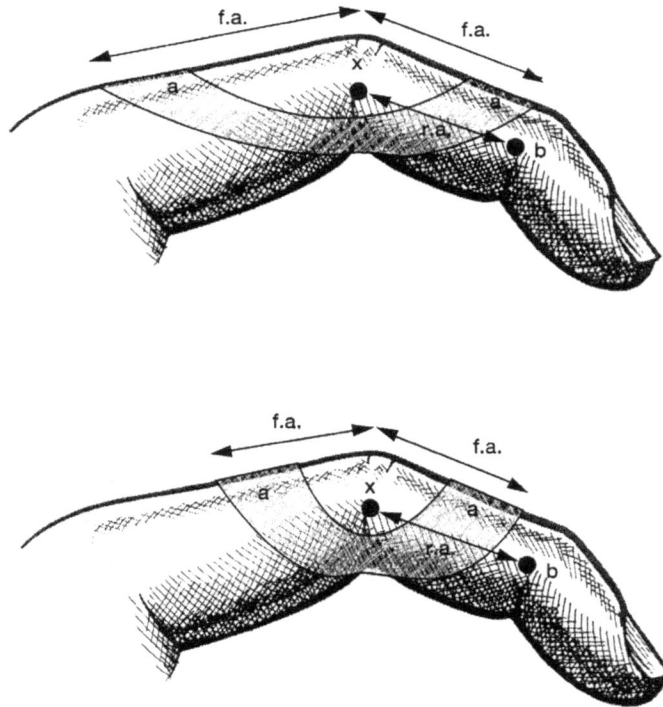

Figure 6: Mechanical Advantage. x = joint axis of proximal interphalangeal (PIP) joint; a = position of force application; b = joint axis of distal interphalangeal (DIP) joint, f.a. = force arm, r.a. = resistance arm. In an orthosis to flex the PIP joint, the proximal and distal components provide the forces to resist the extension force applied through the resistance arm. By lengthening the force arms, less force is required through a to maintain a position of flexion.

target, or rotation around an undesired axis. The system in its entirety must be analysed to determine the most appropriate and the most effective placement of forces. For this reason straps are an integral component of the force application of any orthosis.

Another means of applying force is via a coaptation circuit where two opposing forces are applied in the same plane in circumferential orthoses. When the two forces turn against each other inwards they create pressure which can but used to provide pressure to protect stable fractures, repaired digital pulleys, or increase efficiency of flexion mobilizing orthoses.[20]

Force couples can also produce rotary motion around a point or axis of rotation by acting in opposing directions at separate points around the axis. In forearm mobilization orthoses (see Figure 9 of Chapter 4) forces are applied in opposite linear directions but in the same direction of rotation.

Torque

Torque, defined as the rotational effect of a mechanism, is an essential consideration in mobilizing orthoses. The terms moment or moment of force are also used interchangeably with torque. Torque is the product of the applied force multiplied by the perpendicular distance from the axis of rotation to the line of application of the force.

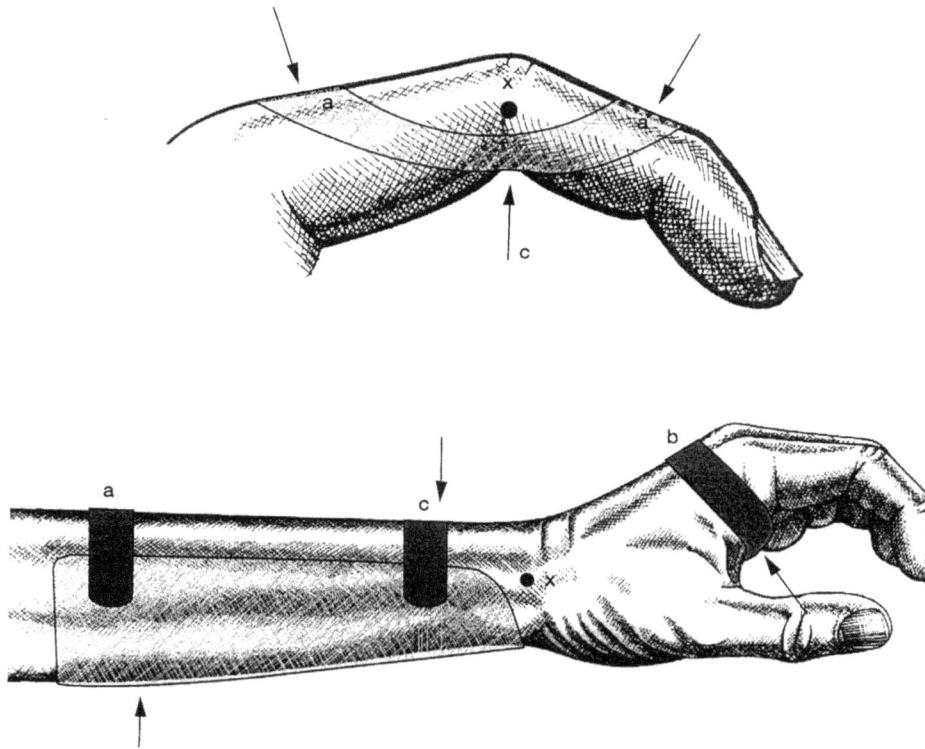

Figure 7: Direction of Force Application. x = joint axis; a, b, c = positions of force application. In order to effect motion or position at the targeted tissues at x, force needs to be applied in the directions designated at a, b and c.

Torque = force x distance

The perpendicular (i.e. shortest) distance from the axis to the line of application of the force is described as the moment arm (Figure 10).

There are three methods to maximize torque:
- Apply greater force.
- Apply force further from the axis.
- Apply force perpendicular to the lever.

Torque effects in mobilizing orthoses are discussed later in this chapter.

Pulley Action

A pulley provides a method of changing the direction of a force to improve its angle of application. It allows a force generated from any means and position to be redirected to the desired target to produce movement in the desired direction or to increase effective rotational force. Outriggers used in mobilizing orthoses are essentially pulleys.

CLINICAL IMPLICATIONS

The therapist must integrate knowledge from a range of sciences to enable them to formulate a logical, comprehensive and complete method of designing the most beneficial orthosis. The difficulty for therapists, particularly students, novices and those who fabricate orthoses intermittently, is to remember all essential aspects of anatomy, kinesiology, biomechanics, pathology and physiology. This section explains a method, or process of thought, which can be followed to integrate and utilize the previously presented information to design a successful orthosis. Therapists must have knowledge of how to approach and solve isolated one-off problems.

Identify Purpose of the Orthosis

Utilising information from Chapter One, determine which is the desired function of the orthosis - immobilization, mobilization, restriction or to transmit torque. For mobilization orthoses it is necessary to further refine purpose in addressing passive or active motion deficits. Consider the normal muscle, gravitational, and pathological forces that impact on the specific joint/s of the upper limb for which an orthosis is required. Determine if one orthosis can achieve the desired purpose.

Identify the Forces Required to Achieve Orthosis Function

To immobilize or restrict a joint it will be necessary to control all forces acting across the joint. Identify what manipulatory and stabilizing forces are required and to what joints or tissues they should be directed. Minimum of three forces are required.

If mobilizing forces are required identify tissues to which they must be directed. All orthoses that create mobilizing forces require a secure base, which is generally some form of immobilization orthosis.

Identify Appropriate Force Placements

Utilising concepts of direction of force application, determine the most effective placement of forces. Consider first the manipulatory and mobilizing forces and then the required stabilizing forces. Using anatomical, kinesiological and functional knowledge, evaluate how the forces are to be applied. Are they to be applied to volar or dorsal surfaces? Are palmar bars, or is dorsal or volar restriction required? Is circumferential force required or can straps apply the required force? The wrist immobilization orthosis demonstrates this dilemma. The choice to achieve this goal includes volar, dorsal, dorsal-volar or circumferential designs. The therapist can only make a decision based on knowledge integrated from a variety of areas.

Generally if an orthosis is to impact on a joint it must traverse it. However, the orthosis may impact on intrinsic forces within the limb that may affect tissues not directly influenced by the orthotic forces. For example, tension in multi-joint muscles may influence joints proximal or distal to the applied orthosis forces. These effects may need to be controlled or, indeed, may be beneficially utilized, by the orthosis forces to achieve the desired outcome.

Design the Application of Manipulatory Forces

The application of manipulatory forces should be considered as a lever system where the axis is the axis of the joint on which the therapist wishes to impact. The resistance is the part of the limb that must be positioned and the force is applied by the orthosis in opposition to the weight or action of that part.

Using principles of mechanical advantage, the longer the force arm the greater the advantage. The length is restricted only by the necessity to protect anatomical function. For example, movement of joints distal to the orthosis must not be compromised.

Principles of minimization of pressure must be addressed. As the length of the force arm at best will still only approximate the length of the resistance arm, large force will be exerted between the force arm (the orthosis) and the resistance arm (the limb). That is, there will be large compression forces on the tissues of the limb. In order to minimize pressure, the force should be distributed over the largest possible area.

Design the Configuration of the Stabilizing Forces

To impact upon a joint, the orthosis must traverse that joint to the proximal region of the limb. This proximal component of the orthosis gives rise to the required stabilizing forces. By virtue of being approximated to the orthosis base by some means (commonly a strap), the joint to which the manipulatory or mobilizing forces are to impact gives rise to a corresponding point on the orthosis base

around which rotary forces are directed. This point becomes the axis of a first class lever.

In order for the system to be in equilibrium, force torque must equal resistance torque. The resistance (the limb), in applying force to the resistance arm, will attempt to rotate the lever around its axis and, in so doing, will rotate the proximal end of the orthosis, or its stabilizing strap, into the limb. The longer the force arm, the lesser the force applied by the limb to the force arm (the proximal orthosis) and at the same time a smaller force is applied by the orthosis to the limb. This becomes an issue of pressure minimization - pressure reduces as the surface area of application increases.

CLINICAL APPLICATION
In summary:

1) Direction of force application has implications for:
   a) Directing forces to targeted tissues.
   b) Creating desired rotary motion.
   c) Preventing undesired motion.

2) Mechanically advantageous levers maximize the force arm length in relation to the resistance arm length to:
   a) Minimize force and pressure on tissues.
   b) Prevent unwanted rotation.
   c) Prevent component failure and material fatigue.

3) Systems in equilibrium have force torque counterbalanced by resistance torque and therefore prevent undesired motion.

ADVANTAGEOUS APPLICATION OF MOBILIZING FORCES

Mobilizing orthosis forces produce motion by applying tension to target tissues. These orthoses can be used to either:

1. Address deficits in *passive* ROM, where static, static progressive or dynamic orthoses apply tension to shortened tissues at the end of available range, or

2. Address deficits in or facilitate *active* motion, where dynamic orthoses apply tension to maintain a joint position from which movement in the opposite direction is allowed or encouraged.

In designing the most beneficial mobilizing orthoses the therapist must consider how to direct the mobilizing force to targeted tissues, the quantity of force to be applied, and duration of that force. For serial progressive and dynamic orthoses there are additional considerations as to the type of outrigger and traction system.

OPTIMIZING ROTATIONAL FORCE AND TORQUE EFFECT

A thorough understanding of how to apply force to optimize rotational and torque effects is essential when designing the outrigger incorporated in mobilizing orthoses. A tension force applied to a body component may be resolved into two components, the rotational force and the translational force. To maximize the rotational force the tension must be applied at 90° to the longitudinal axis of the bone distal to the joint being mobilized.

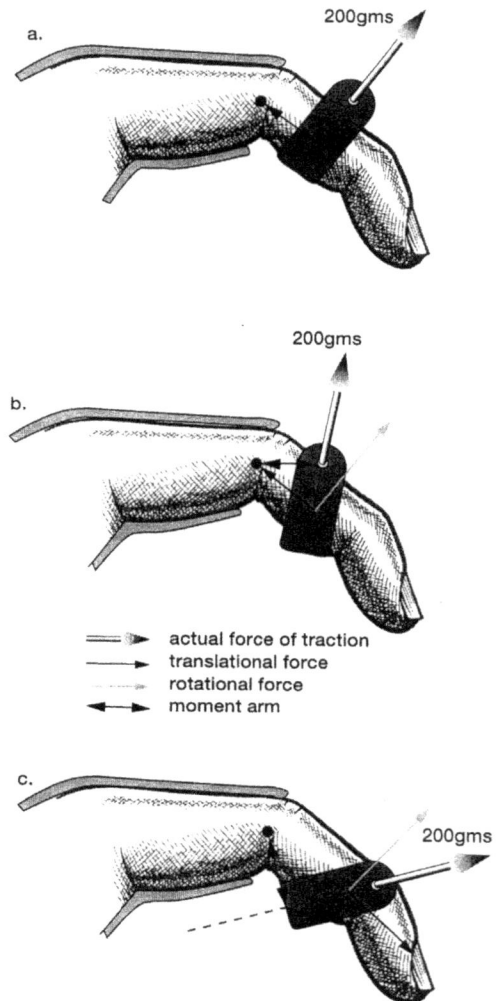

Figure 8: Resolution of Forces. When force is applied to a limb part, it may produce a number of effects on the axis (the joint). With a force designed to extend the PIP joint, the force arm being acted on is the longitudinal axis of the middle phalanx between the PIP joint axis and the point of application of the sling. When the traction force is applied perpendicular to the force arm (a), the length of the moment arm equals the length of the force arm. When the actual force of traction is applied at less (b) or greater (c) than 90°, the moment arm no longer equals the force arm, but is shorter. The traction force is partially resolved into rotational effect, and partially into translational force.

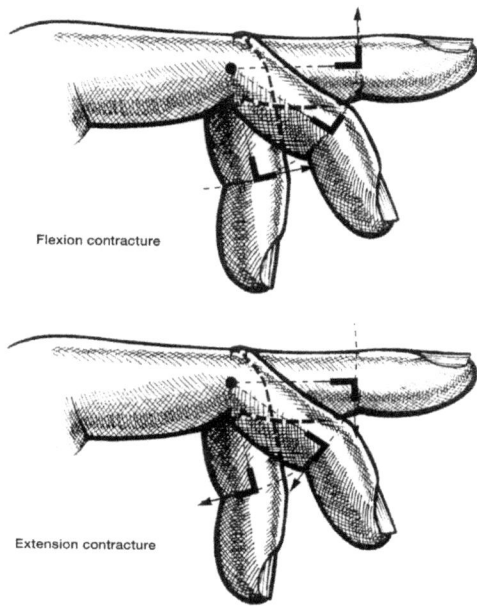

Flexion contracture

Extension contracture

Figure 9: Modification of Angle of Force Application. As force must be applied at 90° to prevent resolution into translational force, it is critical the application angle of traction force is modified appropriately as the joint contracture resolves.

In this situation, all the tension is converted to rotational force, the moment arm is equal to the force arm (Figure 8a). When the tension is applied at an angle greater than 90° some of the rotational force is lost to translational force that will tend to distract the joint. Similarly when the tension is applied at an angle less than 90° some of the rotational force is lost to the translational force that will tend to compress the joint. Where a force is applied at greater or less than 90°, the moment arm is shortened (Figures 8b and 8c) and consequently torque is reduced.

This resolution of forces is demonstrated in Figure 8. Therefore as improvement is made, modifications are required to the outrigger to maintain an appropriate line of pull (Figure 9). The therapist must educate the patient to note the angle of pull and return to the clinic for modification should it not be at 90°.

The outrigger length will also determine torque effect, by varying the distance from the joint axis to point of application of traction sling. Torque is the rotational effect that is applied to the shortened tissues at the joint. Torque is the product of the applied force multiplied by the perpendicular distance from the axis of rotation to the line of application of the force. If the same tension (force) is applied via a sling perpendicular to the lever, the distance from the axis of the joint to the point force is applied will determine the torque. Two orthoses with the same force applied at different distances from the axis will produce different torques (Figure 10). For example 100 grams of force applied 2 cm from the axis of the joint will produce 200 Ncm torque. However, if that force is applied 3 cm from the axis of the joint the torque is 300 Ncm, 150% the original torque. Torque is expressed in Newton centimetres, which indicates that both distance and force are critical issues. Potential to maximize torque is limited in the fingers by the length of the phalanges, however increasing the distance force is applied from the wrist or elbow axes can be a very effective method to increase torque without increasing pressure to the skin.

MECHANICAL RESISTANCE

Resistance is often in the form of oedema or adhesions. In injuries where joint alignment is compromised, periarticular structures produce resistance to normal glide. Where there is mechanical resistance to a mobilizing force attempting to gain ROM in joints, the force will act on the point of least resistance. The force will cause rotation around an inappropriate axis (Figure 11b) unless additional applications of force direct the mobilizing force to the desired joints and restricts mobilization of inappropriate joints (Figure 11c).

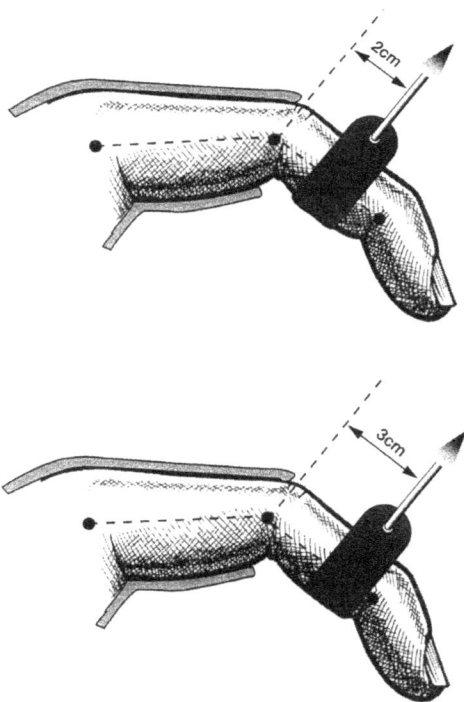

Figure 10: Position of Force Application – Torque Effect. Increasing the distance from the axis that the force is applied will increase torque.

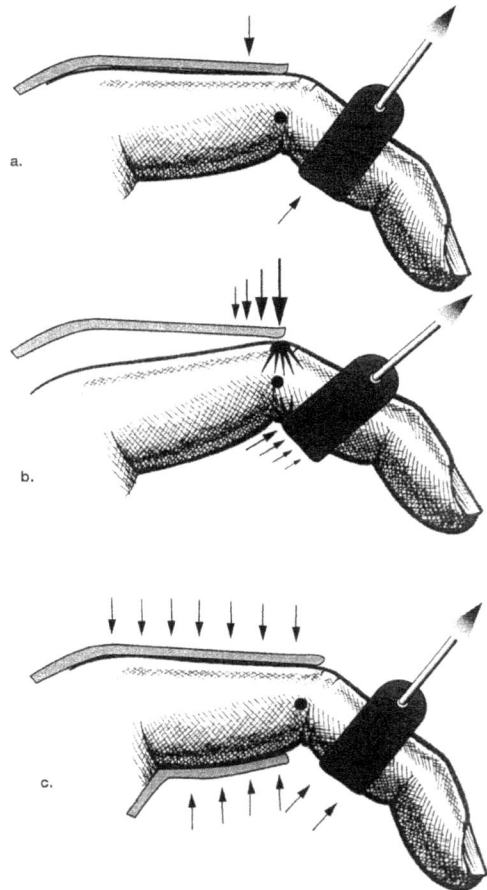

Figure 11: Direction of Application of Mobilizing, Manipulatory and Stabilizing Forces.(a) Perpendicular application of mobilizing force maximizes torque.(b) If forces are only applied at the sling and the dorsal orthosis component (indicated by arrows in a), rotation will occur around an undesired axis (the distal end of the dorsal restrict). Pressure will increase in magnitude towards the proximal edge of the sling and the distal edge of the dorsal component, and shear stress will occur in the finger at those points. The same situation will result when the sling does not pull at 90°, or when there is mechanical resistance at the PIP joint.(c) A reactive (stabilizing) force is required (volar orthosis component) to prevent unwanted movement and direct the applied mobilizing force to the target tissues. Pressure is now evenly distributed along the orthosis components.

OUTRIGGER DESIGN

For static progressive and dynamic orthoses an outrigger is the lever used to direct the traction at the required angle to targeted tissues. The axis is the distal point of anchorage to the orthosis base, the resistance arm is between this point and the sling suspension, and the force arm is the distance between the distal anchorage point and the proximal anchorage point (Figure 12).

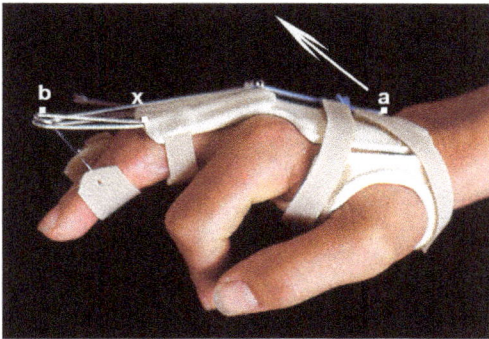

Figure 12; Attachment of the Low-Profile Outrigger to the Orthosis Base. The outrigger and it's attachment is a first class lever (axis at x, force arm at x - a, resistance arm at x - b). When the orthosis is designed with mechanical disadvantage, the downward force at b results in rotation around axis x, and movement in the direction indicated at a.

Although some of the resistance force is absorbed by the traction component, there is still significant resistance applied to the resistance arm (the outrigger) by the part being acted upon. This resistance force must be counteracted by an equal force on the force arm (the orthosis base) to create a system in equilibrium. To create mechanical advantage, the force arm needs to be as long as possible. Where the force arm is short, a system of mechanical disadvantage exists and it is unlikely the outrigger bond or the proximal base will be able to generate enough

force to balance the resistance torque. The result is either the proximal bond fractures, or the orthosis rotates around the lever axis, lifting the proximal base away from the hand or forearm. Design the orthosis with the shortest possible resistance arm and the longest possible force arm. There is no mechanical advantage in putting bends in the extension arms of the outrigger. It makes the outrigger more difficult to fabricate and the bends become potential axes of motion i.e. they are a site of potential fatigue.

Outrigger design should be chosen carefully with specific consideration to the mechanical advantages of the suspension of the traction system. Mobilizing orthoses designed to address passive ROM deficits generally use a low-profile outrigger that uses a pulley to redirect the line of pull, locating the traction along the length of the orthosis. The length and height of the outrigger is determined by pulley position for optimal rotation that can be as low as 1-2 centimetres above the tissues in the case of digits. Frictional drag will occur at traction pulley interface and must be considered when determining the force the traction system will apply.

Outriggers need to be adjusted with gains in passive ROM so that the pulley maintains the perpendicular line of pull of the traction force; otherwise there is a loss of corrective force that is translated to a compression force to the joint. Austin et al.[1] used mathematical modelling to demonstrated minimal differences between changes in line of pull of the traction force from a high as compared to low-profile outrigger with a change in ROM up to 30°. Findings suggest when the angle of applied force deviates from 90° the reduction in the corrective forces is small, however larger shear forces emerge.

High-profile outriggers have a place when the objective is to assist active motion in supple joints in one direction, allowing the patient to move joints in the opposite direction. For example following MCP joint replacement surgery the requirement is for traction to direct MCP joints in extension and radial deviation whilst still allowing motion of the joints into flexion. High-profile outriggers require less strength to oppose traction force than low-profile outriggers.[3,8] In diagnoses where patients are encouraged to move intermittently in the direction opposite to the dynamic traction maintaining the 90° angle of pull throughout the whole ROM is not critical as the force in the traction is augmenting active muscle action to reach a predetermined position. The compression forces associated with large deviations from the 90° angle of applied force are of short duration.

In orthoses designed with high-profile outriggers the *elastic traction component is attached directly to the outrigger* with height determined by the length of the elastic traction required. As high-profile outrigger designs tend to have low patient acceptance due to aesthetics and negative impacts on function; therapists tend to use medium profile outriggers with a pulley and traction directed along the length of the orthosis - a hybrid of the two principles.

PULLEY

In low and medium profile outriggers the outrigger length will determine position of the traction pulley. A pulley provides a method of changing the direction of a force to improve its angle of application. It allows a force generated from any means and position to be redirected to the desired target to produce movement in the desired direction or to increase effective rotational force. Thus force can be generated by either static lines or elastic bands along the length of orthoses which is then redirected via the pulley to the required 90° angle to targeted tissue. The pulley is a high point of friction.

QUANTIFICATION OF FORCE APPLICATION

Numerous authors[2,4,9,11,13] recommend tension forces between 100-300 gm. for the small joints of the hand, with fewer recommendations of around 1,000gm. for the elbow.[7] However this figure relates to the compression force applied to underlying tissues by the mobilizing traction or distal orthosis component, and not the torque applied to the shortened tissues in the vicinity of the joint. The ability of tissue to tolerate this compression is certainly an issue, but critical to clinical efficacy is what quantity of force is translated to joint tissue, and what is the tolerated and beneficial range. Type of tissue to which force is applied is another consideration. It is likely different tissues (ligament, capsule, muscle, tendon, young or old scar) have different beneficial ranges and they respond at different rates to applied forces. Physiological aspects such as vascularity or type and configuration of collagen may also have an influence.

If force is used to elongate tissues beyond their normal elastic limit, microscopic tears of fibres and cells will occur, inducing an inflammatory reaction. Fibrinogen deposition as a result of this inflammation has the potential to create an even greater limitation in motion. More information is needed to determine the safe upper force parameters for tissues, clinical observation and judgement must be used in the meantime.

Orthoses used to address passive ROM deficits either

1. Exert a constant but dynamic tension on the restraining structures to mobilize shortened tissues and gain greater end ROM, or
2. Exert a constant but non-dynamic tension to position tissues at end range so do not allow movement in the direction opposite the traction.

The essential difference between the two types of orthoses relates to the properties of the force application or traction unit and potential for movement. Dynamic traction units are constructed from elastic materials or springs while static progressive units are constructed from rigid inelastic materials such as fishing line, cord, Velcro®, screws or fixed hinges. Chapter one addressed the differences in tissue response to these two types of traction and potential advantages/disadvantages of each. However the therapist determines the quantity of force applied by either type of traction. In both instances quantity

of force required to position tissues at the predetermined position can be measured by using a Haldex® or spring gauge (Figure 13).

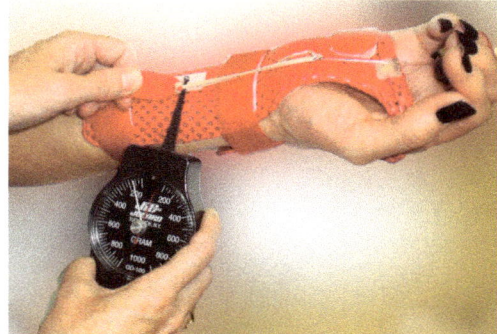

Figure 13: Determining Tension Applied By Traction System. The orthosis is fitted and cuffs positioned appropriately. The required tension is applied via the Haldex® or spring gauge at end of the traction system elongating the elastic band. The tensioned elastic traction is then anchored to the orthosis at that point. (Courtesy Celeste Glasgow).

The dynamic, or force, component of orthoses can be elastic bands or thread, mercery thread (elastic thread with a woven polyester coating that limits over stretching) or springs. These components have two variables, length and tension. Quality and thickness of the material determines its potential to generate tension, while length determines the potential elongation and distance through which tension can be generated.

Determining the right ratio of length to tension in elastic traction components is integral to orthotic design. Selection of an appropriate rubber band and then setting its stretched length are the two critical phases in creating dynamic traction. How to determine force potential of various thicknesses and lengths of elastic bands and thread is discussed in Chapter 3.

Table 1: Summary of Mobilizing Options

	Passive Motion Deficits		Active Motion Deficits
Type of mobilizing force	Dynamic	Serial Progressive	Dynamic
Application of force options	Elastic traction unit or springs. Hinges are used to control joint motion only.	Traction unit non elastic, Velcro®, turnbuckles or hinges used to create force.	Traction - elastic or elastic combined with inelastic components.
Type of Outrigger	Low-profile	Low-profile	High or hybrid profile
Force of Traction	Determined by tissue tolerance to pressure, potential to spread force over large surface and potential to use torque. Fingers 100-300gm Larger joints up to 1,000gms		Determined by resistance of target tissues in achieving desired resting posture, combined with muscle capacity to actively overcome resistance of traction and move into desired position or alignment.

Dynamic components of orthoses are prone to fatigue or failure due to their composition and the manner in which they are used. Hysteresis is the loss of energy that occurs in an elastic material from repeated loading and unloading. Length change from a sustained force may also occur when material quality is poor or the force exceeds the elastic capacity of the material. This is referred to as creep, or deformation under constant load. Elastic bands are prone to creep and therefore require monitoring and adjustment to achieve a consistent force. When structural fatigue occurs, length-tension relationships of materials become inconsistent and are unreliable. Monitoring the stretch' length of elastic bands will ensure correct tension continues to be applied by the orthosis.

There is no literature that provides information on how much torque is required to lengthen a given cross sectional area of living tissue. To date, discussion has focused on the pressure that can be applied to the skin and subcutaneous tissues and then translating this into raw force units. However two orthoses with the same force applied at different distances from the axis will produce different torques (Figure 10). It is therefore torque parameters that must be investigated, not force.

Where the force is applied to move a joint through an arc of motion to substitute for paralysed muscle, or in case of tendon repairs to substitute for the tendon that needs protection, the force is being applied to supple joints. The force applied to the segment need only be sufficient to move the segment to the desired position or alignment overcoming tissue resistance and effects of gravity.

The science of force application in orthotic fabrication remains under investigation. How much force will produce results without risking compromise to tissue integrity or function? How is force measured? How much force actually reaches the targeted tissues?

DURATION OF FORCE APPLICATION

Mobility and flexibility of connective tissues that surround a joint may be affected by pathology associated with disease or trauma, by restricted mobility due to injury to other regions of the limb, or by prolonged immobilization. Connective tissue demonstrates elastic and viscous properties. Elastic properties allow recovery of shape and dimension after deformation. Viscous materials yield continuously under load and do not recover after unloading, commonly referred to as plastic deformation. When a force is applied to connective tissue in order to gain greater motion, some of the elongation occurs in the elastic tissue elements and some in viscous elements. Thus when stress is removed, the elastic deformation recovers whilst plastic deformation remains.[4,5] The stress must be applied for sufficient duration to produce synthesis of new tissue. Lengthening then becomes the result of tissue growth and not just deformation.[6]

Timing of force application therefore becomes a critical issue when mobilizing orthoses are used to correct deformity through the application of gentle forces. These forces cause tissue growth with an associated increase in passive ROM. Flowers and LaStayo[10], Prosser[15] and Glasgow et al.[11, 12, 13] demonstrated an association between duration and intensity of force application and resolution of finger joint contractures. Increased duration, or prolonged moderate tension, is recommended when restoring passive motion in finger joints. High stress short duration loading has a significantly higher risk of exceeding pain limits or producing evidence of tissue tearing. Refer to Chapter One for more detailed information on contracture resolution.

CLINICAL APPLICATION

1. Determine purpose of mobilization orthosis and required components.

Purpose will determine the type and force required in the traction and thus the profile of outrigger. Table 1 provides a summary of outrigger and traction systems required in addressing active and passive motion deficits.

2. Produce Maximal Torque from Applied Force - Ensure Perpendicular Application of Traction from Outrigger

Optimize torque by applying forces at 90 degrees to the long axis of the bone distal to the joint to be mobilized to:

(a) Maximize the length of the moment arm and ensure the total magnitude of the applied force is converted to rotational force.

(b) Prevent loss of force to translational force (joint compression or distraction).

(c) Minimize shear forces on tissues.

3. Manipulate Torque - Modify Distance of Force Application from Joint Axis

Force applied at a greater distance from the joint axis will produce greater torque on the target tissues. This is achieved by adjusting the outrigger length or point of attachment of mobilizing traction. Clinical judgement must be used to determine whether it is appropriate to increase or decrease torque. Increasing the torque allows smaller forces to be applied, particularly where tissues are vulnerable to pressure.

4. Use Pulleys

Pulleys are used to improve force application by adjusting angle of application optimizing rotational force.

5. Apply Appropriate Stresses to Modify Tissues

Mobilizing orthoses apply two types of stress - compression at the site of force application and tension at the site of contracted tissues. The dose of stress, as determined by force applied by traction, spring or hinge must be sufficient to cause a therapeutic effect on the tissues under tension. However, an excessive dose may produce complications such as pain and inflammation, not only in the tissues under tension but also in the compressed tissues at the site of force application.

6. Determine Dose Of Intervention

Maximizing total time spent at end range is the critical principle for lengthening of tissues and resolution of contracture. Identify the hours per day that are available to apply the force to the relevant tissues. The 'dose' of treatment is the summation of the force of the traction system, multiplied by the time the joint is held at end range each day, multiplied by the total number of days intervention is worn. It is determined by tolerance of the patient and the requirement for function or other treatment of the hand.

To date research on finger joints has shown total end range time to be associated with contracture resolution.[10,11,12,13,15] However findings also suggest there is a daily limit to the number of hours patients can find to wear some orthoses.[12,13] Duration of intervention will be determined by resolution of contracture. Therapists need to encourage patient persistence with interventions that often require many months to achieve desired ROM.

UTILIZATION OF MECHANICAL CHARACTERISTICS OF MATERIALS

CONTOUR

Thermoplastic materials are thin and when they are in flat sheets they have little ability to resist bending. By curving and contouring the surface, the mechanical characteristics of the material are changed and it has greater strength to resist externally applied forces. A thin piece of metal may be easily bent if it is levered over a hard object, but if the same piece of metal was turned into a pipe, it is very difficult to bend. In the clinical situation where the material must resist forces applied by the limb to maintain a prescribed position, and where enlarging the orthosis for strength is contraindicated for anatomical or functional reasons, contour is used to provide the necessary strength.

FRICTION

Friction is the force tending to prevent one body or object sliding on another. When a force is applied to an object that attempts to move the object, the force of friction prevents the object from moving (referred to as 'limiting friction'). If the force attempting to cause movement is strong enough, it overcomes the limiting friction and the object moves. Friction continues to operate to oppose the moving force and the objects exert an equal and opposite force on one another (referred to as 'normal reaction'). They do not slide freely they 'rub'. Friction may be beneficial where it prevents unwanted movement or creates traction to enable work. It may be detrimental when it diminishes the efficiency of a machine or when one surface abrades another. There are instances when it is better to increase friction and other times when the aim is to diminish friction. In both instances, it is usually a fine balance between the two to achieve beneficial results.

No surface is completely smooth but has depressions and projections. It is the interlocking of these tiny projections in the surfaces in contact that cause friction. Friction is consequently dependent on the type of surface, the size of surface area in contact, and the normal reaction between the objects (the force holding the two together).

Friction between the orthosis and the limb is useful to prevent the orthosis from migrating and is achieved by increasing the contact surface area (fit and contour) and increasing the normal reaction (for example by applying straps). When forces that attempt to move the orthosis (as may occur when grasping the hand) cannot overcome the friction, the orthosis and skin will move as one and the subcutaneous tissues will be exposed to sheer stress. If there is potential movement it is better to provide an interface between the orthosis and the limb so the movement occurs between the orthosis and the interface. Similarly friction caused by movement of the orthosis on the limb will cause irritation to the skin. An interface layer between the two surfaces can assist in this regard. A removable hand sock will address this need. (This is the same principle as wearing socks with shoes.)

Low-profile outriggers are reported to require up to 40% more strength from the patient than do high-profile outriggers to initiate and maintain active motion opposite to the dynamic assist direction of pull.[14] There is a similar loss in the amount of force that is generated by the dynamic force component that is transmitted to the target tissues. This is directly attributable to frictional drag at the traction system and outrigger pulley interface.[3,14] Loss of force secondary to friction between dynamic components of the orthosis and the outrigger or pulley plays a major role in influencing the amount of distal force applied.[14] Numerous attempts have been made to improve the drag and minimize friction from the traction-pulley interface. It is desirable to use a free and frictionless bar on the outrigger.[2,6] However, cost is a consideration in use of accessories such as wheel pulleys.

MATERIAL FATIGUE

In creating mechanical advantage in orthoses by increasing the length of the force arm (refer to Figures 6 and 7), there is a corresponding increase in the length of the moment arm around 'x' and therefore less force is required to produce a given amount of torque. Orthoses with longer proximal components are more prone to bending and therefore to material fatigue and fracture at the point adjoining the joint axis than are those with short proximal components. As mechanical advantage must not be compromised, the orthosis must be strong enough to withstand this rotational force. In the case of wrist orthoses, this point is also the narrowest part of the orthosis. Contour, including rolling edges, adds the required strength. Reinforcement may be necessary in some materials with low inherent strength.

SUMMARY

The design of successful orthoses is dependent upon a sound understanding of biomechanical principles. Pressure minimization, advantageous application of forces and beneficial use of material characteristics are the critical principles to be utilized.

References

1. Austin GP, Slamet M, Cameron D, Austin NM. A comparison of high-profile and low-profile dynamic mobilization splint designs. Journal of Hand Therapy. 2004;17(3): 335–43.

2. Bell-Krotoski JA, Breger-Lee DE, Beach RB. Biomechanics and evaluation of the hand. In: Hunter J, Makin E, and Callahan A editors. Rehabilitation of the Hand. 4th edn. St Louis:CV Mosby; 1995. p. 153–184.

3. Boozer JA, Sanson MS, Soutas-Little RW, et al. Comparison of the biomechanical motions and force involved in high-profile versus low-profile dynamic splinting. Journal of Hand Therapy. 1994;7: 171–182.

4. Brand PW. Mechanical factors in joint stiffness. Journal of Hand Therapy 1995;8: 91–96.

5. Brand PW, Hollister A. Clinical Mechanics of the Hand, 2nd edn. St Louis: CV Mosby. 1992

6. Brand PW, Thompson DE. Mechanical resistance. In: Brand PW, Hollister A Clinical Mechanics of the Hand. 2nd edn. St Louis:CV Mosby; 1992. p. 92–128.

7. Chinchalkar SJ, Pearce J, Athwal GS. Static progressive versus three-point elbow extension splinting: a mathematical analysis. Journal of Hand Therapy. 2009;22: 37–42.

8. Fess EE. Splints: Mechanics verse convention. Journal of Hand Therapy. 1995;8:124–130.

9. Fess EE, Gettle KS, Philips CA, Janson JR. Hand and Upper Extremity Splinting: Principles and Methods, 3rd ed. St Louis: Elsevier Mosby. 2005

10. Flowers KR, LaStayo P. Effect of total end range time on improving passive range of motion. Journal of Hand Therapy. 1994;7: 150–7. Reprinted in January 2012.

11. Glasgow C, Fleming J, Tooth LR, Hockey RL. The Long-term relationship between duration of treatment and contracture resolution using dynamic orthotic devices for the stiff proximal interphalangeal joint: a prospective cohort study. Journal of Hand Therapy. 2012;25(1): 38–46.

12. Glasgow C, Fleming J, Tooth LR, Peters S. Randomized controlled trial of daily total end range time (TERT) for Capner splinting of the stiff proximal interphalangeal joint. American Journal of Occupational Therapy. 2012;66: 243–248.

13. Glasgow C, Wilton J, Tooth L. Optimal daily end range time for contracture resolution in hand splinting. Journal of Hand Therapy. 2003;16(3): 207–18.

14. Gyovai JE, Wright Howell J. Validation of spring forces applied in dynamic outrigger splinting. Journal of Hand Therapy. 1992;5: 8–15.

15. Prosser R. Splinting in the management of proximal interphalangeal joint flexion contracture. Journal of Hand Therapy. 1996;9(4): 378–86.

16. Sangeorzan BJ, Harrington RM, Wyss CR, et al. Circulatory and mechanical response of skin to loading. Journal Orthopedic Research. 1989;7: 425–431.

17. Sapega AA, Quedenfeld TC, Moyer RA et al. Biophysical factors in range of motion exercise. The Physician and Sports Medicine. 1981;9: 57–65.

18. Strickland JW. Biologic basis for hand and upper extremity splinting. In: Fess EE, Gettle KS, Philips CA, Janson JR. Hand and Upper Extremity Splinting: Principles and Methods, 3rd ed. St Louis: Elsevier Mosby. 2005; p.87–103.

19. Thompson DE. Dynamic properties of soft tissues and their interface with materials. Journal of Hand Therapy. 1995;8: 85–90.

20. Van Lede P, van Veldhoven G. Therapeutic Hand Splints. A Rational Approach. Volume 1. Antwerp:Provan. 1998.

3

MATERIALS AND METHODS

INTRODUCTION

Design and fabrication of orthoses requires a high degree of technical and practical competency. This chapter provides the information necessary to put into practice the skills to build and maintain a competency base. The information presented covers practical issues related to the physical environment and to the materials and equipment used in a fabrication of hand orthoses.

WORKING ENVIRONMENT

In designing an effective working environment (either a new clinic or re-organisation of an existing one), ergonomics, safety and efficiency must be considered.

OCCUPATIONAL HEALTH AND SAFETY

ERGONOMIC DESIGN

The available work area must be designed to allow easy but safe movement from equipment to patient. Very few therapists have the luxury of designing the ideal area, thus design concepts and principles must be successfully incorporated into the available area. The three critical areas of patient, heat source and work area are best organised into a triangular configuration. Secondary areas can be arranged around this plan. Equipment, tools and materials must be positioned to provide easy access and speed of use. All work surfaces should be at ergonomically recommended heights (900 mm for standing, approximately 700 mm for sitting). The width of workbenches should be 450-600 mm, with frequently used tools positioned above the workbench ideally placed between 900 mm and 1500 mm (1800 mm maximum).

The position of the patient and the therapist for fabrication must be considered to maximize comfort and effectiveness (Figure 1). The most common position for application is with the patient's elbow supported on a surface with the elbow flexed and the hand elevated (forearm mid prone). Irrespective of the patient and therapist's position, it is critical that the therapist is at the correct height to work safely on the patient's limb and is able to easily move around the limb (e.g. by mobile stool) to view and work on all aspects of the orthosis.

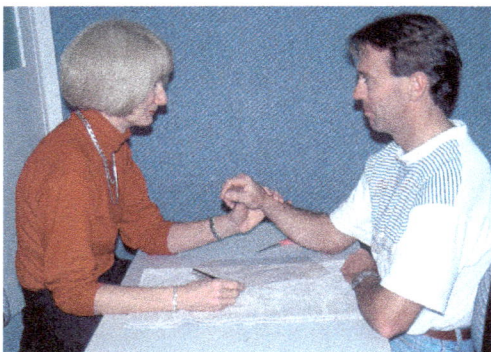

Figure 1: Ergonomic Therapist - Patient Position. The therapist on the left is easily able to examine and treat the patient's upper limb. She is also in an ideal position to communicate with and respond to the patient.

HAZARDS

There are a number of safety hazards in the environment. Close proximity of water and electricity, toxicity of plastics when heated, heat sources and sharp tools pose risks for the therapist and patient. Additionally, the repetitive and physically stressful nature of orthotic fabrication predisposes the therapist's upper limbs and spine to misuse and overuse injuries. Good working habits, adequate worker fitness and training and diligent application of occupational health procedures are essential to maintain a healthy working environment.

HYGIENE

There exists a high risk of cross infection in hand therapy practices. Standard infection control procedures[3] should be adhered to - hand washing before and after treatment, using gloves in the presence of wounds, wiping down tools and surfaces etc. The frequency of cleaning equipment used to heat water to activate thermoplastic material is dependent upon size. For large units heating water to 70°C for 100 minutes will allow for weekly rather than daily water changes. Orthoses, particularly those worn by patients with open lesions or exfoliative skin conditions, should be cleaned prior to any adjustments being undertaken. Tea tree oil has an antibacterial action and can be used in the heating pan without altering any properties of thermoplastic material.

AESTHETIC CONSIDERATIONS

Consideration must also be given to the aesthetics of the environment. Therapists are treating patients who are often in pain, fearful or with chronic conditions. A pleasant, calm environment, without compromise to impressions of professional quality, will assist in putting patients at ease.

ENVIRONMENTAL ISSUES

Therapists should consider environmental factors in the choice of thermoplastic materials. Some products are biodegradable and/or recyclable (e.g. Orfit®). Minimizing waste in use of thermoplastic and synthetic products has both environmental and fiscal benefits.

FISCAL CONSIDERATIONS

A successful practice requires effective accounting systems and methods. An efficient method of inventory and stock replenishment should be used.

Factoring the true cost of an orthosis, whether it be custom made or prefabricated, should include the time and expertise of the therapist, cost of materials, practice overheads, and depreciation on equipment and plant. Numerous attempts to achieve acceptable fabrication of an orthosis are very expensive in terms of the therapist's time, particularly if the result is unsuccessful. A prefabricated orthosis may appear to be expensive, but it requires less therapist time

to prescribe and fit. However there is cost involved in carrying stock, or alternatively supplying on demand.

The true cost of an orthosis can only be measured once it successfully achieves the objectives for which it was designed. Financial outlay in material terms only, disregards the cost of labour time to manufacture, repair or replacement of the orthosis, for both the patient (such as lost work time to attend therapy) and therapist. Additionally the patient may incur "expense" in terms of suffering physical and psychological costs with an orthosis that fails to achieve its objectives or (in extreme cases) inflicts damage.

EQUIPMENT

The major items of equipment are heating sources, both wet and dry, to render low temperature thermoplastic materials malleable. Hot water in a quantity sufficient to heat the majority of orthotic patterns must be regulated to the temperature appropriate to the materials being used. Large and deep electric frypans are adequate for most forearm/hand orthoses; purpose designed hydrocollators and Suspans provide larger quantities of hot water.

There are a variety of heat guns available for hot air. Free standing table models or hand held models can be used for heating patterns, for spot heating for remoulding and to heat Velcro® adhesive and material surface for strap application. Funnel attachments are available

Table 1: Tools

Tool	Use	Advantage	Recommended Types
Scissors and sharpener	Cutting materials	Accurate, neat smooth finish, proficient use requires practice	Blunt nose surgical, Fiskar many sizes
Shears	Cut patterns from large sheets of cold thermoplastics	Fast, reduces waste, strong not precise	
Stanley trimmer	Cutting straight lines in large sheets of cold thermoplastics	Easier, less stress than scissors	
Hole punch	Punching holes in thermo-plastics, Velcro®, strapping materials	Neat, fast, even, smooth edge	Single hole punch, revolving leather punch
Pliers	Bending, cutting outrigger metals	Safer, stronger, faster, more precise, less stressful than by hand	Square nose, round nose
Small vice	Bending outriggers	Safer, stronger, faster, more precise, less stressful than by hand	Bench press or small vice
Riveter	Securing 2 part rivets	Less expensive than adhesive Velcro®, still required for some attachments	Hand press or bench mounted
Wax pencil	Marking thermoplastic material	Visible, removable and aes-thetically preferable to pen	
Jigs	Making wire springs, bending outriggers	Safer, stronger, faster, more precise, less stressful than by hand	
Spatula	Removing thermoplastics from hot water pan or tank	Safer technique, minimizes damage to heating source	
Large plastic syringe or baster	Applying hot water to specific locations on orthosis	More precise means to reheat in order to modify a small area of an orthosis	

to reduce the size of the hot air stream. Good tools suited to the therapist's requirements increase the efficiency of orthotic fabrication. Tools must be well maintained, including regular sharpening to decrease the physical stress to the therapist's muscles and joints. Tools dedicated to orthotic fabrication prevent frustrating losses effecting productivity, prevent contamination with unacceptable substances, and ensure maintenance of good condition. Table 1 lists essential tools and their uses.

Table 2: Low Temperature Thermoplastic Materials

	Plastic based/plastic like	Rubber based /rubber like	Translucent materials plastic like
Product examples	NCM Clinic NCM Preferred Orthoplast II Polyflex II Polyform Sansplint XR	Ezeform Leodisplint Multiform Isoprene NCM Spectrum NCM Vanilla Orfit Eco Orthoplast Synergy Tailorsplint	Aquafit™ NS Aquaplast-T Encore Orfit Classic & Non Sticky Reveals Colour ranges in these materials lack translucency
Rigidity	Moderate, depends on thickness	Excellent	Excellent, determined by orthosis design and material thickness
Mouldability	• Excellent stretch and drape • Finger tips can make impressions • Requires minimal force to mould • Used with gravity assistance	• Low, minimal drape so can be used against gravity. • Requires some force to mould • Can be secured with bandage	• Excellent elasticity and stretch • Sticky surface on materials eliminates need for securing during moulding • Thickness determines mouldability
Conformity	High – excellent for intricate designs	Low – ideal for larger orthoses	Excellent using stretch qualities.
Elastic memory	None	No elastic memory but poor stretch means original shape can be approximated on reheating	Good memory, suitable for multiple remouldings

MATERIALS

THERMOPLASTICS

Thermoplastics are plastic and plastic like materials that are affected by heat. They are divided according to their activated temperature. High temperature thermoplastics (HTTP) are generally used by orthotists in fabrication of durable long lasting orthoses. This involves a three-stage process requiring a plaster cast of patient's hand, fabrication of a positive mould and finally moulding on the plaster model. Low temperature thermoplastics (LTTP), which soften at 60°-70°C (140°-160°F), can be moulded directly onto the patient's limb saving time and allowing cheaper orthosis fabrication techniques.

An understanding of the properties of various materials is required for selection of the most appropriate material for a particular orthosis for a client. It allows the therapist to work with and take advantage of these properties for easy, accurate fabrication. In the same way that different types of clothes are made from different types of fabric so it is with orthoses. The specific properties of each material lend themselves to the most appropriate design and construction techniques. As the variety of LTTP materials used for orthotic fabrication continues to grow it is appropriate to consider materials as having rubber-like, plastic-like, or combinations of plastic and rubber properties.[5] Product information is available online from commercial suppliers and therapists are encouraged to test products to determine the basic properties and their personal preferences for the patient population requiring orthoses. Table 2 provides a guide to properties of thermoplastic materials.

FEATURES OF LTTP THERMOPLASTICS

General Characteristics

LTTPs have different properties when cold and when heated. The features when cold give some indication of the properties of the orthosis once fabricated and include such things as thickness, rigidity and the presence of perforations. This has implications to the patient and how they will use the orthosis.

The properties of the LTTPs when heated suggest how that material will respond during the fabrication process. This has relevance to orthotic design and what the material is suitable for, the fabrication techniques that can be used, and the unique needs of the client (e.g. the aged, children, or the presence of wounds).

Time, chemicals and temperature can influence the elastic and plastic qualities of LTTPs. Product storage and care instructions should be followed to ensure good shelf life prior to fabrication and longevity of the orthosis following fabrication.

Activation Temperature

The temperature at which LTTPs become pliable is referred to as the activation temperature. It is important to note this temperature and set the thermostat of the heating pan accordingly, as the properties of some materials may change if overheated.

Too high an activation temperature may contribute to materials loosing properties such as the ability to reach true pliability when heated, stretchability (e.g. Orfit®), or become over stretched (e.g. Sansplint XR® / Polyflex®), or lose rigidity when cold. Colour changes may occur in some materials. Materials that are transparent when heated may lose this characteristic and remain opaque. These problems may also occur with some materials if they are reheated several times.

With a lower activation temperature there is a lower the risk of burns to both the therapist and patient. This is an important consideration for those patients with fragile skin, particularly children, the elderly and post trauma in the presence of grafts and burns. However, too low an activation temperature will decrease the working time for moulding as the material cools and hardens in a few minutes. Activation of the whole piece of thermoplastic is recommended to ensure even moulding to the contours of the hand.

Mouldability

Once heated, materials exhibit varying degrees of rigidity and mouldability. Materials can be graded along a continuum from those that drape easily requiring very little moulding to those that have little drape and require more forceful moulding by the therapist. Highly drapable materials (e.g. Sansplint XR® / Polyflex®) are recommended in acute phase post injury or in the presence of significant pain when the patient's tissues cannot tolerate any force being applied during fabrication. Highly drapable materials require gravity to assist moulding with little effort from the therapist to achieve a precise mould to the contours of the limb. However, this material is difficult to use without the assistance of gravity, as bandaging is not recommended. Caution is required when handling this type of material as it can be easily stretched and the surface of the material marks very easily.

More rigid materials (e.g. Ezeform / Tailor-splint) require greater force and constant pressure to achieve good conformity during moulding. These materials are used for large orthoses where bandages are used to secure material to the limb to facilitate moulding. The moulding temperature is determined by the material thickness, degree of perforations, and presence of adhered lining. Moulding time is the period the product retains its optimum elasticity and plasticity before it begins to cool. It is the period when there is a difference between the activation temperature and room temperature.[4] Moulding time can be increased by increasing the room temperature, or decreased by application of cold water, cold spray or ice packs. In the hardening period of LLTPs, when material is no longer stretchable but still flexible, any force applied by the patient moving or manipulation of the orthosis when removing from the limb can distort the shape. Hardening is complete once material returns to its pre activation temperature.

Elastic Memory

A material that has the ability to return to its original size and shape when reheated has elastic memory. Thus orthoses can be completely remoulded to accommodate changes due to reduction of oedema or changes in range of motion as in the case of serial orthotic intervention. It also has benefits for the novice as mistakes are easily rectified by reworking the same piece of material. Also remoulding is possible, saving expense in material outlay when repeated orthotic application is required over time.

When using material with elastic memory, like those in Orfit® and Aquaplast® ranges, partial melting can result in significant changes in contour and shape that can distort the original design. It is better to become proficient at achieving all desired characteristics in one mould, something that can only be achieved by practise. LTTPs with excellent memory tend to take longer to harden so ensure the material is completely hard before removing from the limb.

Coating and Self-Adherence

Many of the materials have a coating on the surface that prohibits self-adherence when activated. This lessens the risk of the thermoplastic material adhering to itself, the patient or dressings when activated during moulding. Cut edges will still adhere. Coatings have to be removed with solvents or sandpaper prior to attempting to adhere another orthotic component such as an outrigger or straps. Greater attention is required when using coloured materials to ensure bonds are secure.

Materials without a coating are referred to as self-adherent. They simplify orthotic fabrication through eliminating the need for bandaging as they adhere to the patient or to themselves when used circumferentially. Straps and other components adhere without requiring solvents or bonding agents.

Self-adherent material must remain wet while moulding to prevent the material from adhering to itself and other products. Gauze, Micropore™ or stockinette can be used over postoperative dressings so the thermoplastic adheres to that and not the dressing.

Transparency When Heated

Polyester based materials within the Orfit® and Aquaplast® product range become transparent when heated, which is often claimed to be advantageous as anatomical landmarks and skin blanching can be seen whilst moulding, however the benefit in reality is negligible. Transparency allows the therapist to easily determine when the material is activated, saving time and avoiding the risk of overheating.

Perforations

Transpiration of water via the skin is an ongoing process. Therefore, the application of thermoplastic material that prevents the normal evaporative process may lead to accumulation of moisture with maceration of the skin. Materials with perforations may be cooler, drier and more comfortable as they allow the skin to breathe only in those locations with holes. If orthoses are to be effective in reducing the temperature and allowing evaporation the holes need to be sufficiently large and spaced at close intervals.

One disadvantage of maxi perforated thermoplastic materials is that skin may be pushed through the perforations and cause shear at the edges. Perforated materials should not be stretched during fabrication, otherwise the holes may be enlarged and strength properties lost. Perforated materials have been shown to break down in areas of high stress.[1] The edges of perforated materials must be smoothed or rolled as cutting causes uneven and sharp edges to be formed.

Coloured Options

Colour is an option in various ranges of thermoplastic materials. Patient acceptance is generally high with colours selected according to vocational demands or preference. The properties of the materials do vary from the original with some variability between colours. Novice therapists are encouraged to trial a small piece of material to familiarise themselves with the material properties particularly mouldability and bonding prior to use. Cost of coloured material can be higher than neutral colours. Practice fiscal issues will determine range of coloured materials available for patient selection.

How To Test LLTP Properties.

As the number of LTTP materials is constantly increasing testing the properties of materials is encouraged. Using a small sample experiment using the following procedures, reactivating the LTTP by returning to hot water after each test.

Heat one:

- How long does it take to be fully activated?
- Does it go transparent when activated?
- On removing from the water place across dorsum of slightly flexed wrist - does it drape and contour the shape, or do you need to apply some pressure?
- Does gravity affect material?
- Do you leave fingerprints on the material surface?
- How long does it take to go completely hard?

Heat two

- Does it return to original shape?
- Once reactivated wrap around part of your finger MCP joints and gently press two corners together - does it bond to itself?
- Can you snap bond apart once material is cold?

Heat three

- If bond did not come apart note activation temperature between single and double layers of material.
- Cut section off - do edges bond together along cutting line?

Heat four

- Gently stretch and mould material over thumb index finger webspace or over flexed finger MCP joints. Does material conform to convex and concave surfaces well?
- What impact has remoulding had on material?

NEOPRENE®

Commonly referred to as wetsuit material, this material comprises an internal rubber layer of various thickness and external nylon layers in a range of colours. It is cut and sewn to fabricate orthoses. The material does not limit motion and is bulky, hot and not well tolerated in warm climates. Breathoprene™ and Comforprene™ are latex free variations on neoprene with towelling and nylon linings to increase comfort and resolve sweating issues. Contour is achieved by the pattern design and rigidity gained by additional reinforcement from thermoplastic inserts. This material is commonly used for orthoses for very young children where the bulk of the material offers enough restriction to position joints, as a means to maintain warmth surrounding a joint (for example post healed fractures); and for persons with arthritis because of the gentle support and warmth. Iron-On™ Seam Tape Hook and Loop Velcro® limit the need for sewing pieces together and allow for quick fastening.

LEATHER

Three millimetres thick stiff, natural leather is used for work-based orthoses to immobilize the wrist in environments where thermoplastic materials cannot be used (in the presence of heat and petroleum based chemicals). The basis of patterns is similar to that for neoprene. Wet leather is moulded directly to the limb and bandaged, then allowed to dry for approximately 24 hours. Straps are riveted or glued. The leather can be sealed and polished.

PLASTER OF PARIS

Plaster bandages are a cost effective, easy method of fabricating circumferential serial orthoses, especially for the elbow and PIP joint. It allows tissue to breath so it does not macerate the skin and it can be used over lacerations and ulcers. Finger plasters are applied without underlying protection. Larger plasters require cast padding. The plaster is rolled on without any compression until the required thickness is achieved and then smoothed off with moistened hands giving particular attention to the edges. Small plasters can be soaked off; larger plasters require bivalving with a plaster saw.

Plaster, in bandage form, is gauze impregnated with plaster (calcium sulphate). Plaster setting involves an exothermic chemical reaction that results in the hydration of calcium sulphate to produce gypsum. The rate of this reaction is largely dependent upon the amount of water incorporated in the dry plaster and the temperature of this water. For application, the plaster should be saturated with water but not "dripping" wet. Excessively dry or wet plaster yields poor crystallisation. Ideally, the dipping temperature should be between 25°C - 30°C (77°F - 86°F). Curing time is dependent on temperature, humidity and most importantly adequate air circulation around the cast. Strength (gypsum crystal interlocking) depends upon the speed of setting, the water content and the amount of motion during cure. During setting, water is incorporated into the gypsum crystals resulting in cast expansion. This expansion enhances intimate moulding to anatomical contours. Excess water gradually evaporates and most is lost within four hours.

Thus for best casting results:
1. Use water between 25° - 30°C (77° - 86°F).
2. Apply material smoothly with the minimum number of layers possible.
3. Prevent motion during setting.
4. Do not insulate from free access to air by placing a bandage, towel or bandage over a freshly applied plaster.

SYNTHETIC 'PLASTERS'

The unbreakable nature, colour options and waterproof qualities of synthetic plasters make them a popular, but more expensive, alternative to Plaster of Paris. A variety of resin-based synthetic materials such as rigid fibreglass or semi-rigid non-fibreglass (Soft Cast) are available. Handling requirements during fabrication; rigidity, flexibility and texture of the finished casts; and process of removal by either unwrapping the bandage, or cutting through layers with scissors or an oscillating saw; differ in each case. Often a combination of casting materials are used to achieve a mouldable cast, with the strength of Plaster of Paris and the lightness of a synthetic material.

LYCRA®

Lycra® has long been used in the manufacture of pressure garments for oedema control and scar management. Incorporation of various Lycra® fabrics into flexible wrist orthoses has been reported in the literature. Lycra® offers the potential to manufacture orthoses with a range of mobility and rigidity. Where multiple joints are involved rigid materials would prevent movement to the point of loss of hand function, where as a Lycra® orthosis can be fabricated to allow the appropriate movement in prescribed joints. The elastic nature of Lycra® can offer enough support for unstable joints in rheumatoid arthritis when total restriction is contraindicated or functionally unacceptable.

Lycra® is available in a range of strengths, weights and colours. It breathes but can become hot to wear. To make a garment, a pattern is required and the pieces are overlocked together. Numerous brands of prefabricated and custom made Lycra® based orthoses are available.

STRAPPING MATERIALS

Straps are required to provide stability and to secure the orthosis to the body in the prescribed position. Distal movement of the orthosis, especially rotation, will compromise the desired outcome and can be controlled with appropriate choice and application of strapping to correctly distribute forces. Velcro® is perhaps the most common form of strapping material but other options are available.

Velcro®

Velcro® is available in various widths, with or without elasticity, in various colours and with or without adhesive backing. Although both hook and pile Velcro® is available with adhesive backing, only adhesive hook Velcro® is generally required for orthoses. Choice of colour should reflect consideration of aesthetics and the patient's preferences. Low-profile pile Velcro® is available for finger based orthoses, however it does wear more quickly. Choice of width reflects functional considerations and surface area required for optimal pressure distribution. (usually 20mm hook and 25 or 50mm pile is used, dependent on circumferential or dorsal/volar orthosis design).

Elasticated pile Velcro® is a softer texture compared to non-elastic pile Velcro® and can thus make a more comfortable strap that accommodates variation in arm circumference. Caution is required, however as securing straps too tightly can compromise vascularity.

Velcro® is a brand name and is a good quality product. Cheaper products with similar properties are available, however durability and performance is directly related to cost.

Betapile™

When skin is fragile, Betapile™ may be used in conjunction with hook Velcro®. It is available in various widths and consists of brown-brushed nylon bonded to two sides of 5mm thick foam. Betapile™ has slight stretch and therefore cannot be used where a firm strap is required.

Cotton or Dacron Webbing with Velcro® Tabs

These materials are tough, durable and non-elastic. Hook and pile Velcro® and buckles must be sewn on. The straps can only be attached to the orthosis with rivets. Webbing is advised when straps must be long lasting and strong.

PRINCIPLES OF STRAPPING DESIGN AND APPLICATION

Consideration of strap application must be included throughout the design process to ensure a professional, aesthetically pleasing, and functionally acceptable product. The position of application should be carefully determined prior to actual application, for once most straps are attached they are difficult to remove and inappropriate positioning may render the orthosis ineffective or unusable.

Biomechanical Considerations

Adherence to biomechanical principles of orthotic design, as described in Chapter 2, is essential. Critical issues pertaining to strap application are:

1. Straps apply at least one critical component of the force couple exerted by the orthosis to maintain the correct position. Thus strap width must be generous.
2. The angle of application must allow for the tapering shape of the forearm. Thus straps sit flush with the skin providing firm, equal pressure distribution.
3. Straps are unable to contour to concave or convex surfaces. Bony prominences are convex in more than one plane therefore uneven pressure results when straps are applied. Elastic Velcro® does not solve this problem.
4. The position of application of straps should maximize the mechanical advantage offered by the orthosis. An orthosis that requires a proximal component to be two-thirds the length of the forearm should not be compromised by a proximal strap positioned only halfway along the length.

Anatomical Considerations

1. Apply straps acknowledging the architecture of the hand changes with motion. Movement should not be impaired by strap width or location.

2. Protection of circulatory integrity. Straps are liable to impair lymphatic and venous drainage or compromise arterial status unless width allows adequate distribution of pressure and placement does not jeopardise critical structures.

3. Protect skin integrity. Consider fragility of the skin and tolerance to wear when choosing strap material, placement and width. Permeable materials allow water and air exchange and thus lessen the risk of maceration but are harder to keep clean and pose an infection risk (the thermoplastic is not permeable and can be disinfected).

Functional Considerations

1. *Prescription of amount of Velcro®.* Prescribe in accordance with the requirements of the patient and the therapist's objectives. Too much Velcro® may prove difficult for those patients with diminished hand function to undo. Small amounts are acceptably strong and secure. Make the hook Velcro® a little thinner and smaller than the associated pile Velcro® as this will result in the hook being completely covered by the pile, particularly for those patients with diminished manipulation skills. Full coverage of hook Velcro® is essential, as exposure may result in skin irritation or trauma, or snagging against other materials.

2. *Ease of application and removal.* Consideration must be given to the patient's bilateral upper limb function when determining the orientation of straps for the direction of fastening and unfastening to enable the patient to apply the orthosis independently. Patients with diminished hand function may need to sweep the opposite wrist or forearm around the orthosis to fasten or unfasten straps, or even need to use their teeth. The ends of the pile Velcro® must be slightly longer than the underlying hook to afford full coverage and give adequate grip to unfasten. Those with bilateral injuries or diminished manipulation skills require strap adaptations or modified prehension patterns to simplify the task of fastening and unfastening. Alternatively there may be occasions when straps are applied to make orthosis removal more difficult as is the case with young children.

3. *Comfort and function.* In firmly securing the orthosis to the hand, comfort should not be overlooked, as this will significantly affect duration of wear. The hook Velcro® should be applied onto the thermoplastic, facing away from the patient's skin, with the pile Velcro® applied at the edges of the thermoplastic facing towards the skin. This prevents discomfort, irritation or trauma to the patient's skin from the rough hook material.

4. *Durability.* The straps should withstand the constant wear the orthosis will receive.

Aesthetic Considerations

The strapping components should be of the same colour and of a colour to match or complement the thermoplastic material. If multiple colours are available the patient should be given the choice to ensure the finished orthosis is aesthetically acceptable. The ends of both the hook and the pile Velcro® should be cut to the desired length and curved for neatness.

LINING MATERIALS

Rather than automatically lining orthoses as standard procedure, lining should only be prescribed if it is essential. All linings have advantages and disadvantages that can limit the life of the orthosis. Many adhesive backed lining materials are very difficult to apply and remove so consider this fact prior to application. Linings essentially fall into three categories - fabric surface products, foams and gels. Fabric products are used for comfort acting as a skin thermoplastic material interface. However they absorb moisture and cannot be cleaned easily. Closed cell foams have potential to disperse pressure but have a limited life span as structure does break down over time. Gel products can mimic subcutaneous fat so are an effective lining to disperse pressure. See Table 3.

INDICATIONS FOR USE OF LINING MATERIALS
Comfort.

Plastic materials are not comfortable to wear next to the skin, particularly if heat or perspiration is a problem. Skin maceration may result. Orthoses are often lined to minimize this problem but these linings quickly become soiled with perspiration and grime. If the lining becomes wet it will remain so for extended periods, risking skin integrity. The lining is difficult to clean, and once wet, difficult to remove. Replacement is expensive, time consuming and often difficult. To increase the comfort of shoes we wear socks or stockings. 'Hand socks' can be purchased ready-made or in stockinette or tubular padding bandage rolls that can be cut to length. They are made in combinations of cotton and polyester and products that wick moisture away from the skin. Arm protectors, used to prevent injuries for elderly persons, are effective linings for elbow orthoses.

Linings are either closed cell or open cell in structure. Liquids, perspiration, odours and bacteria do not penetrate the surface of closed cell materials but they do not breathe. They are however, easier to clean. Open cell materials breathe but will absorb liquids and so are unhygienic. Also they easily stain and become odoriferous.

To Enhance Pressure Distribution.

The addition of lining increases pressure as opposed to decreasing it, and should not be seen as a means of improving the fit of a poorly designed and fabricated orthosis. If lining is deemed necessary to improve pressure distribution, allowance should be made for it in initial fabrication. Some linings are adhered to the thermoplastic prior to heating and moulding but they significantly affect the qualities of the thermoplastic. Linings that do not bottom out have the ability to absorb shock and reduce shear stress. Any lining that bottoms on compression (squeeze between thumb and finger to test) is inappropriate to address pressure or shear. A sock or stockinette liner decreases shear as movement occurs between the orthosis and the liner rather than the skin. All linings minimize orthosis migration by increasing friction between the orthosis and skin but therefore

Table 3 Lining Materials

Material	Description	Options	Durability	Availability
Splint/orthosis liners with or without inserted thumb	Tubular fabric made of various fabrics such as cotton, terry-like polyester with and without spandex. Edges finished	Available in two widths related to hand size, and short or long lengths	Hand washable, durable	Available individually or in packets of 10
Tubular padding and linings. Sold as cast padding or protective padding	Tubular fabrics and fabric mixes of cotton, polyester, jersey. Density of material dependent upon product	Available in various widths related to hand/limb circumference for adults and children. 10 metre rolls cut to required length	Hole is cut for the thumb. Raw edges require finishing if used for extended periods of time. Polyester products are more durable than cotton	Cost effective option for short duration intervention Polyester products more expensive than cotton
Cotton or felt padding self adhesive	Soft surface fabric adhered to orthosis post fabrication. Thin used for comfort and protecting fragile skin rather than pressure dispersion.	Various thicknesses 2-6.4mm	Stretchable and easily adhered to orthosis shape. Not easy to clean, absorbs moisture & potentially bacteria. Adhesive can make replacing lining difficult	Sold in sheets of various sizes
Closed-cell foam padding self adhesive	Water resistant so can be applied to thermoplastic and moulded to form custom padded orthosis.	Two thicknesses 3.2mm and 6.4mm	Closed cell will not bottom out impermeable to moisture so easy clean. Do not allow air exchange. High durability. Adhesive make replacement difficult	Sold in sheets of various sizes
Gel Pads & Sheeting medical grade mineral oil gel	Visco-elastic properties allow gel to move with skin. Ideal for interface with hard thermoplastic materials when extra protection is needed to protect and cushion the skin against pressure and shear forces	Wide range of products used in Podiatry and Prosthetic practice	Washable reusable. High durability, excellent adhesion that allows gel to be replaced. Cannot be used on open wounds	Wide variety of adhesive pads. Sheets economical size (10cm squares) can be cut to required shape

require careful monitoring of the skin for shear problems. Orthoses should not be partially lined as this alters the skin/orthosis interface and causes areas of shear stress.

Strategic placement of padding or gel may be used to resolve potential pressure issues, particularly over the bony prominences on the dorsum of the hand and wrist. Proprietary gel products designed to protect, cushion, soften, and moisturize the skin against abrasion and shear forces associated with wearing a prosthesis are ideal products to use when significant forces are transmitted from orthosis to hand and hand to orthosis. To achieve effective pressure distribution a piece of adhesive backed padding, gel or substitute such as stiff exercise putty, is shaped and attached to the skin creating an inverse mould in the orthosis. Once the orthosis is moulded the product is then reversed and attached to the orthosis. It is best to use a substitute if the shape to be padded is not reversible. This requires careful removal of mould to act as a pattern to shape padding or gel being mindful that the adhesive surface contacts the inside of the orthosis.

Maintenance of Skin Integrity

Clients with sensitive skin may require the orthosis to be lined. Lining is a special consideration in orthotic fabrication for persons with an allergy to thermoplastic materials, with fragile skin such as in rheumatoid arthritis or post skin graft, or with sensory loss who cannot feel skin irritation.

PRESSURE MEDIA

Where pressure needs to be applied to skin to modify a scar, an orthosis is unable to conform to the scar surface to give even pressure distribution. Linings likewise have inadequate conformability and may be contraindicated for some scars. Pressure media such as Silastic® elastomer or Otoform K2 may be utilized under the orthosis, creating true congruity and offering a beneficial side effect in softening the scar. These media can also be used for precise positioning of joints of the hand within the orthosis, in cases of rheumatoid arthritis and severe trauma.

MOBILIZING HARDWARE

HOOKS

Although there are many devices available from suppliers to tether and align mobilizing traction, paperclips, safety pins, and dress hooks and eyes are economical and convenient. Clips, pins and hooks are bent at 90° to create a point of attachment, or a pulley guide, for the traction system then heated and embedded in the thermoplastic (some require a small piece of thermoplastic bonded over the top).

OUTRIGGERS

Outriggers require ease of adjustment to ensure angle of pull of traction remains at 90°. Outriggers may be constructed from a range of materials.

1. Metal. Outrigger wire, brass welding rod or stainless steel rod (3.2, 2.4 or 1.6mm diameter) is cost effective, aesthetically acceptable and easy to bend, cut and modify. Paper clips and safety pins of various sizes make quick effective outriggers for small or single finger orthoses. These metals are bent using vices, pliers and jigs. In low-profile traction systems a narrow small strip of thermoplastic can be attached to larger metal outriggers to allow holes to be punched and act as pulleys. Embed metal eyes into the proximal curve of the holes to reduce friction against the nylon thread. Flat aluminium strips, available in 12mm and 20mm widths, form effective outriggers for forearm and elbow mobilizing orthoses.

2. Thermoplastic. In order to achieve the desired strength, a roll or several layers of material bonded together, is required. The design is extremely bulky in large orthoses and therefore unattractive and expensive.

3. Orfitubes®. The traction is completely encased within a tube. Expense is an issue however aesthetically they are very acceptable. Orfitubes® are cold formable to the desired length of the orthosis. Maximum length of elastic traction can be used as no pulley is required.

4. Outrigger kits are available from hand therapy suppliers. Kits include all the metal rods, finger cuffs and traction components. Cost is an issue. Benefits relate to ease of adjustment to ensure correct line of pull, however aesthetically there is minimal gain.

FORCE COMPONENTRY

The mobilizing, or force, component of the traction system in dynamic mobilizing orthoses can be elastic bands or elastic thread, mercery thread, Thera-Band® tubing, or springs. These components have two variables

1. Tension. Quality and thickness of the material determines its potential to generate tension. This tension is translated to force applied to tissues.

2. Length. Length determines the potential elongation and distance through which tension can be generated. This distance is critical for allowing full-prescribed range of motion.

When mobilizing traction is used in an orthosis the therapist needs to know how much tension is generated when the component is stretched to a predetermined point. When the same amount of force is applied to components of differing thicknesses and lengths, different elongation results. Greater elongation occurs in longer elastic bands when compared to short bands. Similarly, thinner elastic bands elongate more than thick bands. If the components are stretched to a similar length, the tensions generated vary widely. This is clinically significant as it demonstrates that the component has an optimal range of lengths at which it can exert useful tension. Short bands produce larger tension with less excursion than do longer bands, which make short bands inappropriate in many applications.

Elastic bands, tubing and thread all have a life span so it is important to use quality products to ensure consistent length and tension. Corded elastic, commonly referred to as hat elastic, is available in various strengths and is a useful alternative to rubber bands as the cord protects the elastic from being overstretched.

Determination of Length-tension of Elastic Traction

The design of the orthosis must accommodate the desired excursion of the mobilizing traction not vice versa. Where the objective is to address deficits in passive range of motion (PROM) and influence tissue length, the critical issue is low force applied over a long time. In these orthoses, the appropriate force is determined to be that which will maintain the joint at it's end range and is of the correct magnitude to impact positively on tissue change (see Chapters One and Two). Low-profile orthoses use a longer base to accommodate the lower force traction system. When the orthosis is designed to facilitate a prescribed active range of motion and the patient is required to move against the orthosis traction in a repetitive manner (e.g. to achieve the therapeutic objective of minimizing adhesion formation), higher profile outriggers are used to allow for excursion and recoil of dynamic components. A distinction must be made regarding the therapeutic rationale and outcome objectives for mobilizing traction as this will modify the determination of force range.

Passive Range of Motion Deficits

The traction unit for a low-profile orthosis consists of the cuff, an inelastic component (usually nylon thread or fishing line) and an elastic component (either elastic thread, elastic bands, springs, Thera-Band® or stretch Velcro®). The nylon thread need only be long enough to yield full excursion through the pulley, allowing the longest possible mobilizing component. This system permits flexibility in the choice of dynamic component, as there exists a greater range of safe length to desired tension. As each dynamic component has a different length-tension curve, therapists must be familiar with the relationship in components they use.

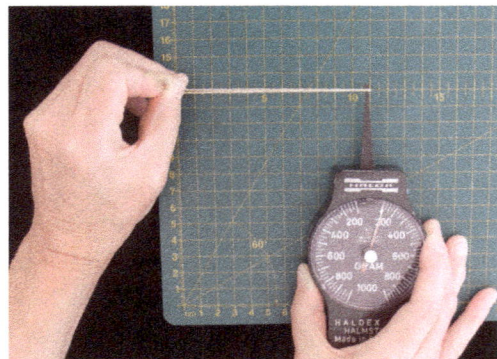

Figure 2: Plotting length-tension curves for dynamic components. Using a Haldex® Gauge (or other calibrated force gauge) and a means to measure length, plot force used at various points of elongation of the dynamic component. Testing commonly used elastic in this way will guide selection of an appropriate size elastic band.

Elastic bands are the most common dynamic component used and come in various lengths and thicknesses. The resting length of the band is measured, a known force, for example 200gm, is applied and the increase in length recorded (Figure 2 and 3). Thus when this band is applied to the traction unit it must be stretched to this recorded length. Elastic bands constantly stretched will gradually lengthen so do not regain their original length

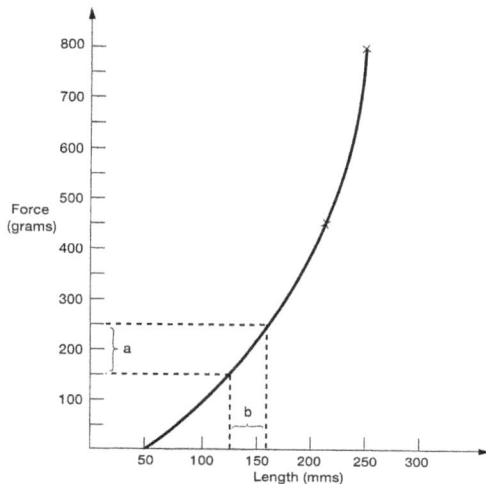

Figure 3: Length - Tension Curve of a 50mm Elastic Band. This graph demonstrates the curvilinear relationship of length and tension force in a 50mm elastic band. This curve is used to determine the correct application of dynamic traction to achieve the desired force application. For example, if the range of force required is 150-250gms, identify this on the vertical axis (notated by a). Project these values across to the curve, and then down to the horizontal axis (notated by b). The range identified by b is 125-162mm. Therefore, the excursion of the elastic band which will achieve the desired force range equals 125-162mm. Traction must be applied with the band elongated to 125mm. This component will allow 37mm linear range of movement at the targeted joint.

once tension is removed. This 'creep' will contribute to the elastic band loosing some force over the original stretched length. For this reason it is necessary to monitor elastic components and change as creep occurs. In low-profile (horizontal traction) the outrigger is used as a pulley with loss of some force to friction acknowledged. The suspension sling is attached to nylon thread that runs through the pulley and then attaches to the mobilizing component. This sits horizontal to the orthosis and is tethered proximally. Elastic bands may be secured to a hook or attached to Velcro®. Velcro® allows for an easier

adjustment of tension, allowing modification during initial applications or with creep in the elastic band over time. Patients must be educated if they are to be responsible for modifying tension in traction systems.

A Haldex® Gauge enables therapists to determine the desired force applied by dynamic traction once applied to the joint. Cuffs are secured to the digit or hand, threaded through the outrigger, the elastic band stretched until the desired force is recorded on the gauge (see Figure 13 Chapter 2). The point of anchorage of the traction or the length of the nylon cord is adjusted to the required length. When using serial progressive principles the Haldex® Gauge applies a predetermined force to the traction moving the joint to end position. Traction is then secured to the orthosis base maintaining position.

Facilitation of Active Range of Motion
Two measures determine the force required when traction is used to facilitate movement. The first is the minimum force required to maintain the joint in the prescribed position, overcoming gravity and resistance of the involved tissues (Figure 4). The second determines if the antagonist muscle group is able to generate sufficient force to over come the resistance of the traction to move to the desired end range of motion. An elastic band is required that can generate that tension to achieve the prescribed position but has sufficient elongation to allow movement through the required range of active motion. A clinical decision may be required in the event of the antagonists being unable to

oppose the minimum force. Modifications may be required to the therapeutic regime to address this issue. Once length and tension of elastic traction has been determined, it may be attached directly to the outrigger, therefore determining the height of the outrigger. If a hybrid outrigger design is being used the elastic band is anchored to the orthosis base and attached to finger cuff via nylon cord threaded through the outrigger pulley. The nylon cord must be long enough so that the elastic band is not caught in the pulley during full movement in flexion. Metal outriggers can be adjusted once fitted to the orthosis to ensure a good line of pull, however traction will not be perpendicular throughout the whole range of movement.

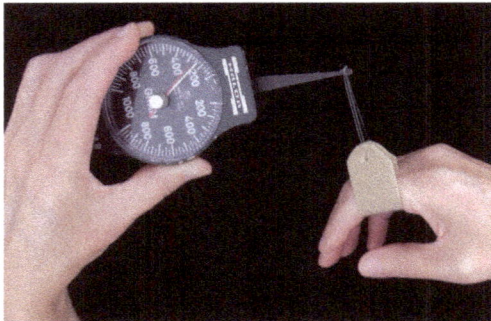

Figure 4: Force Range Requirements. Using a force gauge, measure the amount of force required to maintain the joint in the prescribed position. If the therapy objectives require joint motion, measure the force the patient can generate against the gauge to achieve this joint motion.

Finger Cuffs

Cuffs in mobilizing orthosis are used to apply force to the fingers to address either passive or active motion deficits. Selection of material requires the same consideration as other orthotic components, with regard to skin integrity. Cuffs must be durable, comfortable and resist stretching. Velcro®, suede or leather may be chosen. For strong functional loops (e.g. orthoses used for radial nerve palsy) leather is appropriate. Suede is softer and more compliant and is a better choice for patients with frail skin. Biomechanical principles must be adhered to, specifically pressure distribution and the avoidance of shear stress.

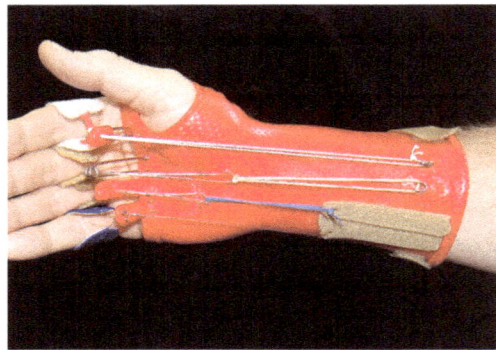

Figure 5: Examples of finger cuffs and mobilizing traction. Index finger Velcro® cuff with width maintained by a small piece of thermoplastic material, stainless outrigger with thermoplastic pulley, corded elastic traction secured to dress hook; middle finger Betapile™ cuff, stainless steel out rigger and pulley, nylon and elastic traction secured to paper clip hook; ring finger Velcro® cuff, thermoplastic outrigger with pulley, nylon cord and elastic band secured via Velcro®; little finger Fabrifoam® loop, paper clip supported by thermoplastic with dress hook eye reinforcing pulley, non elastic nylon and Velcro® traction.

Cuffs that have a single point of attachment to the traction unit tilt easily and exert shear and lateral pressure on the digit. Cuffs that are attached to the traction unit on either side tend to tilt less and are more comfortable due to lower lateral pressure. If a single piece of nylon line is threaded through the holes on both sides of the cuff and then knotted, the length of the traction can be adjusted to equal lengths while attached to the mobilizing force without the need to untie it from the cuff. A small piece of thermoplastic material can be use to bridge the finger cuff. This maintains the required width minimizing potential for medial/lateral compression and increases ease of application. Figure 5 illustrates several types of finger cuffs and traction options.

When a cuff is to be applied to a DIP joint adhesive backed Dycem matting can be attached to the inside of the cuff which will provide grip and traction to the nail and prevent the cuff from slipping. Alternatively the cuff can be made from Fabrifoam®.

Constructing the Mobilizing Component for a Single Digit

1. Identify the components to be used in the traction system.
2. Design and fabricate the appropriate orthosis base to stabilize the body part and provide a base for attachment of the outrigger.
3. Apply selected straps to secure the orthosis but not to obstruct construction or placement of the outrigger.
4. Fabricate the outrigger.
   a. Roughly measure the length of outrigger material required (the minimum is the length of the bones proximal and distal to the joint to be mobilized). When using metal a pulley is constructed at the midpoint by coiling with pliers.
   b. A piece of thermoplastic material, with a hole for the pulley, can be a quick effective short outrigger.
   c. Make a digit cuff and attach nylon thread.
   d. Secure the orthosis to the hand and place the cuff on the digit.
   e. Place the outrigger on the orthosis with the nylon thread through the pulley. Mobilize the joint to its end range using the tension on the cuff. Adjust the position of the outrigger to achieve a perpendicular pull by the traction system on the digit. Mark the location of the outrigger on the orthosis base. Trim the excess length off the outrigger and contour it to the orthosis base. Secure the outrigger on the orthosis base by bonding on an additional piece of thermoplastic material.
   f. Adjust length of nylon thread to the length of mobilizing component i.e. accommodating tension length of elastic traction or length of non-elastic component.
   g. Heat a small dress hook and secure it to the orthosis base at the point predetermined by the length tension required by elastic traction. Adhere hook Velcro® to the orthosis base if using pile Velcro® to secure non-elastic traction.
   h. A pulley, to maintain traction alignment close to the orthosis base, can be made from the 'eye' of a dress hook or bent paper clip secured to the orthosis base.

Constructing the Mobilizing Component for Multiple Digits

A single outrigger is used for several digits where the contributing pathology and the deficits in joint range of motion in each digit are similar. Where there is a disparity in either of these factors, individual outriggers are made to address each digit.

1. Identify the components to be used in the traction system.
2. Design and fabricate the appropriate orthosis base to stabilize the body part and provide a base for attachment of the outrigger.
3. Apply selected straps to secure the orthosis but not to obstruct construction or placement of the outrigger.
4. Fabricate the outrigger.
    a. Roughly measure the length of the outrigger required (the minimum is the width of the digits involved plus twice the length of the hand and/or forearm orthosis base).
    b. Make digit loops and attach a length of nylon thread to each loop.
    c. Secure the orthosis to the hand and place a loop on the most radial digit involved.
    d. Bend the outrigger at approximately 90° at the distal radial corner allowing sufficient length for the radial arm to contour the orthosis base.
    e. Mobilize the most radial digit involved to its end range using the tension on the cuff. Determine the length of the outrigger from the orthosis base to the intersection of the traction to achieve a perpendicular pull on the digit. This location is marked. The outrigger metal rod is then shaped to contour the radial side of the orthosis base. The outrigger is then shaped to accommodate the width of the involved digits following the architecture of the hand. The ulnar arm of the outrigger is shaped similarly to that of the radial arm. Again location on the orthosis base is marked. The excess length of the outrigger is trimmed prior to securing it to the orthosis base with additional thermoplastic material. The protective non-adhesive coating on some thermoplastic materials must be removed prior to bonding the outrigger.
    f. A thin piece of thermoplastic material is then moulded over the distal end of the outrigger. The position can be varied through an arc of 180° to ensure the correct angle of pull on the traction. A hole is punched in this thermoplastic material, to create the pulley for each digit.
    g. The 'eyes' of dress hooks are heated over the heat gun and positioned in the thermoplastic around the holes to minimize friction and prevent the traction cutting through the thermoplastic material.
    h. A small dress hook is melted into the thermoplastic at the proximal end of the orthosis.
    i. Thread the traction through the

corresponding hole in the outrigger then attach the mobilizing component to the nylon thread. Secure traction to the orthosis base with a dress hook or hook Velcro®.

Spring Wire

The principles used to choose spring wire are the same as those for elastic bands. Strength is determined by thickness and quality of steel wire, while stiffness is determined by the diameter and number of coils.[4] Piano wire, commonly used to make finger springs, is manufactured from carbon steel. It is available in various gauges (thickness) that relate to the load required.

Springs can be made using a jig or pliers, or purchased from hand therapy suppliers. Coil springs should be loaded in the same direction the coil is made, with the middle of the spring aligned to the axis of the joint. Spring arms, long enough to allow joint movement, are inserted into the thermoplastic of the orthosis.

Commercial Components

Commercially available hinges consist of two plates hinged to allow movement in one plane. They have a form of locking device to either restrict movement to a specific range or sustain the joint at a predetermined range. The locking device provides a convenient adjustment of the orthosis joint position by the therapist or patient. They come in kits of various sizes suitable for the finger, wrist, and elbow joints with either screws or mouldable plastic to allow attachment to custom made

thermoplastic components. Mobilizing hinges are available for larger joints with pretension springs that can be adjusted to sustain a specific range, or to return to a predetermined range should the patient move against the spring. Several brands of hinges are available from major hand therapy product suppliers with considerable variability in cost, strength and durability. Hinges can be used multiple times and recycled within a hand clinic.

METHODS

PATTERN DESIGN

Pattern design is an integral part of prescription, requiring concurrent analysis of material choice, fabrication technique and essential componentry. Essentially the problem is similar to dressmaking in that a three dimensional orthosis is manufactured from a two dimensional material.

There is a direct correlation between the precision of the pattern taken and the outcome of the orthosis. Taking a good pattern is the first stage of successful orthotic intervention. Specific patterns are discussed in the appropriate chapter. It is vital to read all the instructions with the diagrams and have an understanding of the procedure prior to commencing. Pattern making, similar to all aspects of orthotic fabrication, is a skill to be practiced.

Methods Of Pattern Making

The requirements for patterns vary with the material. The type of material used will govern the choices available in pattern making. The more rigid materials require more precise patterns.

In order to take a pattern you will need a piece of paper towel or plastic sheet, pencils, pens, ruler, scissors and tape measure. Plastic sheet, often found in the thermoplastic sheet material packaging, is more resistant to tearing and is therefore more appropriate for use with children or non-compliant patients, and taking larger patterns.

1. Landmark, Pattern and Apply

This is the more precise design technique. Identify appropriate landmarks and shape the pattern using those landmarks. This pattern must be cut out from the paper or plastic and applied to the limb to check the fit prior to transferring it to the thermoplastic material. If the pattern is inaccurate or incorrect it will have direct implications to the success of orthotic fabrication.

2. Rough Pattern, Stretch and Mould

The unique properties of highly malleable thermoplastic materials allows stretch and contour without loss of properties. A rough pattern only is required, and this is stretched and pulled into position. Excess material is trimmed post moulding. If these materials are stretched too far, they become thin and lose strength. They should be stretched slowly to avoid this occurring.

FABRICATION TECHNIQUES

Cutting Thermoplastic Material

Shears are generally used to cut cold thermoplastics. Straight lines can be cut on sheets of thermoplastic by scoring it with a Stanley trimmer along a straight edge and then bending it to snap open the scored line. When cutting heated thermoplastics use single, long strokes with scissors to ensure smooth edges. This is particularly important when cutting around curves.

Cutting Hot Seams

Many orthoses, such as cylindrical orthoses and hand-based orthoses, can take advantage of properties that allow a neat seam to be created. Materials need to be drapey and stretchable, and be either self-adherent or adherent with pressure or on cutting. The material is pulled around the limb and the two edges adhered or held together where the seam is desired. Holding the scissor blades parallel and close to the skin surface, cut with long, smooth strokes. The cut edges will bond together to form a flat neat seam. For the neatest results, care should be taken to ensure the material is pulled together and cut in a straight line, usually aligning with some limb axis. The seam may need reinforcing with a thin strip of thermoplastic dry bonded over the top.

Moulding Over Joints

Materials with a high degree of stretch and drape allow orthoses that traverse angulated joints to be fabricated without seams to conform at the joint margins. The material is anchored either proximal or distal to the joint with a circumferential mould. The material can then be gently stretched over the joint, with the lateral aspects stretching less than the central aspect. This is particularly useful for elbow orthoses.

Creating Holes

In materials with a high degree of stretch and drape, creating openings for digits requires only a small hole punched with a leather punch when material is cold. Ensuring the material is activated gently enlarge the hole, rolling the edge over smoothly to the appropriate size. Soft, gentle and slow strokes are advised in materials without elastic memory to avoid over stretching the hole and thinning the material. Creating holes in less mouldable materials that are 'plastic like' (refer to Table 2) requires a larger hole to be cut, roughly 2cm in diameter. The edges of the hole are then teased back and semi folded along the entire circle circumference before bonding the plastic back on itself to create an even thumbhole.

Circumferential Orthoses

Materials that are self-adherent enable therapists to fabricate circumferential orthoses easily. A non-exact pattern is used, the material is pulled around the hand or arm and the edges lightly pinched together. No bandage or wrap is required as the material holds itself on the limb. This saves time allowing the therapist to easily see and evaluate the orthosis whilst working. Bandaging is not required and this is beneficial for the patient who cannot tolerate a lot of handling. If the material is only lightly pinched together, it is easily pulled apart to release the patient.

The orthosis may be finished either by hot seaming (e.g. cylindrical finger orthosis), by creating an opening where fasteners will be attached (e.g. wrist gauntlet), or both (e.g. hand-based thumb orthosis). Circumferential orthoses by design are very strong and a thinner material can be used and still achieve a high degree of rigidity and therefore immobility in the body part.

Attaching Straps

Using adhesive backed hook Velcro® is the easiest and quickest method to secure straps. Cut the Velcro® to the length required and round the corners. Ensure the area on the orthosis where Velcro® is to be attached is clean. Peel off the backing, gently heat the adhesive with a heat gun (hold the Velcro® with scissors or pliers to prevent injury) and attach to the orthosis at the correct location and angle. Press it on firmly ensuring there are no air bubbles. If this method is unsuccessful in securing the Velcro®, the surface of the thermoplastic can be spot heated with the heat gun, being careful not to distort it. The Velcro® is also heated and then pressed into place. Some materials with coating may require solvents or bonding agents to aid the process of adhering.

Thermoplastic materials such as Orfit® and Aquaplast® can be heated till the surface is shiny, then the pile Velcro® applied directly to the material. Do not overheat the material or distort it with the pressure used to apply the strap. In materials where this is not possible, use hook Velcro® on both sides of the orthosis to attach the pile Velcro®.

In circumferential orthotic designs the seam join of the two edges of thermoplastic material can be used to reinforce and secure the Velcro® straps. Non-adhesive loop Velcro® straps are attached to one side of the orthosis by gently spot heating a small area of the orthosis edge, sticking the loop Velcro® backside down onto the orthosis. The small thermoplastic edge is heated and then rolled back over securing the Velcro®. The strap may also be secured to the seamed edge by spot heating the seam with the heat gun and folding the strap down so that it will attach to the adhesive backed hook Velcro® on the adjacent side of the orthosis. Images of orthoses throughout this text illustrate various methods to secure Velcro® to thermoplastic material.

For some materials, the adhesive backed strapping will not remain secured to the orthosis. Cut a small moon from either side of the strap then secure by adhering a piece of thermoplastic material over the section of Velcro® or webbing. Although this type of attachment is bulkier than a rivet the advantage is the inside surface of the orthosis remains smooth. This method is also useful when adhesive Velcro® and rivets are not available.

In some situations it may be necessary to consider using bandaging to secure the orthosis. For example, nursing home patients may have fragile skin intolerant of straps, may pick at and pull off the straps or injure themselves on the Velcro®, or pile straps may continually be lost. In the case of children, bandaging an orthosis on the limb may be an efficient means of securing it.

D-rings may be used to make it easier for the patient to put on the orthosis, particularly when weakness is a problem. D-rings enable the patient to secure the orthosis more firmly. They are also useful where there is insufficient surface area on the orthosis to secure straps. The D-ring must be placed so its total surface is over the orthosis and not in contact with the skin.

Applying Lining

1. Apply all straps to the orthosis prior to lining it.
2. Retain the pattern from the orthosis and use it to outline the lining material. Ensure the pattern is positioned so the adhesive back will adhere to the correct surface of the orthosis.
3. For lining materials that have some "give" allow approximately 1 cm around each edge, allow 2 cm for non-stretchy lining materials.
4. Apply the lining material to the orthosis in small sections. Do not take the whole backing sheet off at once.
5. Orientate the lining to the orthosis at the wrist and then work proximal and distal.
6. Avoid wrinkles or overlapping the lining material, as this will cause pressure.
7. Trim the lining material to the edge of the orthosis, allowing a few millimetres overhang. Dry heating the exposed adhesive and adhering it over the edge of the orthosis prolongs the life of the linings attachment (it doesn't prolong the life of the lining itself).
8. The lining should be changed regularly as it becomes soiled.

PATIENT PREPARATION PROCEDURES

Introduction

Discuss the purpose of the therapy session, the intended procedure and the expected outcomes, both short and long term. Clarify the patient's intended goals and identify fears and anxieties. Inform the patient of the possibility of pain or discomfort particularly in post-operative cases. Reassure the patient that the procedure itself should not cause pain. This is important as fear, anticipation of pain or lack of precautions can jeopardise the procedure. If the patient is a child, a few minutes spent at this point relaxing and having some fun, making a small orthosis from scrap material for the child's favourite doll or teddy, or letting them play with the thermoplastic material will save a lot of time later when an uninformed and tense child becomes non-compliant. If the child is unsettled, it is better to proceed quickly with as little fuss as possible.

A time frame for review of the orthosis is determined by the pathology and expected course of therapy intervention. Arrangements are necessary for after hours appointments or for referral to other practitioners where patients live far from the clinic

Evaluation

Obtain a complete clinical picture by thorough evaluation of the patient and their hand.

Clinical Decision Making

Decision-making is a collaborative effort between patient and therapist. Issues to consider are discussed in Chapter 1. Identify the therapy and orthotic requirements and objectives. Determine the extent of limb involvement and appropriate positions for joints involved in the orthosis. Identify design, material, strapping and lining options and select the most suitable. Identify precautions for therapist and patient.

Patient Instruction

Describe the procedure of application and moulding of the orthosis and instruct the patient of your expectations of them during the procedure (this includes where and how to hold the limb, and to not grasp the material, or assist unless asked to do so). Advise that the material should be warm, not hot.

Environment and Equipment Preparation

Ensure the work area is clear of extraneous products. Wound dressings should be protected during orthosis fabrication or changed immediately after the procedure. Gather all essential items and organize in a tidy and accessible manner.

Pattern Taking

In order to create patterns, a therapist needs the ability to see a pattern in two dimensions transformed into a three-dimensional object. Take the pattern and ensure correct fit before cutting it from the sheet of thermoplastic. Cut out the material and heat.

Patient Preparation

While the material is heating, protect susceptible tissues. Pad out bony prominences and position the patient's limb for the fabrication procedure. Small pieces of lining material or exercise putty can be moulded over protuberances prior to fabrication of the orthosis. Support at risk tissues such as tendon repairs or MCP arthroplasties. Protect grafts, flaps, pin sites and wound dressings. Acrylic fingernails bond very easily to plastic based materials such as Orfit® so cover if there is any risk of adherence prior to orthosis fabrication.

Orthosis Fabrication

Mould orthosis according to requirements. Evaluate, check position, fit and pressure and correct or modify as appropriate. Trim excess, roll or smooth edges, apply outriggers, straps and lining (if any). Place back on the limb and conduct a final evaluation.

Patient Education

Educate the patient regarding wearing regimes, including daily schedule, time span, weaning off, activities to avoid while wearing the orthosis, activities requiring removal of the orthosis, how to complete activities with orthosis on and concomitant therapy requirements. Give the patient information on care of the orthosis, including cleaning and protection from sustained heat. Advise the patient to return if problems are experienced (e.g. red areas, altered sensation, broken components) and document follow-up or review appointments. The responsibility for the review process must be formalized (i.e. who is responsible for setting dates and conducting the review) with the therapist taking primary responsibility for their work. It is unethical to deliver treatment without some form of acceptable follow-up. It is advisable to issue a patient handout with all this information covered, including the therapist's name and a contact phone number.

Restoration of Therapeutic Environment

It is essential for safe and efficient work practices, let alone for professional presentation, to restore the environment to its original state. Clean and, if necessary, disinfect tools and equipment and return to the correct storage position. Soiled towels and bandages should be stored for laundering, and fresh stocks replenished. Dressings, swabs and disposable packs should be disposed of appropriately. Clean surfaces of all waste materials and mop up any water spills. Make note of any stock re-ordering which is required.

CONCLUSION

Pride should be taken in all aspects of designing, fabricating and finishing off an orthosis. It represents visible evidence of the therapist's quality of work and will become part of the patient's personal presentation. Quality fabrication is a result of sound knowledge of material characteristics and properties, and the ability to handle those materials to achieve maximum performance. As with the development of all technical skills, competency and efficiency is improved with practice. A well organised, safe and efficient work environment assists in this process.

References

1. Breger-Lee DE, Burford WL. Properties of thermoplastic splinting materials. Journal of Hand Therapy. 1992;5: 202–211.

2. Breger-Lee DE. Objective and subjective observations of low-temperature thermoplastic materials. Journal of Hand Therapy. 1995; 8:202–211.

3. Standards Australia/Standards New Zealand. AS/NZS 4187:2003. Cleaning, disinfection and sterilising reusable medical and surgical instruments and equipment, and maintenance of associated environments in health care facilities. Sydney: Standards Australia International Ltd.

4. Van Lede P, van Velderhoven G. Therapeutic Hand Splints. A Rational Approach. Volume 1. Mechanical and Biomechanical Considerations. 1998. Antwerp:Provan.

4

ORTHOSES/SPLINTS TO ADDRESS THE ELBOW AND FOREARM

INTRODUCTION

Normal use of the hand depends upon a well functioning elbow joint, as it is the critical link in lengthening and shortening the upper limb. Stability is crucial to ensure effective transmission of forces by the upper limb. However mobility is essential to function as it allows the forearm, wrist, and hand to be positioned in space. Morrey et al[21] determined normal functional range of elbow motion is 30°-130° with 100° rotation: 50° in supination and 50° pronation. The elbow presents a challenge to therapists as it is a notoriously unforgiving joint in disease and following trauma.[7] A systematic approach to patient assessment is recommended to determine the stability, irritability, mobility, and function of the elbow in order to implement effective treatments for positive outcomes.[17]

ANATOMY OF THE ELBOW AND FOREARM

The elbow complex consists of the ulnohumeral and the radiohumeral articulations, with close associations to the proximal radioulnar (PRU) joint. Whilst commonly considered a hinge joint, due to its primary motion of flexion-extension, accessory movements of abduction, adduction and axial rotation are well recognised.[22] The centre of rotation of the elbow remains an issue of discussion with most authors agreeing there are centres of rotation that correspond to a line from the inferior aspect of the medial epicondyle through the centre of the lateral epicondyle.[1, 28]

The obliquities between the proximal humeral shaft, the trochlea, and the distal ulna shaft define the carrying angle. In the frontal plane, this valgus angle averages 10°-15° in men and 15°-20° in women, however the angle is not evident in pronation.[20,30] There is considerable individual variation so therapists are encouraged to refer to the contralateral side rather than with 'normal angles'. The changes in the carrying angle, from extension to flexion in the frontal plane, have implications to the use of articulated orthoses. The axis of motion of the elbow and the degree of rotation of the forearm, and the alignment of the axis of the hinge, requires careful attention to avoid misalignment.

Stability is afforded the joint by the congruous articular surfaces and the soft tissue constraints. The trochlear notch of the olecranon articulates with the conical trochlea of the humerus and is the primary determinant of bony stability. The radiohumeral joint also contributes to lateral stability and force transmission through the elbow. The ulnohumeral, radiohumeral and PRU joints are enclosed within a common fibrous capsule reinforced by the medial and lateral collateral ligaments. Of these the medial ligament is the most important due to the orientation of functional stress. The medial collateral ligament consists of anterior and posterior bundles that contribute to stability in different ranges of motion. Anterior fibres are taut in flexion and extension and the posterior fibres are taut only in flexion.[19,23] The flexor pronator muscles also contribute to stability. The lateral collateral ligament is uniformly taut throughout elbow motion, because it attaches to the lateral epicondyle at the axis of rotation.[19] The anconeous muscle contributes to lateral stability along with wrist and finger extensor musculature.

Whilst functionally distinct joints, the proximity of the ulnohumeral to the radiohumeral and to the PRU joints, implies that injury to one joint may have consequences for the mobility of the others.

Rotary motion occurs at the proximal and distal radioulnar (DRU) joints in the actions of pronation and supination. The axis of rotation is through the centre of the radial head and capitulum, and along the line extending through the base of the ulna styloid (Figure 1). While most authors agree that the radius rotates in an arc around the ulna during pronation-supination, the contribution of the ulna to this movement is still an area for discussion. The two radioulnar joints are coaxial. While greater motion is seen at the distal joint as the radius rotates about the ulna, it must be remembered that except when either of the bones is misaligned, the radius rotates through the same arc of motion at the PRU and DRU joints. Wrist and hand orthoses applied to a forearm surface must allow for the changing dimensions of the forearm during rotation. Maximizing range of forearm rotation is a therapeutic goal commonly addressed by orthotic intervention following fractures to the radius and or ulna.

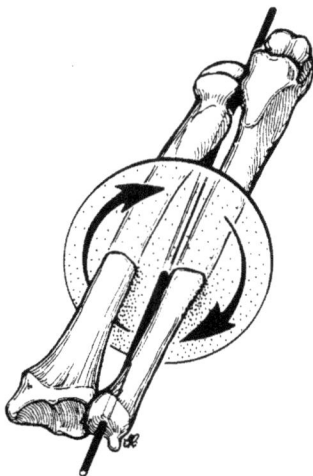

Figure 1: Axis of motion for pronation-supination. This axis is located along the entire length of the forearm. Traction applied at a 90° angle could approximate 360° curve (from Collello-Abraham, 1990, p.1135).

Rotation of the head of the radius about its axis occurs within the fibro-osseous ring formed by the annular ligament and the radial notch of the ulna. The unique shape of the proximal radius and the head of the radius mean that rotatory movements are

also accompanied by lateral movement, and distal tilting of the radius. The flexibility in the annular ligament permits this movement.

The DRU joint is the head of the ulna articulating on the concave sigmoid notch of the radius. While the joint surfaces are well adapted to each other, the joint geometry varies with the relative length of the ulna to the radius. Stability of the distal joint is due to the triangular fibrocartilage complex (TFCC), the radioulnar ligaments, and the capsule. The TFCC consists of a cartilaginous central portion (the disc), surrounded by thick dorsal and volar radioulnar ligaments, the ulnar collateral ligament, the meniscus homologue, the extensor carpi ulnaris sheath, the ulnolunate and lunotriquetral ligaments. Translocation of the ulna, dorsally during pronation and volarly during supination, is checked by the dorsal and volar DRU joint ligaments thus preventing dislocation. Instability, impingement, and incongruity are common problems of the DRU joint, which impact upon the functional range available for rotation. The wrist joint is isolated from the radiocarpal joint, except when there are deficits in the triangular fibrocartilage secondary to trauma or degeneration.

Tremendous forces are transmitted across the elbow joint by the action of powerful flexor and extensor muscles. Elbow flexion is achieved by biceps brachii, brachialis, and brachioradialis with triceps the extensor. Brachialis muscle is implicated in post-traumatic contracture of the elbow due to its location on the anterior capsule of the elbow. Haematoma and scar tissue in the muscle are possible causes of heterotopic ossification (pathologic bone deposited within the muscle) associated with capsular contracture.[5]

Laterally the wrist and hand extensor musculature arise from the supracondylar ridge and lateral epicondyle. Medially the flexor pronator group arise from the medial epicondyle. By their location proximal to the elbow joint, the wrist extensor and flexor musculature have a small moment arm for rotation at the elbow, but a significant contribution to joint stability. Epicondylitis, a common clinical presentation with pain in the region of either the medial or lateral epicondyle, is exacerbated by resisted action of muscles arising from the involved epicondyle.

The major nerves to the hand traverse the elbow joint and, with the exception of the ulnar nerve, are generally protected by the muscles through which they traverse. Attention should be focused on the ulnar nerve, in its path around the medial epicondyle, to ensure that it is not compromised by pressure from any form of orthotic intervention.

ORTHOSES TO IMMOBILIZE THE ELBOW

Orthoses are used following bone and soft tissues injuries to protect healing structures and optimize positions of immobilization.

Elbow immobilization can be achieved with or without immobilization of forearm rotation. Circumferential designs offer the greatest immobilization and are required following some injuries in the vicinity of the elbow, while posterior application is recommended for orthoses to immobilize the elbow for rest.

The choice of thermoplastic material has implications to design and fabrication technique. Non-stick materials are easier to handle in large pieces; however, require the additional step of bandaging to secure the material to the limb. Materials with a sticky surface require careful handling when being removed from the heating pan, but stick to the patient's limb once placed eliminating the need for bandaging. An assistant may be required or the patient instructed how to assist during fabrication.

Orthoses to address the elbow (Figures 2 and 3) use a series of length and circumferential measurements as illustrated in Figure 4.

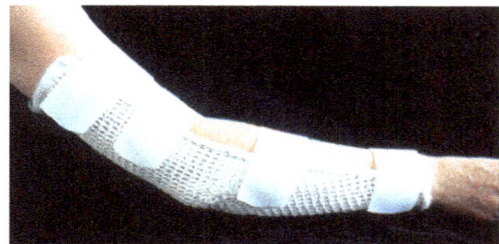

Figure 2: Posterior Elbow Immobilization Orthosis. This orthosis is generally used to rest and support the soft tissues.

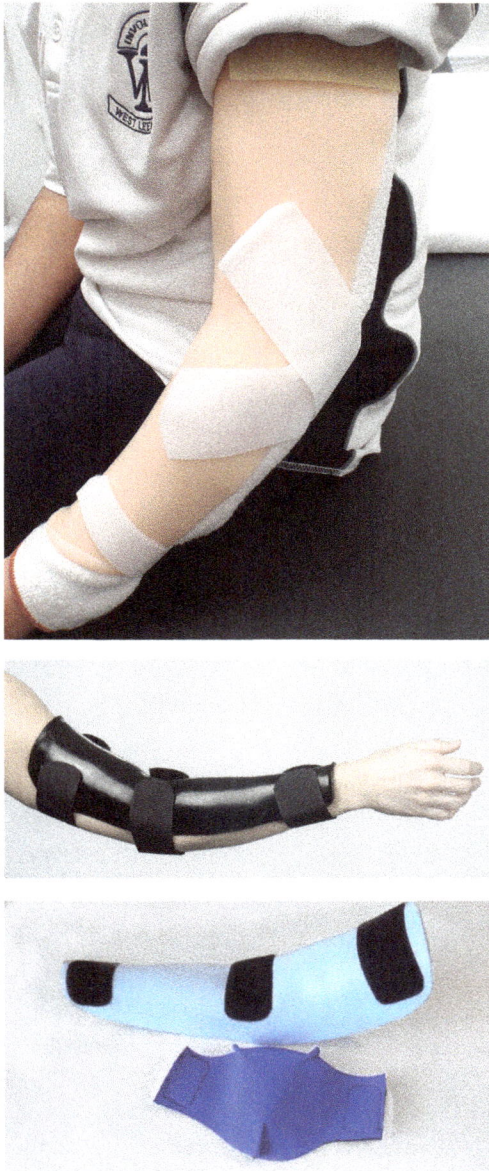

Figure 3: Anterior Elbow Immobilization Orthosis. Orthoses applied to the anterior surface to minimize risk for pressure problems at the elbow. Strapping is an important component of the lever system with various options illustrated. (Lower two images courtesy Michael Fitzgerald)

ELBOW IMMOBILIZATION ORTHOSIS (ANTERIOR OR POSTERIOR SURFACE)

When the elbow is immobilized at angles less than 70° flexion, the properties of stretch and mould are used to contour the material to the arm. However, if the angle is greater than 70° flexion, a dart may be required in the thermoplastic material at the elbow to ensure contour. This can be done by pinching the excess thermoplastic material together during moulding. Do not cut dart material off if orthosis is to be remoulded several times to accommodate swelling or changes in joint angle.

Large elbow orthoses require longitudinal strength to achieve their objective to immobilize tissues. Therefore thicker materials are combined with contour to mechanically achieve strength required.

Numerous bony prominences require padding prior to fabrication. Where the biceps muscle is also tight, as in the case of an elbow contracture, care should be taken to avoid pressure on the tendon.

Procedure To Make A Pattern

Measurements required for this orthosis are taken with the arm in the position it will be immobilized (Figure 4):

1. Length axilla-elbow-wrist proximal to the ulna head.
2. Circumference at the axilla.
3. Circumference at the wrist proximal to the ulna head.
4. Circumference proximal to the elbow

93

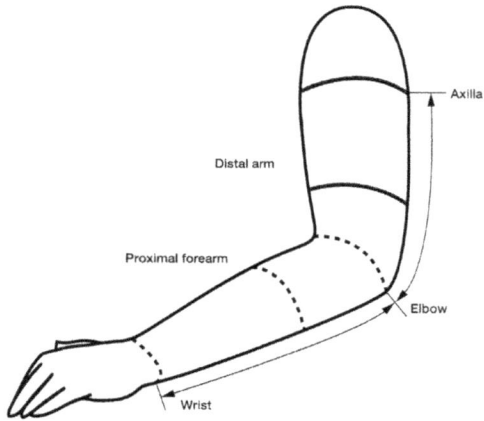

Figure 4: Elbow Orthosis Measurement. Location of circumferential and length measurements required to make a pattern for an elbow orthosis.

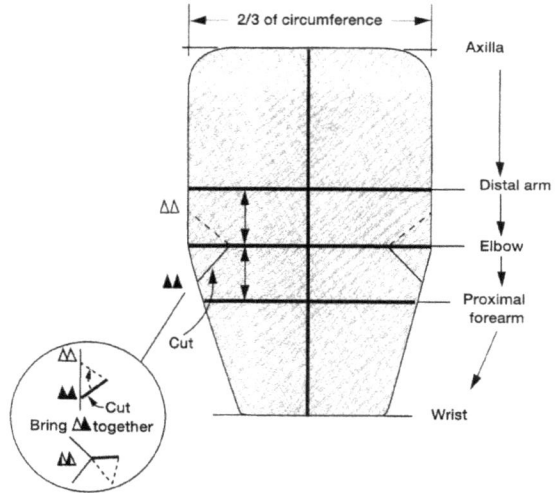

Figure 5: Elbow Immobilization Orthosis Pattern .

(one third the length measurement of the upper arm).

5. Circumference below the elbow (one third the length measurement of the forearm).

Measurements may provide all the information necessary to cut out required thermoplastic without making a formal pattern. The more rigid the thermoplastic material used the more precise the pattern required. To formalize the pattern:

1. Draw a vertical line in the centre of your pattern material the length of the arm (Figure 5).

2. Square three lines through this at the level of the axilla, elbow, and wrist. Mark the points where the circumferences were taken proximal to the elbow and distal forearm then insert the related circumferences. For circumferential orthoses, use the full measurement, with two-thirds the measurement for anteri-

or or posterior orthoses.

3. Darts may be required in orthoses applied to the posterior surface. In that case mark the depth of two 'V' shaped darts at the elbow (refer to inset Figure 5).

4. Apply the pattern to the patient's arm; make any adjustment to the pattern prior to transferring it to the thermoplastic material.

Fabrication Procedure

Owing to the large piece of thermoplastic material involved in this pattern some planning is required to avoid difficulties. When removing the material from the heating pan ensure that it is supported along the length to avoid stretching. Anterior application is easiest by placing the material on the arm aligning the elbow crease with the elbow component. For posterior application, it may be easier to lay the patient down, either supine or prone, and use shoulder movement to position the arm and forearm so that gravity can be used to assist application. For circumferential orthoses, apply the anterior surface then bring the posterior component around to bond on either the medial or lateral borders. Once thermoplastic material is secured reposition the arm to the side of the body so that the medial surface is moulded between the arm and the chest.

Once thermoplastic material is completely cold, mark edges that need to be adjusted, particularly under the axilla and at the distal forearm. Rolling edges along length of orthosis not only addresses comfort but also adds strength.

The strapping system is a very important component of the force used to immobilize the elbow in the orthosis. The middle force can be two wide Velcro® straps proximal and distal to the joint, a crisscross type of strapping pattern over the posterior aspect of the elbow just proximal to the olecranon, or a wide neoprene strap with darts sewn at proximal and distal ends contoured to the elbow, minimizing pressure from being directly applied over the bony olecranon (Figures 2 and 3).

ORTHOSES TO MOBILIZE THE ELBOW

Deficits in passive range of motion (ROM) of the elbow are a common complication of injury to the joint and surrounding soft tissues. Factors contributing to passive ROM deficits should be identified in consultation with the medical team prior to initiating orthotic intervention. The terms 'extrinsic' and 'intrinsic' are used to describe contracture for purposes of planning intervention. Extrinsic causes include contracture of the joint capsule and ligaments, muscle contracture, adherence, extra-articular osteophytes, and ectopic ossification. Intrinsic causes include intra-articular adhesions, incongruity, osteophytes, loose bodies, and chondral defects.[10] Whilst the patient may present with extrinsic and intrinsic components to the contracture, therapy interventions usually address only the extrinsic components. The high propensity for contracture, even following relatively minor trauma, increases the importance of prevention. Principles of application of mobilizing orthoses to address deficits in passive ROM are discussed in Chapter One.

Forceful manipulation of the joint can be counterproductive by tearing tissue and stimulating further contracture. Therefore, by applying a small force to extend the tissues for a prolonged period of time using mobilizing orthoses, gradual lengthening of tissues can be achieved. Resolution of elbow contractures may take many months of orthotic intervention so therapists need to consider protocols that are sensitive to the patient's life style demands and encourage participation in interventions that may be uncomfortable and interrupt daily activities.

Serial static and static progressive mobilizing principles are the foundation for the majority of elbow mobilizing protocols. Outcomes of case series using a specific orthosis and wearing protocols all report positive outcomes over many weeks,[2,3,11,12,13,26] however comparative studies are limited. Lindenhovius and colleagues[16] in a prospective clinical trial compared commercially manufactured static progressive and dynamic orthotic interventions in 66 persons with posttraumatic elbow stiffness. They found there were no significant differences in improvement in motion from wearing a dynamic orthosis applying low force for 6 to 12 hours a day, or static progressive orthosis applying high force twice daily for 30 minutes. Evaluation over twelve months identified no differences between cohorts in terms of motion, improvement of motion, or disability rating on Disabilities of the Arm, Shoulder and Hand (DASH). Cost and availability of these commercial mobilizing orthoses can be prohibitive. With limited research evidence to guide practice the choice of orthosis should be determined in consultation between the patient, surgeon/ physician and therapist.

Following assessment and determination of an objective for mobilization of the elbow, the therapist must consider the choices in the design taking into consideration the pathology and the specific needs of the patient. The design choices are:

- Serial static orthoses are made of one piece of thermoplastic material moulded over the anterior, or posterior surface of the arm and forearm

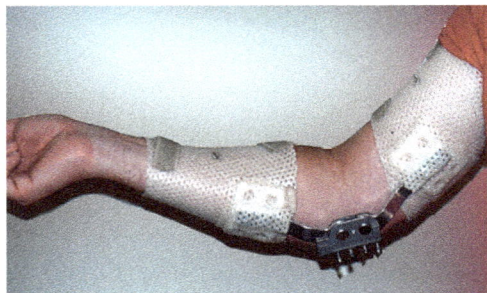

Figure 6a: Elbow Mobilization Orthoses Hinged Elbow Orthosis. Mobilizing force applied via hinge aligned of the axis of the joint. Four screws in this style of hinge allow for adjustment of joint position or restriction of joint range.

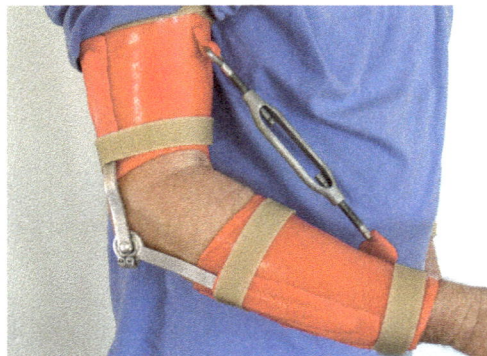

Figure 6b: Elbow Mobilization Orthoses Hinged Elbow Orthosis. Mobilizing force applied via turnbuckle with hinge controlling axis of rotation, thereby eliminating any compressive force being transferred to the joint.

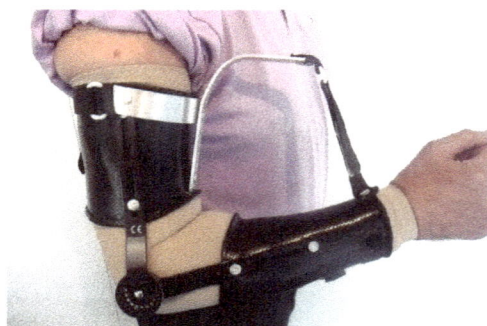

Figure 6c: Elbow Mobilization Orthoses Hinged Elbow Orthosis. Mobilizing force applied via Velcro® using aluminium rod to create outrigger, with hinge controlling axis of rotation. (Courtesy Michael Fitzgerald)

depending upon passive ROM deficit. The therapist progressively remoulds it as motion increases. This orthosis uses three points of pressure to create the mobilizing force so strapping is a vital component. Pattern for this orthosis is the same as that used for anterior/posterior immobilization orthosis. It is important that the thermoplastic material used has sufficient strength, memory to return to original pattern shape when reheated, and can withstand multiple remouldings.

- Static progressive orthoses generally have a hinge, aligned with the axis of elbow joint motion, to either:
  - (a) Create the mobilizing force that is applied via the arm and forearm cuffs. The hinge transfers the rotational component of the force to the elbow joint thus minimizing any potential compressive forces associated with changing line of pull (Figure 6a), or
  - (b) Control rotation created by the force from the turnbuckle, Velcro® or non-elastic strapping (Figure 6b and 6c).
- Dynamic Orthoses use a hinge aligned with the axis of elbow joint motion to control rotation created by elastic or Thera-Band® traction.

The angle of joint motion deficit is the primary determinant of intervention design. Mathematical modelling by Chinchalker et al.[6] and Szekeres[25] considered resolution of forces in elbow orthoses to provide some guidelines

for therapists as to choice of orthotic intervention. The ideal force acts perpendicular to the longitudinal axis of the radius/ulna with minimal rotation lost to joint compression (refer to biomechanical principles Chapter 2). In resolution of extension deficits Chinchalker et al.[6] demonstrated when the arm is flexed; force components from a turnbuckle screw in the static progressive extension orthosis provide the greatest rotational/compressive ratio. In the later stages of therapy when the goal is terminal elbow extension applying an adjustable posterior strap directly over the elbow joint, to produce an opposing force to the two forces produced by the turnbuckle, will develop greater rotational force. Thus a static progressive orthosis is an effective option in applying force to flexion contractures of 30°or less.

Regaining end range flexion presents a challenge to the therapist, as it is often difficult to apply an effective line of force application that does not result in compression forces being translated to the joint. Compression can be a source of pain that may limit adherence to a wearing regime. Flexion deficits up to 110° can be addressed using a hinge attached to the orthosis to fix the axis of rotation, thereby minimizing compression forces created by turnbuckles, elastic/non elastic strapping to the joint. For patients trying to gain terminal flexion, a thermoplastic cuff around the forearm with force directed via elastic/non elastic strap to the upper humerus or chest can be adequate despite the compressive forces through the elbow.[25] Forces transmitted through the elbow joint while wearing a flexion cuff are not optimal so this method of mobilizing the elbow into flexion is recommended when the patient is able to achieve greater than 110° of flexion and when its application does not cause pain.[6]

Commercial hinges purchased from hand therapy suppliers are commonly used. Size and strength of the hinges will determine whether one or two are required to efficiently position the joint at end range. The hinge is adjusted to sustain end range position by manipulation of screws or locking devices (Figure 6). Where deficits are evident in both flexion and extension a hinged orthosis can be used to address deficits in both directions.

Hinged orthoses are a cost-effective means of addressing elbow contractures. Although the hinges are expensive, they can be adjusted as the joint accommodates to changes in ROM. If the patient is responsible, he or she may be educated to do this, thereby reducing cost of consultation with the therapist. Recycling hinges also reduces cost. If the hinge is only required to control rotational forces the hinge can be made from two pieces of thermoplastic material connected by a screw rivet.

Pattern and Fabrication Procedure

The hinged elbow orthosis, as illustrated in Figure 6a, uses circumferential cuffs for the arm and forearm. This provides a large area to contact for pressure dispersion minimizing potential for straps to cut into soft tissues. Circumferential thermoplastic cuffs are not necessary, however migration or tipping of the orthosis can be problematic requiring firm wide non-slip strapping. Area of force application should be contoured thermoplastic, anterior surface for extension and posterior surface for flexion, with strapping located on opposite surfaces.

1. Length and circumferential measurements are taken using locations identified in Figure 4.
2. Thermoplastic cuffs are moulded around the arm and forearm. Ensure openings of both cuffs are aligned longitudinally. After initial moulding mark the location of the hinge/s on medial and lateral borders using a wax pencil, prior to removing cuffs from the arm. Mark any edges that need to be trimmed to allow for movement to end range. This is particularly important when mobilizing into flexion.
3. Remove thermoplastic components from the arm and secure the hinges to the cuffs with hinge rivets or any additional pieces of thermoplastic material.
4. Apply straps to both cuffs.
5. Apply orthosis to the arm and check hinge alignment and all edges. Flare all edges to ensure no shear pressure.
6. If mobilizing force is to be created via turnbuckles, elastic/non elastic strapping this is then attached on the surface appropriate to the direction of force. Turnbuckles are available in various sizes, with size dependent upon ROM to be gained.
7. If the patient is to modify the orthosis angle, they must be instructed in the following:
   (a) When to wear the orthosis. This will

be determined by lifestyle. Some patients are better able to tolerate the orthosis during the day whilst others can comfortably wear the orthosis during sleep. Prior to wearing this orthosis during sleep, the patient should have worn it for extended periods during the day to ensure no complications.

(b) When to change the angle. This will be determined by compliance of tissues to lengthen in response to the gentle stress applied. It is recommended that patients wear the orthosis for upwards of six hours per day for several days with 'no awareness of pulling or tension in the tissues' before increasing passive range by several degrees.

(c) The procedure to change the angle. It is important that the patient has the necessary tools and has demonstrated competence in the procedure prior to leaving the clinic.

(d) Precautions. Attempting to increase the angle faster than the tissues can accommodate may result in injury to tissue and further scarring. The patient must understand risks of incorrect use of the orthosis. Patients using orthoses to regain elbow flexion must also be educated regarding signs of paresthesia associated with traction or compression on the ulnar nerve.

ORTHOSES TO RESTRICT MOTION IN THE ELBOW

Restriction of elbow motion is often used to promote safe healing of injured or repaired structures around the elbow, for example fractures, tendon repairs and tendon transfers. The presenting pathology, combined with recommendations from the upper limb surgeon, will determine the limits of motion to specific degrees in the arc of extension/flexion. Articulated elbow orthoses use the stops in the elbow hinge (Figure 6a) to restrict the range of motion. Fabrication of this orthosis follows the procedure described for a hinged elbow orthosis in the previous section.

ORTHOSES TO IMMOBILIZE THE FOREARM

Forearm immobilization or restricted ROM may be indicated in the management of injuries to the radius, ulnar, or proximal or distal radioulnar joints. Immobilization of the forearm can only be achieved when both proximal and distal joints are addressed. For this reason it is necessary to include the wrist and the distal humerus. Thus orthoses that immobilize the forearm generally immobilize the wrist and restrict motion at the elbow; due to insufficient strength in low temperature thermoplastic materials to control proximal forearm rotation.

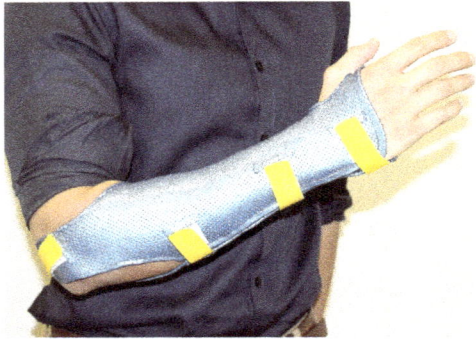

Figure 7a: Forearm Immobilization Orthoses.
Orthosis Muenster style is circumferential in the distal forearm, wrist and hand with allowance at the proximal end for some degrees of active elbow flexion. (Courtesy Stuart Wilson)

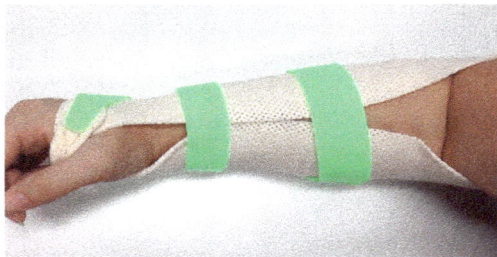

Figure 7b: Forearm Immobilization Orthoses.
Orthosis Sugartong style applies thermoplastic moulded on both dorsal and volar surfaces of forearm and hand, traversing posterior aspect of the elbow. (Courtesy Cathy Merry and Maryanne Simpson)

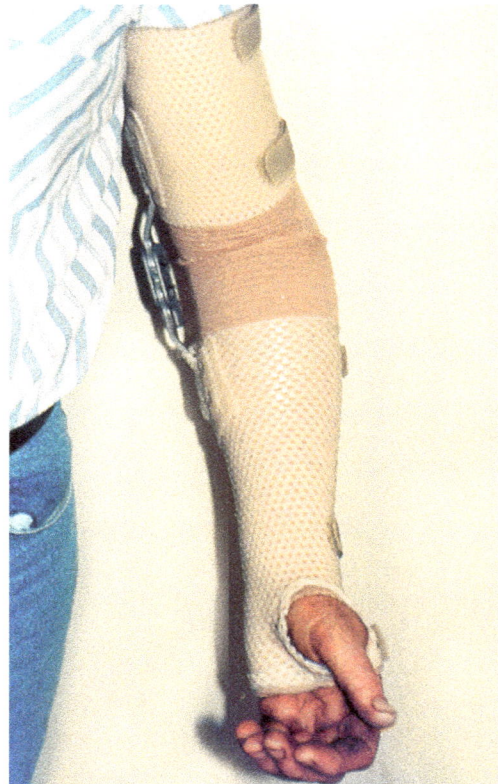

Figure 7c: Forearm Immobilization Orthoses.
Orthosis elbow hinge allows freedom of flexion extension motion, but prevents forearm rotation when attached to wrist immobilization orthosis.

Two styles of immobilization orthoses are commonly used. The Muenster style replicates the cast of the same name in which the forearm is immobilized by circumferential immobilization of the wrist and inclusion of the elbow till just proximal to the humeral condyles limiting elbow extension but allowing some degrees of elbow flexion (Figure 7a). The Sugartong style (so named because the finished orthosis looks like tongs used for sugar cubes) extends from proximal to finger MCP joints along dorsal forearm, around the posterior aspect of the elbow incorporating medial and lateral humeral condyles, and along volar forearm to mid palm region (Figure 7b). In a comparative study using healthy subjects Slaughter et al.[24] found both orthoses allowed some active pronation and supination when the participants used maximal force to rotate the forearm against the orthosis. The Sugartong orthosis was found to be more restrictive in pronation.

Fabricating orthoses that immobilize the forearm present a unique challenge. The therapist must manage large pieces of thermoplastic material whilst controlling multiple joints. To achieve the desired function of the orthosis the therapist must control the position of the wrist, forearm, and the elbow during moulding.

FOREARM IMMOBILIZATION ORTHOSIS - CIRCUMFERENTIAL APPLICATION (MUENSTER STYLE)

This orthosis is very similar in its construction to the wrist immobilization orthosis that is extended past the elbow. It uses the principle of contour to provide rigidity, with thickness of thermoplastic material determining the resistance to deformation associated with active forearm movements. Climatic and vocational demands will determine the type of material, its thickness and the degree of perforation.

Using gravity to assist fabrication the opening is placed along the ulnar border of the hand and forearm. This also allows for easier access. However it is important that the ulnar aspect of the hand is well supported to prevent ulnar deviation of the wrist.

Measurements for this orthosis pattern are all taken with a tape measure (Figure 8).

Procedure To Make A Pattern
The hole for the thumb is located in the middle of the material.

1-2   Circumference around the heads of the finger MCP joints.

3-4   The length from the head of the index finger metacarpal to the carpometacarpal joint of the thumb.

4-5   Length between carpometacarpal joint of the thumb and anterior aspect of the elbow position in 90° flexion.

1-6, 2-7 The length from the head of the little finger metacarpal to the olecranon.

6-7   Circumference of forearm.

Fabrication Procedure

1.   Position the limb with the elbow at 90° flexion, forearm in desired position of rotation with wrist in neutral or slightly extended. Ensure the thumb is in a position of opposition. Bony prominences around elbow and wrist require padding prior to fabrication.

2.   Heat the whole piece of thermoplastic material to ensure even moulding. If it is too large for the water heating source soften one half then fold over a piece of paper towel to prevent two sides sticking. Remove the material from the water supporting as much of the material as possible. Lay it on the table enlarge the thumbhole and roll edge, roll edge around the elbow. If material has cooled reheat carefully maintaining rolled edges prior to application to the patient.

3.   Position material hole over thumb, then along forearm, press together the edges (XXXXX) on the posterior aspect of the elbow, then distal edges around hand. Once the thermoplastic material is secured, your hands are free to mould the rest of the orthosis.

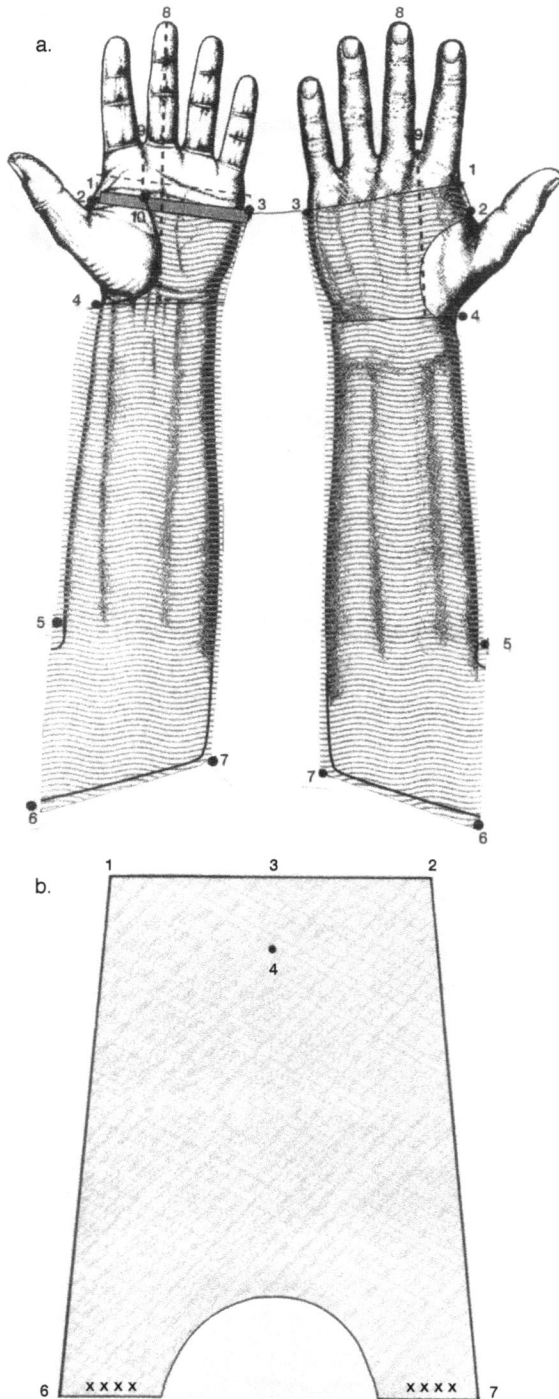

Figure 8: Forearm Immobilization Orthoses Patterns
(a) Sugartong style orthosis (b) Muenster style orthosis

4. Ensure good contour is achieved around the elbow, wrist and palmar arch and thenar eminence.

5. When the material is cool, but before it goes completely hard, separate the bonds. Mark the edges that need to be rolled, ensuring clearance for movement of the fingers at the MCP joints, the thenar eminence, olecranon and some degrees of elbow flexion. Then remove the orthosis from the arm.

6. Trim any excess material along seam.

7. The distal end is also rolled back to provide a rounded edge allowing full motion at the MCP joints. The component in the web space between the thumb and index finger must have a smooth round edge to minimize problems of friction.

8. Four straps are applied (hand, wrist, forearm and posterior aspect of the elbow).

FOREARM IMMOBILIZATION ORTHOSIS (SUGARTONG STYLE)

Fabrication of this orthosis is achieved using a long narrow piece of thermoplastic material that has some elasticity, good rigidity and memory. Materials like Orfit® or Aquaplast® are used however perforations can be problematic if stretched and distorted.

Procedure To Make A Pattern

The pattern covers volar and dorsal surfaces of the forearm and hand as illustrated in Figure 8a. It is based upon two measurements.

1. Width of the hand.

2. The length from distal palmar crease of the hand, along forearm, around elbow and back to the dorsum of the hand.

The thermoplastic material is cut and heated.

Fabrication Procedure

1. The arm should be positioned so that the hand is supported with clearance under the forearm and elbow. Position the elbow, forearm and wrist joints in the desired immobilization positions. Pad out the ulna head and all bony prominences around the elbow prior to fabrication.

2. Remove the thermoplastic material from the heating source taking care to support the length of the material so that it does not stretch.

3. The centre is applied to the posterior aspect of the elbow, with two ends stretched gently along volar and dorsal aspects of the forearm with edges bonded together on medial and lateral aspects of the hand just proximal to the distal palmar crease. Once thermoplastic is secured on the limb at proximal and distal ends mould to ensure good conformity around all joints and along the entire length.

4. Roll distal end on palmar surface to clear distal palmar crease, mould around the thumb eminence and through the webspace.

5. When completely cold mark the edges that need to be adjusted, ensuring clearance for movement of the fingers at the MCP joints, the thenar eminence, and some degrees of elbow flexion prior to

removing the orthosis from the arm.

6. Very gently reheat the edges and roll. The rolled edge decreases shear stress and improves comfort whilst also providing reinforcement.

7. Attach three straps, one at each end of the forearm, and one to secure hand component and immobilize the wrist.

This design allows elbow flexion greater than 90°. Deficits in elbow extension common on removing the orthosis are addressed with active and passive movement.

FOREARM IMMOBILIZATION ORTHOSIS – ARTICULATED ELBOW HINGE

Immobilization of the forearm can also be achieved with the wrist immobilized in an orthosis that is circumferential, an arm cuff and a hinge connecting the two. The hinge allows freedom of elbow movement in flexion and extension, but stops all forearm rotation by incorporating the distal radioulnar joint in the wrist immobilization orthosis (Figure 7c).

ORTHOSES TO MOBILIZE THE FOREARM

Deficits in supination of the forearm present a greater functional limitation than deficits in pronation. Abduction and internal rotation of the shoulder will compensate for pronation.

However no other movement can substitute for supination. Rotation of the forearm occurs at the coaxial proximal and distal radioulnar joints. The axis of rotation of the forearm is found the length of the radius and ulna. A force applied at any point along the length of these bones to effect rotation, will affect both joints equally. The two styles of orthoses commonly used to mobilize the forearm in directions of pronation and supination can be made using serial progressive or dynamic principles depending upon type of traction applied.

DESIGN INCORPORATING ELBOW AND WRIST ORTHOSES

The design is simple to make and has high patient acceptance in comparison to other designs. It consists of an anterior elbow immobilization orthosis and a circumferential wrist immobilization orthosis (Figure 9a). To create torque that maximizes the rotatory component, force is applied perpendicular to the axis of motion. As forearm rotation normally occurs in a circular motion through approximately 180°, traction can be applied to affect a rotary torque at any point through this arc. The area of force application is determined by the size of the wrist immobilization orthosis. The hand is included in the forearm orthosis as much of the pathology affecting forearm rotation also has an impact upon the wrist. Also, inclusion of the hand increases the area for distal anchorage and patient comfort. Velcro® is commonly used for strapping with non-elastic pile chosen when using serial progressive principles, or elastic pile Velcro® or elastic bands with dynamic principles.

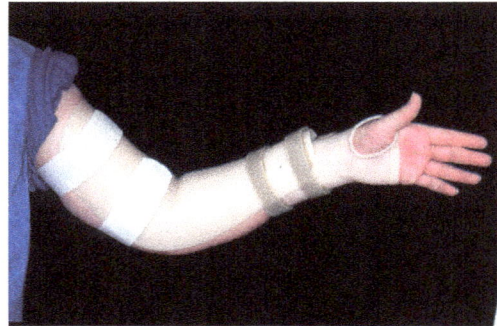

Figure 9a: Forearm Mobilizing Orthoses.
A serial progressive orthosis combines a circumferential wrist immobilization orthosis and an anterior elbow immobilization orthosis with force applied by a two Velcro® straps.

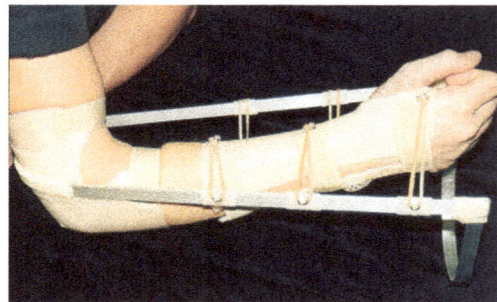

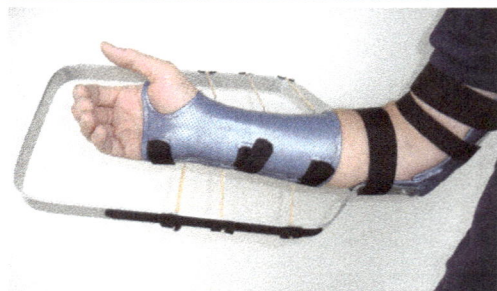

Figure 9b: Forearm Mobilizing Orthoses. Dynamic pronation - supination orthosis applies force via a wrist immobilization orthosis to an aluminium frame in clockwise or counter clockwise directions to effect rotation of the forearm. Elastic bands can be secured to aluminium via hooks or Velcro®. The top orthosis outrigger suspends the forearm within the cradle of the orthosis. The bottom outrigger requires the patient to correctly position the orthosis to minimize potential lost of rotational force through friction contact with the surface on which the arm rests. (Bottom image courtesy Michael Fitzgerald).

Procedure For Fabrication

1. Make a circumferential wrist immobilization orthosis (instructions for the pattern and fabrication procedures page 125-6)

2. Make an anterior elbow immobilization orthosis (instructions for the pattern and fabrication procedures page 93). When moulding this orthosis, just prior to the material going completely hard slightly increase the circumference of the forearm component to allow for the wrist immobilization orthosis underneath. Secure straps to the arm component.

3. Two rotational straps are essential to achieving end range when applying rotation force. Attach two pieces of adhesive backed hook Velcro® in a circumferential direction to the wrist immobilization orthosis, one at wrist and the other at mid forearm level. A long piece of pile Velcro® is then attached wrapping around the forearm in the direction of rotation required. These are referred to as rotation straps.

4. Secure the elbow orthosis in place. Take the rotation strap on the wrist orthosis and wrap around over the anterior surface of the elbow orthosis. Mark the location and then apply the adhesive backed hook Velcro®.

To use the orthosis, the patient takes the rotation strap, rotates the forearm in the direction of the deficit to end range and then secures first strap to the elbow orthosis. The second strap can then be used to readjust the tension to achieve end ROM. As the tissues accommodate the position the rotation straps can be tensioned to increase the degree of rotation. This orthosis is the mobilizing orthosis of choice for younger children due to its low-profile appearance and ease of application, and for adults when the wearing regime includes application during sleep.

DESIGN INCORPORATING OUTRIGGER

The procedure to fabricate a dynamic pronation supination orthosis (Figure 9b) was first described by Collelo-Abraham.[9] Aesthetics of this orthosis, as well as ease of fabrication, are increased considerably by the used of aluminium flat rod to make the outrigger. Aluminium rod is available from large hardware stores in several widths.

Procedure For Fabrication

1. Make a circumferential wrist immobilization orthosis (instructions for the pattern and fabrication procedures page 125-6).

2. Make a short posterior elbow immobilization orthosis (instructions for the pattern and fabrication procedures page 93). The length above and below the elbow needs to be sufficient to stabilize the elbow in 90° flexion but not interfere with rotation of the forearm.

3. Two styles of aluminium outrigger are illustrated in Figure 9b. The length of the flat aluminium rod (15mm or 20mm width) is determined by a series of length and width measures using a tape measure: double the forearm and hand lengths, plus additional width to either

traverse across the hand or around the posterior aspect of the elbow. The outrigger that suspends the forearm within the cradle of the orthosis requires a second piece of aluminium (approximately 25cm in length) to be bonded to the main frame using two pieces of thermoplastic material. Locate centre of the rod and bend to the desired outrigger shape contouring around the elbow as illustrated in Figure 9b.

4. Position outrigger rod in alignment with the longitudinal axis of the forearm and mark location on the elbow orthosis using a wax pencil. Secure rod to the orthosis with a piece of thermoplastic material or rivets. Pad or protect the rivet sites to ensure they cannot cause pressure on the inside of the elbow orthosis.

5. Apply adhesive backed pile Velcro® along the outside of the flat aluminium rod the length of the wrist immobilization orthosis; or secure hooks with small pieces of thermoplastic.

6. Apply a minimum of three metal anchor loops, made from dress hooks or paper clips, along both medial and lateral aspects of the wrist immobilization orthosis.

7. An appropriate size elastic band is secured to each metal loop. It is then connected to a piece of hook Velcro® which is wound in direction of pronation or supination and secured on the aluminium outrigger. Adhesive Velcro® along the aluminium rod is a quicker method to secure rotational elastic bands than hooks illustrated. A minimum of six Velcro® elastic bands are required. Force couples are applied in opposite directions to create rotational force in either pronation or supination by securing medial and lateral traction to the Velcro® attached to the outrigger (Figure 9b).

NON-ARTICULAR ELBOW ORTHOSES

Orthoses used to address the symptoms of lateral epicondylitis are in a unique nonarticular category. They are designed to reduce the stresses on the common forearm extensor muscle origin. The orthosis consists of a non-elastic band several centimetres wide which is secured by a Velcro® strap looped through a 'D' ring. Numerous brands are available from thermoplastic material suppliers and retail through pharmacies. It is proposed that the band provides a counterforce to the forearm musculature, decreasing the capacity of the muscles to contract, thereby decreasing the stress on the injured muscle fibres.[14,15,27,]

The literature reports wide variability in the success of orthoses to address the symptoms of localised pain in the region of the lateral epicondyle of the humerus, and strength of grip and functional tasks due to pain with attempted muscle function.[8,14,29] The criterion for prescription of counterforce orthoses for persons with lateral epicondylitis is based upon subjective symptoms of pain and impaired function. The nonarticular proximal forearm orthosis and wrist immobilization orthosis were identified by hand therapists as frequently used treatments with perceived benefits.[18] However systematic reviews suggest evidence is weak with reviews unable to recommend one type of orthosis over another.[4] Modification of symptoms may result from wearing the orthosis, however it is vital that the cause of the problem, and the biomechanics of loading forearm musculature, are addressed in relation to vocational or recreational demands.

CONCLUSION

The elbow and forearm provide important freedoms of movement to the upper limb. Tissues that allow motion through the majority of the available range can achieve orientation of the hand, with sufficient functional motion towards the face, and away from the body. Whilst numerous orthoses are manufactured to rest structures to allow healing, by far the greater role of orthotic intervention in both the elbow and forearm is maximizing the recovery of range of motion.

References

1. An KN, Morrey BF. Biomechanics of the elbow. In: Morrey BF editor. The elbow and its disorders. Philadelphia: WB Saunders; 2000. p. 43–60.

2. Bhat AK, Bhaskaranand K, Nair SG. Static progressive stretching using a turnbuckle orthosis for elbow stiffness: a prospective study. Journal of Orthopaedic Surgery. 2010;18: 76–9.

3. Bonutti PM, Windau JE, Ables BA, Miller BG. Static progressive stretch to re-establish elbow range of motion. Clinical Orthopedics and Related Research. 1994;303: 128–34.

4. Borkholder CD, Hill VA, Fess EE. The efficacy of splinting for lateral epicondylitis: a systematic review. Journal of Hand Therapy. 2004;17: 181–99.

5. Casavant AM, Hastings H. Heterotopic ossification about the elbow: a therapist's guide to evaluation and management. Journal of Hand Therapy. 2006;19(2): 255–66.

6. Chinchalkar SJ, Pearce J, Athwal GS. Static progressive versus three-point elbow extension splinting: a mathematical analysis. Journal of Hand Therapy. 2009;22: 37–42.

7. Chinchalkar SJ, Szekeres M. Rehabilitation of elbow trauma. Hand Clinics. 2004;20: 363–74.

8. Clementis LG, Chow S. Effectiveness of a custom-made below elbow lateral counter force splint in the treatment of lateral epicondylitis. Canadian Journal of Occupational Therapy. 1993;60: 137–144.

9. Collelo-Abraham K. Dynamic pronation-supination splint. In: Hunter, JM, Schneider, LH, Makin, EJ and Callahan, AD, editors. Rehabilitation of the Hand: Surgery and Therapy. 3rd ed. St Louis: Mosby; 1990. p. 1134–1139.

10. Davila SA, Johnston-Jones K. Managing the stiff elbow: operative, nonoperative, and postoperative techniques. Journal of Hand Therapy. 2006;19: 268–281.

11. Doornberg JN, Ring D, Jupiter JB. Static progressive splinting for posttraumatic elbow stiffness. Journal of Orthopaedic Trauma. 2006;20(6): 400–4.

12. Gelinas JJ, Faber KJ, Patterson SD, King GJ. The effectiveness of turnbuckle splinting for elbow contractures. Journal of Bone and Joint Surgery. 2000;82-B: 74–8.

13. Green DP, McCoy H. Turnbuckle orthotic correction of elbow-flexion contractures after acute injuries. Journal of Bone and Joint Surgery. 1979;61: 1092–5.

14. Groppel J, Nirschl R. A mechanical and electromyographical analysis of the effects of various counterforce braces on the tennis player. American Journal of Sports Medicine. 1986;14: 195–200.

15. Jafarian FS, Demneh ES, Tyson SF. The immediate effect of orthotic management on grip strength of patients with lateral epicondylosis. Journal of Orthopedics and Sports Physical Therapy. 2009;39: 484–9.

16. Lindenhovius A, Doornberg J, Brouwer K, et al. A prospective randomized controlled trial of dynamic versus static progressive elbow splinting for posttraumatic elbow stiffness. Journal of Bone and Joint Surgery. 2012;94-A: 694–700.

17. MacDermid JC, Michlovitz SL. Examination of the elbow: linking diagnosis, prognosis, and outcomes as a framework for maximizing therapy interventions. Journal of Hand Therapy. 2006;19(2): 82–97.

18. MacDermid JC, Wojkowski S, Kargus C, et al. Hand therapist management of the lateral epicondylosis: a survey of expert opinion and practice patterns. Journal of Hand Therapy. 2010;23: 18–29.

19. Morrey BF. Anatomy of the elbow. In: Morrey BF editor. The elbow and its disorders. Philadelphia: WB Saunders. 2000. p. xxiii.

20. Morrey BF. Functional anatomy in mechanics of the elbow. In D Kashiwagi editor. Elbow Joint. Amsterdam: Elsevier Science Publishers. 1985, p. 295–303

21. Morrey BF, Askew LJ, An KN. A biomechanical study of normal functional elbow motion. Journal of Bone and Joint Surgery. 1981;63-A: 872–877.

22. Morrey BF, Chao EYS. Passive motion of the elbow joint. Journal of Bone and Joint Surgery. 1976;58A: 501–508.

23. Regan WD, Korinek SL, Morrey BF, An KN. Biomechanical study of the ligaments around the elbow joint. Clinical Orthopaedics and Related Research. 1991;271: 170–179.

24. Slaughter A, Miles L, Fleming J, McPhail S. A comparative study of splint effectiveness in limiting forearm rotation. Journal of Hand Therapy. 2010;23(3): 241–7.

25. Szekeres M. A biomechanical analysis of static progressive elbow flexion splinting. Journal of Hand Therapy. 2006;19: 34–8.

26. Ulrich SD, Bonutti PM, Seyler TM, et al. Restoring range of motion via stress relaxation and static progressive stretch in posttraumatic elbow contractures. Journal of Shoulder and Elbow Surgery. 2010;19(2): 196–201

27. Wadsworth C, Neilsen D, Burns L et al. Effect of the counterforce armband on wrist extension and grip strength and pain in subjects with tennis elbow. Journal of Orthopedics and Sports Physiotherapy. 1989;11: 192–197.

28. Werner FW, An KN. Biomechanics of the elbow and forearm. Hand Clinics 1994;10: 357–373.

29. Wuori JL, Overend TJ, Kramer JF, MacDermid J. Strength and pain measures associated with lateral epicondylitis bracing. Archives Physical Medicine Rehabilitation. 1998;79:832–7.

30. Youm Y, Dwyer RF, Thambyrajah K, et al. Biomechanical analysis of the forearm pronation-supination and elbow flexion-extension. Journal of Biomechanics. 1979;12: 245–255.

5

ORTHOSES/SPLINTS TO ADDRESS THE WRIST AND HAND

INTRODUCTION

The wrist is often described as the key to hand function as it provides a mobile yet stable base for the fingers and the thumb that is independent of forearm position. The challenge for the therapist is to restore function in the wrist where normal biomechanical relationships are disrupted as a result of injury or disease affecting bones, joints, ligaments and muscles. Orthotic intervention is often the treatment chosen to achieve this objective. This chapter will specifically address orthoses fabricated for the wrist and include orthoses to immobilize the whole hand. Orthoses that include the wrist, where the primary function is to address pathology at the distal radioulnar joint, the fingers or thumb, are described in the chapters that address those regions.

Prior to fabricating an orthosis for the wrist it is important to consider the implications to movements of proximal upper extremity joints. The combined joint motion of the upper limb allows an infinite number of movements to facilitate orientation of the hand and limb in functional and vocational activities. Studies on non-injured persons have demonstrated increased humeral elevation and rotation is required to perform usual manipulative tasks when the wrist is immobilized.[4, 14,16] Thus therapists need to consider how a wrist orthosis may impact the quality of motion in the upper extremity, as well as its potential to impact on musculoskeletal pathology that may be present in other parts of the upper limb.

ANATOMY OF THE WRIST AND HAND

This short review of anatomy of the wrist and hand is intended to highlight critical issues of anatomy that impact upon the design and fabrication of the orthoses for this region. Of particular interest is the architectural arrangement of the bones and formation of arches, the inter-relationship between extrinsic and intrinsic musculature to effect motion of the wrist and fingers, and the soft tissue coverings of skin and fascia. Wrist anatomy and biomechanics in health and disease remain an area of much discussion amongst anatomists, surgeons and therapists.

Dysfunction in the wrist is common following disruption of articular surfaces and ligaments resulting in deformity, instability and loss of motion. Restoration of normal anatomy and biomechanics is not possible for many clients. Therefore knowledge of normal anatomy and kinesiology is essential to understanding the changes that have occurred in the injured wrist, whilst an understanding of pathology is essential to determine the appropriate course of therapy intervention.

ARCHITECTURE AND STRUCTURE

Orthotic intervention to rest, position, or to regain mobility in the wrist requires knowledge of the relationships formed by different skeletal structures of the hand. Motion results from the interactions of the carpal bones between themselves, as well as proximally with the articulating surface of the radius and the ulna/triangular fibrocartilage complex, and distally with the bases of the metacarpals. The shape of the articulating surfaces of the carpals combines with strong ligamentous connections to control motion created by muscles that generally insert distal to the joint.

Functionally, the carpals may be considered in proximal and distal rows. The distal carpals have interlocking articular surfaces between themselves and the index and middle finger metacarpals. Thus, the magnitude and direction of movement of the index and middle finger metacarpals is reflected in motion of the distal carpals.[2] The movement of the proximal row is a lot more variable; however, these carpals also tend to function as a unit. The scaphoid spanning both carpal rows plays a critical role in providing stability to what is an inherently unstable arrangement. The inter-relationships between the carpals as the wrist moves through full range are very complex. The articular surface of the distal radius faces ulnarly at an angle of approximately 15° and this means that the axis of flexion-extension is oblique to the axis of

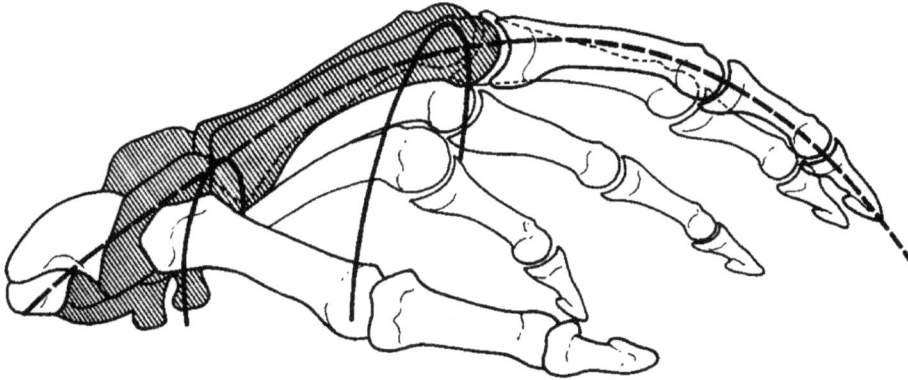

Figure 1: The arches of hand. The longitudinal and transverse arches of the hand are shown inside view. Reproduced from Tubiana (1981, p. 25)

the forearm. Morimoto et al.[17] describes the functional wrist motion from radial extension to ulnar flexion as the 'dart throwing motion'. Most activities of daily living are performed using this motion, which may vary between activities and between individuals. While the biomechanics of wrist motion are beyond the scope of this review, therapists are encouraged to consider the complexity of normal joint and ligamentous arrangements, particularly when designing orthoses to mobilize the wrist joint in the presence of joint pathology.

The wrist normally rests in a few degrees of ulnar deviation, with greater range of motion in ulnar deviation as compared to radial deviation. The articular surface also has a slightly volar tilt contributing to slightly greater motion in flexion than extension. The restraining influence of the ligaments of the radiocarpal and mid carpal joints, the retinacular ligaments of the wrist combined with the wrist muscles, and the agonist antagonist balance of the extrinsic and intrinsic finger muscles, dictate the normal resting positions of joints. These factors also determine joint interaction in functional patterns of motion.

Movement of the wrist occurs about the axes of flexion and extension, and radial and ulnar deviation. Cadaveric studies by Patterson et al.[18] indicate carpal bone kinematics in a healthy normal joint are similar in both simulated active and passive wrist motion. Functionally movements seen in the direction of extension radial deviation and flexion ulnar deviation are the most frequent wrist motions used in activities of daily living.[17] Thus, orthotic interventions designed to address deficits in motion need to consider the multiple planes in which normal motion occurs. Fixed hinges have only one axis of motion, thus any deviation associated with flexion and extension is eliminated. Regaining deficits in deviation may require a second intervention.[10] Alignment of the axis of wrist motion to the axis of the orthosis hinge is critical. Flexible tubing and screw hinges allow some freedom to accommodate the normal requirement for some degrees of deviation.

Fractures of the distal radius and carpals, along with tendon and muscle injury result in swelling and fibrosis that can severely compromise wrist movement. Thus, the position in which the joint is immobilized to allow healing must account for an outcome of stiffness and limited motion, and consider how this position may have an affect on functional use of the hand.

The skeleton of the hand is composed of fixed elements of the distal row of carpals and the index and middle finger metacarpals, surrounded by the other mobile elements of the proximal carpal row and the metacarpals of the thumb, ring and little fingers, and the phalanges to all digits. The architectural arrangement of bones forms a series of arches (Figure 1 and 2). Transverse arches exist at the carpal and metacarpal levels, whilst the longitudinal arches for each finger are formed by the carpals, metacarpal and the mobile phalanges. The depth of the transverse arch at the heads of the metacarpals, and the orientations of the longitudinal arches to the ring and little fingers, change due to the mobility of the fourth and fifth metacarpals at the carpometacarpal (CMC) joints, thus orientating the fingers to the thumb with increasing flexion. With flexion of the ring and little fingers, the heads of the finger metacarpals form an oblique angle to the transverse plane of the forearm. Oblique arches are formed between the thumb and each finger.

The longitudinal axis of the second metacarpal and radius align at rest, with some degrees of deviation at other metacarpals (Figure 3). Deviation of the proximal phalanges on

the metacarpals is evident in ulnar deviation in the index and middle fingers, and radial deviation in the little finger. The progressive decrease in length of the finger metacarpals means the metacarpophalangeal (MCP) joints together form an oblique angle to the longitudinal axis of the forearm.

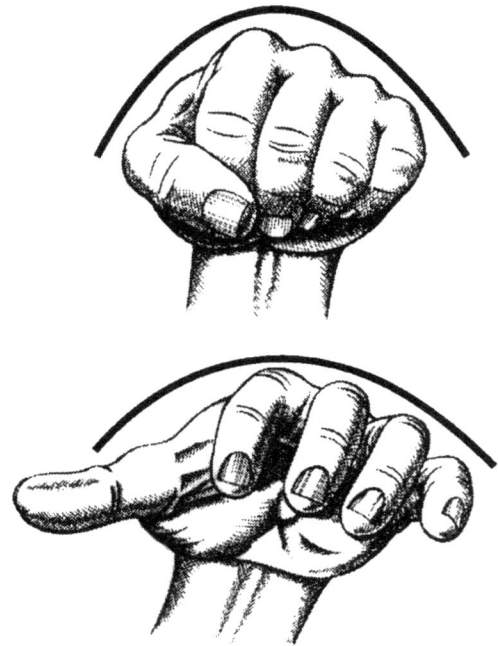

Figure 2: The transverse arch of the hand. At the level of the MCP joints, and also the PIP joints the shape and depth of the arch changes with movements to open and close the hand.

The dynamic structures of the hand, i.e. the transverse, longitudinal and oblique arches, are associated with the two oblique angles created by the changing length and mobility of the finger metacarpals. Thus, joint architecture must be respected in both design and fabrication of any wrist orthosis. Orthoses are generally higher and longer on the radial side.

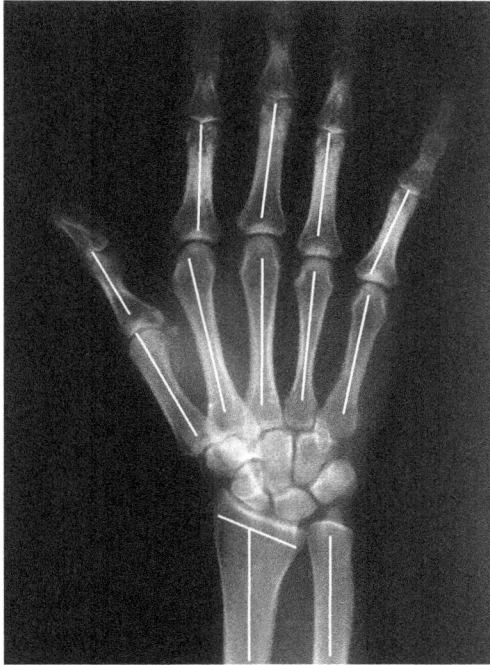

Figure 3: An X-ray of the wrist and hand. Note the normal longitudinal alignment of the bones in the forearm and hand.

MUSCLE FUNCTION

With the exception of flexor carpi ulnaris, whose fibres insert on the pisiform and triquetrium, all wrist muscles insert directly onto the metacarpals. The arrangement of extrinsic finger and thumb muscles, and wrist muscles around the axis of wrist motion provides an agonist antagonist system of forces. Whilst effecting joint motion, the wrist musculature also provides significant stability. The position of the wrist has implications to the function of the thumb

and fingers. The finger flexor muscles are lengthened as the wrist is extended, thus increasing their potential to generate force in grip. Similarly, the finger extensors are lengthened as they cross the greater arc of the flexed wrist, thus passively extending the fingers. The position of the thumb in relation to the fingers is also influenced by the degree of wrist flexion. Wrist extension is a more important motion than flexion due to its association with finger flexion and the fact that many functional tasks require antigravity action of the wrist. Thus, functional orthoses tend to require positions of wrist extension. Substitution of wrist extensor action can be achieved with an orthosis.

Limitations in the excursion of the muscle tendon units that cross the wrist will dictate the positions the distal joints assume as the wrist position is changed. Limited excursion in the flexor digitorum superficialis and profundus will compromise finger and wrist extension. Finger extension is possible with significant degrees of wrist flexion; however, increasing finger flexion is seen with greater degrees of wrist extension. Similarly tightness in extensor digitorum will limit composite flexion of digital joints. The degrees of wrist extension will determine the total digital flexion possible. Passive motion of individual joints can be normal.

Extrinsic finger muscles arise in the proximal forearm with long tendons secured by retinaculum on the dorsal aspect of the wrist, and the retinaculum and carpal tunnel on the volar aspect of the wrist. Inflammation in these regions can affect the glide and function of the tendons with potential to compromise the median nerve in the carpal tunnel. Orthotic intervention is commonly used to limit tendon glide through the retinaculum to facilitate resolution of inflammation.

SOFT TISSUE COVERING TO THE WRIST AND HAND

Any orthoses applied to the wrist and hand must consider the skin and fascial coverings in the areas they traverse. The ability of tissues to withstand pressure has implications to the design.

The skin on the palm of the hand is quite different to that covering the dorsum of the hand and forearm. It has little mobility and is designed to withstand the pressure and shear characteristic of functional grip and pinch. Palmar skin is thick and firmly adhered to the underlying palmar aponeurosis by numerous fibrous connections. Palmar blood vessels and nerves run deep to these structures prior to branching to run medially and laterally to each finger.

Dorsal skin is thin and very mobile. Only a thin subcutaneous sheet of fascia is located superficial to the extensor tendons over the metacarpals. The superficial venous system is visible. Application of pressure to the volar surface of the hand is not associated with the same risks as to the dorsum of the hand. Here the skin, and venous and lymphatic drainage can be compromised, as there is little fascia to disperse pressure being applied through these structures to the underlying bony surface. Bony prominences elsewhere in the hand and wrist present similar risks.

Skin creases are used as a guide to underlying structures for orthosis boundaries. As seen in Figure 4 the location of skin creases does not directly correlate to the underlying joints.

ORTHOSES DESIGNED TO IMMOBILIZE THE WRIST AND HAND

Immobilization of the wrist is undertaken to allow the wrist and associated tissues to rest in a position that minimizes complications associated with inflammation, contracture or paralysis. Immobilization of the wrist, while allowing movement in the fingers and thumb, may facilitate greater functional use of the hand. Studies comparing various custom made and prefabricated designs, and effectiveness of orthotic interventions suggest beneficial effects on wrist pain and functional hand use.[5,8,9,21,22,23,24,27] However no wrist orthosis design fulfils all functional criteria with certain orthoses better suited to specific patient characteristics and functional tasks than others.

IMMOBILIZATION FOR REST

At normal physiological rest the wrist, thumb and fingers adopt a posture that represents a balance of muscular and ligamentous tension in the hand. A 'resting' orthosis aims to restore this balance in the presence of trauma or disease. The resting position, common to the majority of persons, is 10°-20° wrist extension, 20°-45° flexion of the MCP joints, and between 10°-30° flexion of the IP joints.

Hand Creases

distal interphalangeal
proximal interphalangeal
palmar digital
distal palmar
thenar
wrist

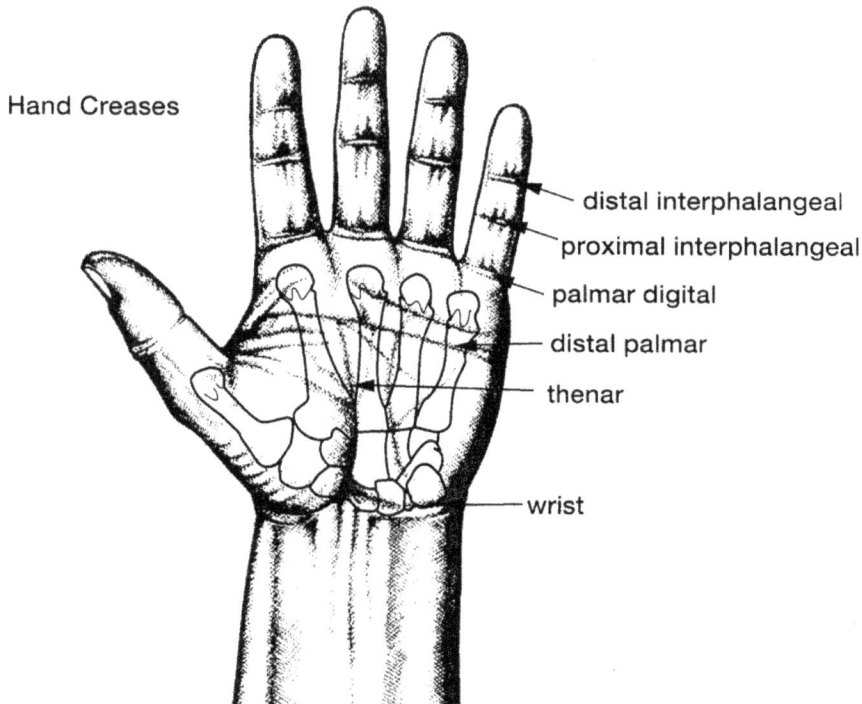

Figure 4: The skin creases of the hand. The skin creases are lines of tethering of the skin and therefore to do not bear a direct relationship to the underlying joints.

The functional position assumed by joints of the hand may vary widely depending upon the vocational, avocational and self care tasks undertaken at any point in time. Therefore adopting one 'functional position' to rest the hand is inappropriate.

Although it may seem a statement of the obvious, a resting orthosis should position the hand in a *resting* position and not a *functional* position. However, on occasions, a position close to function may be chosen for immobilization at rest because this position offers the best functional outcome should mobility not be restored.

Wrist hand immobilization orthoses, or as they are more commonly known resting splints, are one of the most widely used conservative interventions for addressing potential localized wrist and hand difficulties in persons with rheumatoid and osteoarthritis.[1, 9, 22, 27] Published research with various orthoses, wearing schedules and outcome measures have shown differing impacts of resting orthoses/splints on handgrip, pain and function in different phases of these diseases. Therapists are encouraged to consider the unique requirements of the individual and their disease or injury prior to fabricating a 'resting' orthoses. The authors discourage use of diagnostic orthotic protocols in favour of clinical reasoning based upon assessment of the patient, their unique pathology and functional requirements and determination as to whether an orthosis will address their specific needs.

WRIST AND HAND IMMOBILIZATION ORTHOSES

Immobilization of the hand and wrist is achieved with an orthosis applied to the volar surface addressing the wrist, fingers and thumb (Figure 5). It is indicated in the presence of paralysis, pain, inflammation and infection. The position is determined by the pathology of the tissues with specific moulding to achieve a safe position of immobilization in those cases at risk of contracture. Figure 6 illustrates an orthosis design for situations where the thumb CMC and MCP joints are very painful or unstable and require additional support on the anterior surface.

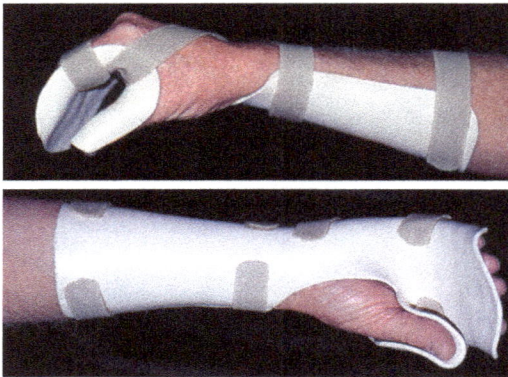

Figure 5: Wrist hand immobilization orthosis. Support for inflamed or painful joints is achieved by an orthosis worn during non-functional periods of rest and sleep. Straps are positioned to avoid bony prominences.

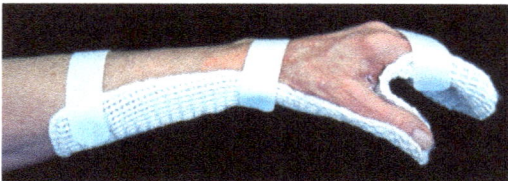

Figure 6: Resting orthosis for the wrist and hand with anterior thumb support. Moulding this orthosis requires particular attention to the thumb position to ensure it is supported on the anterior surface in a resting position of slight CMC abduction and extension.

Orthoses for use with clients with hypertonicity are discussed in Chapter 8. However, if this wrist immobilization orthosis is used in the presence of hypertonicity of the wrist and finger musculature greater attention must be paid to design and location of straps, as these apply significant force to sustain the hand in the orthosis.

Procedure To Take A Pattern

Lay the plastic pattern material on a flat surface and place the patient's hand on top. The wrist should be between neutral and 10° ulnar deviation, the thumb comfortably extended with the fingers very slightly abducted.

The length of the orthosis from wrist to proximal end is generally two-thirds the length of the forearm. This roughly equates to the length of the hand. Mark length with a small dot.

Mark the following points on the pattern referring to Figure 7a.

1-2   Medial and lateral aspects of the hand just proximal to the heads of the finger metacarpals.

3-4   Medial and lateral aspects of the wrist at mid carpal level.

5-6   Medial and lateral aspects of the forearm at length previously determined.

7   Tip of the middle finger.

8   The index and middle finger web.

The width of the orthosis should be half the circumference at the wrist and forearm, and slightly wider at the finger MCP joints so that the material will support the sides of the index

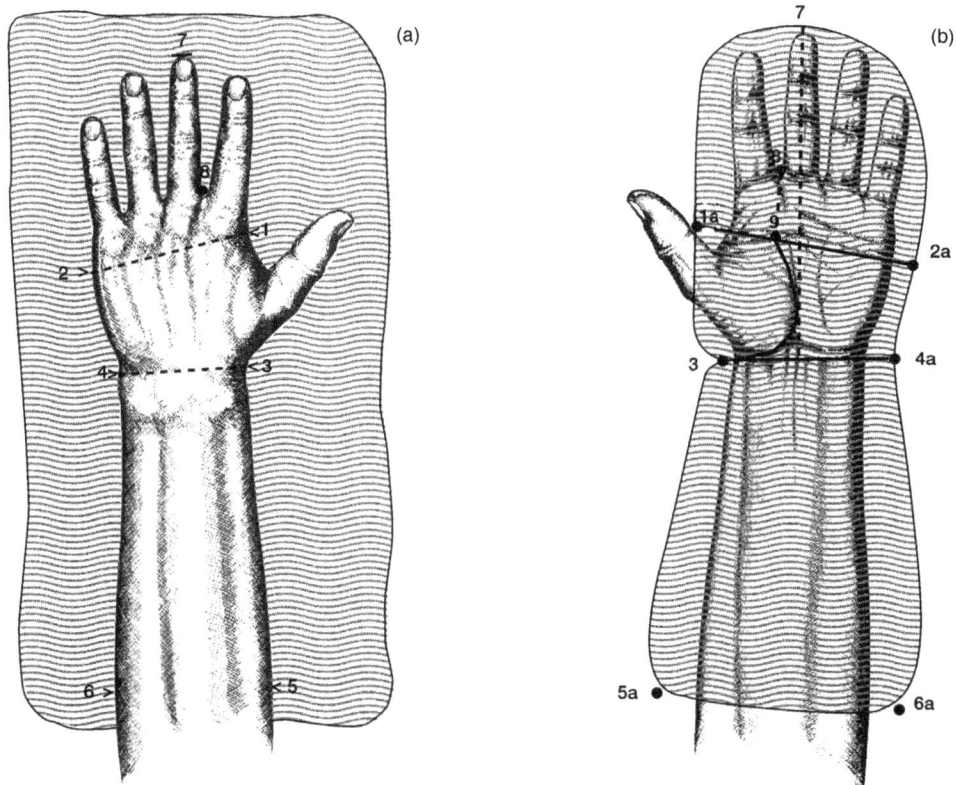

Figure 7: Pattern for wrist hand immobilization orthosis. Landmarks are recorded as per (a) with the completed pattern applied to the volar surface of application (b).

and little fingers. This can be determined by wrapping the pattern material around the hand and marking the desired width at the forearm, wrist and finger MCPs. These width points are indicated on Figure 7b as 1a, 2a, 4a, etc.

Remove the patient's hand. Figure 7b is a volar view of the hand and illustrates how the pattern accommodates the specific landmarks. To follow this diagram work on the wrong side of the material used to take the pattern.

To shape the pattern:
1. Join points 1 and 2 (MCP line).
2. Join points 3-4 (wrist line).

3. Draw a vertical line from point 7 to intersect the wrist line.
4. Draw a vertical line from point 8 to intersect the MCP line - point 9. These lines are used as a guide to determine the location of the thenar crease.
5. Starting at point 7 draw a line around the fingers through points 2a, 4a, and 6a, curve sharply around to 5a then up to 3. The curve though 5a should be shallow to ensure this aspect of the orthosis does not impede elbow flexion.
6. Draw a line between 3 and 9 following the thenar crease so it touches the vertical line from 7 approximately one-third the distance between the wrist line and the MCP line, then curve to point 9.

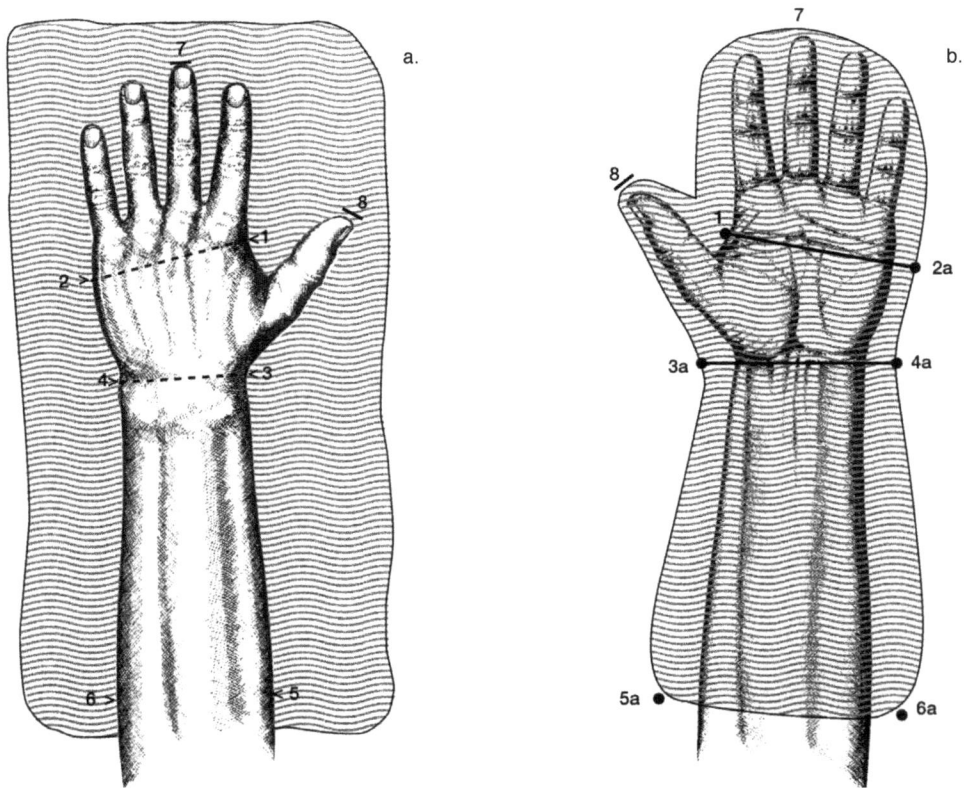

Figure 8: Pattern wrist hand immobilization orthosis with anterior thumb component. Landmarks are recorded as per (a) with the completed pattern applied to the volar surface of application (b).

7. From point 3, draw around the base of the thenar eminence to connect to 1a following on to point 7.

8. Cut the pattern out and check for fit on the patient, prior to transferring it to the thermoplastic material.

Fabrication Procedure

1. The arm should be positioned with the elbow supported, the forearm in a vertical position in mid-pronation-supination, and the wrist in the predetermined position and the rest of the hand relaxed.

2. Heat thermoplastic material and cut out pattern shape. Reheat.

3. On removing the material from the heating source quickly shape the thumb component, particularly the index thumb web space, using your own hand as a mould.

4. Place the thermoplastic material on the patient's hand orientating the alignment at the MCP joint and wrist. Where necessary secure material to the wrist, hand and then forearm using a smooth bandage.

5. When applying orthoses to persons with paralysis of the wrist extensors, a second person may be required to assist bandaging the thermoplastic material to the limb. If no assistance is available bandage the material to the limb at the

wrist first, then loosely bandage around the hand and fingers before sweeping back to secure the forearm component.

6. Now hold the wrist and finger joints in the desired position, while moulding the transverse and longitudinal arches. The thumb component may be moulded at a second stage, if it is not possible to address all components in the first application.

7. When satisfied with the position of the hand in the orthosis a minimum of three straps are applied. Straps are located at the proximal end, in the vicinity of the wrist, and either across the metacarpals or the proximal phalanges.

To design a wrist hand immobilization orthosis that provides support to the volar surface of the thumb the pattern is modified slightly as illustrated in Figure 8. An additional marker is added at the end of the thumb. The fabrication procedure is the same as that described for the wrist immobilization orthosis.

IMMOBILIZATION FOR FUNCTION

Orthoses that immobilize the wrist without involvement of the fingers and thumb may be applied to rest the wrist but generally facilitate functional use of the hand. The angle of immobilization of the wrist is determined in consultation with the patient considering their specific requirements in occupational tasks.

Following assessment and determination of an objective for immobilization of the wrist, the therapist must consider the choices in the design taking into consideration the pathology and the specific needs of the patient. The design choices are:

- **Volar orthoses** support the weight of the hand against the effect of gravity. The palmar skin is well able to tolerate pressure applied by the orthosis. Volar orthoses are designed for primary function in a pronated position. Aesthetically, the majority of thermoplastic material is located on the volar surface with only straps traversing the more exposed dorsal surface. The major disadvantage to this type of orthosis is the presence of hard unyielding plastic in the palm of the hand. This has the potential to compromise gross grip by preventing adaptation of the hand to the shape of the tool or object.
- **Dorsal orthoses** are used for a small population of patients who require wrist support but with greater palmar surface exposed for sensory and friction contact with objects. Perhaps the least supportive of the wrist orthosis designs, dorsal wrist orthoses are popular with persons with rheumatoid arthritis who require support but rarely transmit large forces through their wrists.
- **Circumferential orthoses** provide the greatest amount of immobilization and support. Due to the inherent strength in design they are used in vocational situations where large forces are transmitted through the wrist. This

design also provides uniform pressure dispersion along the forearm and is therefore used in young children who still have considerable subcutaneous fat and for those patients with significant swelling in the hand and forearm that may be compromised by straps.

The use of prefabricated orthoses to immobilize the wrist maybe an appropriate first aid intervention. However the elastic nature of the fabric of most of these orthoses suggests their primary function is to restrict motion and not to immobilize the joint.

WRIST IMMOBILIZATION ORTHOSIS – VOLAR APPLICATION

This is perhaps the most traditional design for wrist immobilization orthoses (Figure 9). It requires a material that is strong and rigid as the component through the wrist is quite narrow. This orthosis is designed to be used in a pronated position therefore should never be moulded to the hand with the forearm in supination. Thermoplastic materials that require a gravity-assisted moulding technique are not recommended.

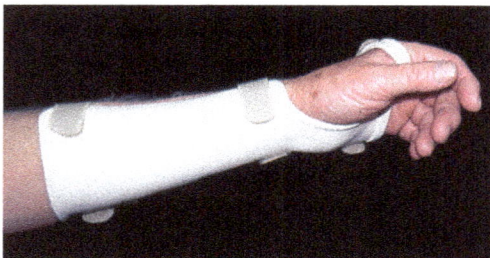

Figure 9: Wrist immobilization orthosis volar application. This orthosis immobilizes the wrist in the required degrees of extension without effecting motion of the fingers and thumb.

Procedure to take a pattern

Lay the pattern material on a flat surface and place the patient's hand on the top. The wrist should be between neutral and 10° ulnar deviation, the thumb comfortably extended, with the fingers very slightly abducted. The length of the orthosis from wrist to proximal end is generally two-thirds the length of the forearm. This roughly equates to the length of the hand. Measure length using a tape and mark with a small dot.

Mark the following points as illustrated in Figure 10a.

1-2 Medial and lateral aspects of the hand just proximal to the heads of the finger metacarpals.

3-4 Medial and lateral aspects of the wrist at mid carpal level.

5-6 Medial and lateral aspects of the forearm at the length previously determined.

7 The tip of the middle finger.

8 The index and middle finger web.

The width of the orthosis should be half the circumference at the wrist and forearm, and to the dorsal aspect of the fifth metacarpal. This can be determined by wrapping the pattern material around and marking the desired width at the MCP, forearm and wrist. These width points are indicated on the diagram as 2a, 4a, etc.

The distal end of this orthosis is extended to wrap around the hand through the web space. Using a tape, measure the width from the dorsum of the little finger metacarpal head across the volar aspect of the finger MCP joints, through the web space to the dorsum

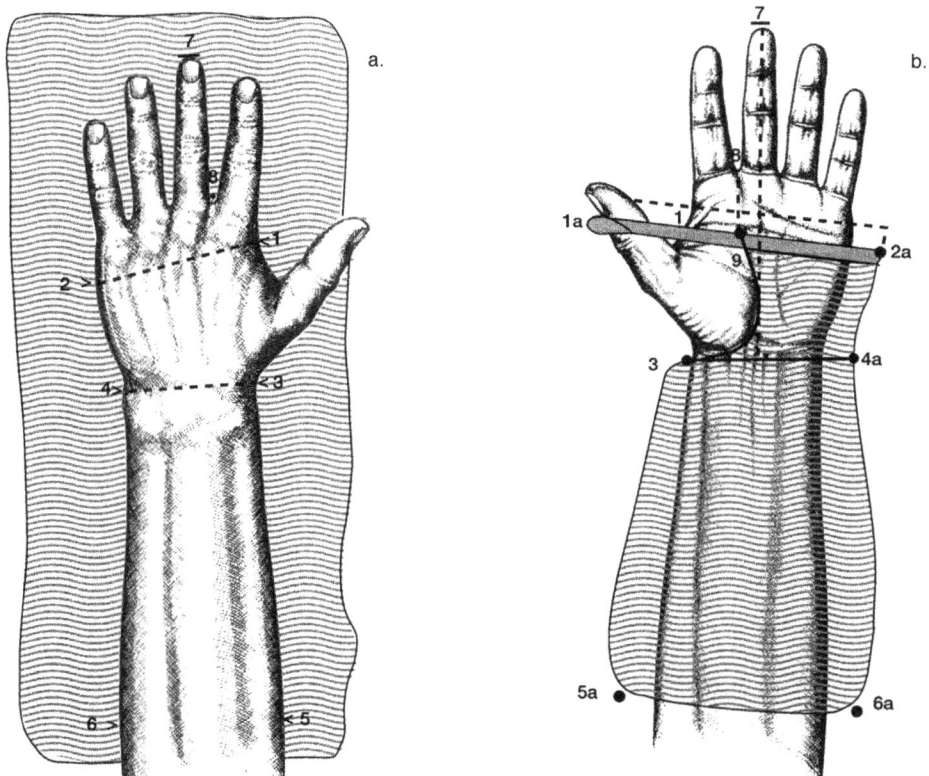

Figure 10: Pattern wrist immobilization orthosis volar application. Landmarks are recorded as per (a) with the completed pattern applied to the volar surface of application (b). Extra length is added to the distal edge as indicated by the dotted line.

of the middle finger metacarpal. This length is used to determine width of the distal end of the orthosis (1a-2a).

Remove the patient's hand. Figure 10b is a volar view of the hand and how the pattern accommodates the specific landmarks. To follow this diagram work on the wrong side of the material used to take the pattern.

1. Join points 1 and 2 (MCP line).
2. Join points 3 and 4 (wrist line).
3. Draw a vertical line from point 7 to intersect the wrist line.
4. Draw a vertical line from point 8 to intersect the MCP line - point 9. These lines are used as a guide to determine the location of the thenar crease.

5. Starting at point 2a, draw a line around the forearm through points 4a, and 6a, curve sharply around to 5a then up to 3. The curve through 5a should be shallow to ensure this aspect of the orthosis does not impede elbow flexion.

6. The line between 3 and 9 follows the thenar crease so touches the vertical line 7 approximately one-third the distance between the wrist line and the MCP line then curves to point 9.

7. Extend the palmar bar using circumferential measurement previously recorded (1a-2a).

8. Add approximately 1 cm across the

121

palmar surface distal to the MCP line. The additional length, indicated by a dotted line, allows the distal end to be rolled back to create a smooth edge.

9. Cut the pattern out and check for fit on the patient, ensuring the forearm is maintained in mid prone or a pronated position. Transfer pattern to the thermoplastic material.

Fabrication Procedure

1. The arm should be positioned with the elbow supported, the forearm in a vertical position in mid-pronation-supination, and the wrist in the predetermined position. Allow room for the changing dimensions of the distal ulna by padding out the ulna head prior to fabrication.

2. Heat the thermoplastic material and cut out pattern.

3. Fold back the component added distal to 1a and 2a to the level of the MCP line, with the exception of the last 2 cm at 1a. This section will provide a flat surface for attachment of a strap. Ensure that the fold is towards the exterior surface of the orthosis as the rolled edge decreases shear stress, and improves comfort whilst also providing reinforcement.

4. Reheat till malleable then apply to the patient's hand. Secure in place with a bandage. Mould intimately around the wrist, the thenar eminence, and the arches of the hand. Flare around the edge of thenar eminence and the proximal edge of the forearm.

5. Attach three straps, one at the proximal end, one in the vicinity of the wrist avoiding direct pressure over the ulna head, and one to the bar at the distal end.

6. Ensure correct fit and that movement of the fingers at the MCP joints and the thumb at the CMC joint in both extension and abduction are not compromised. This small bar can be a point of irritation through the webspace as it is point of force and also significant movement.

WRIST IMMOBILIZATION ORTHOSIS - DORSAL APPLICATION

This orthosis requires a material that is strong and rigid (Figure 11). As the orthosis is designed to be used in a pronated position, gravity assisted thermoplastic materials can be used. These materials are also recommended due to their ability to contour very well to the hand. The ulna head is padded out prior to fabrication.

To support the transverse arch, a rigid thermoplastic component must be incorporated into the design to traverse the palm of the hand proximal to the distal palmar crease. A flexible strap provides no support for the transverse arch. The first pattern described here has an extension on the radial side, which wraps through the webspace across the palm. This style is recommended for dorsal orthoses whose purpose is to facilitate function. A more supportive hinged palmar component is added to this orthosis design when it is used as a basis for mobilizing orthoses or where greater palmar support is required.

Procedure To Take A Pattern

1. Lay the patient's hand on a flat surface and place the transparent plastic pattern material on top. The wrist should be between neutral and 10° ulnar deviation, with the thumb comfortably extended and the fingers very slightly abducted.

2. The length of the orthosis from wrist to proximal end is two-thirds the length of the forearm. This roughly equates to the length of the hand. Measure length using a tape and mark with a small dot.

The following points, illustrated in Figure 12a are common to all models.

1-2 Medial and lateral aspects of the hand just proximal to the heads of the finger metacarpals.

3-4 Medial and lateral aspects of the hand at the thumb web level.

5-6 Medial and lateral aspects of the wrist at mid-carpal level.

7-8 Medial and lateral aspects of the forearm at the length previously determined.

9 The index and middle finger web.

The width of the orthosis should be half the circumference of the forearm and wrist, and support the ulnar aspect of the fifth metacarpal. Wrap the pattern material around the hand and mark the desired width at the fifth MCP joint, forearm and wrist. Width points are indicated on the diagram as 2a, 4a, etc.

Remove the patient's hand and shape the pattern (Figure 12b).

1. Join points 1 and 2 (MCP line).
2. Join points 3-4 (thumb line).
3. Join points 5-6 (wrist line).

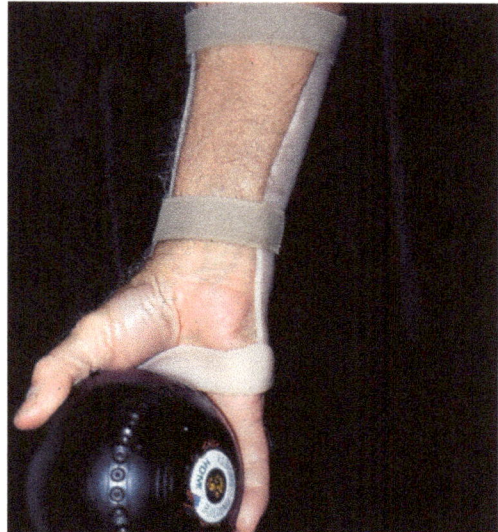

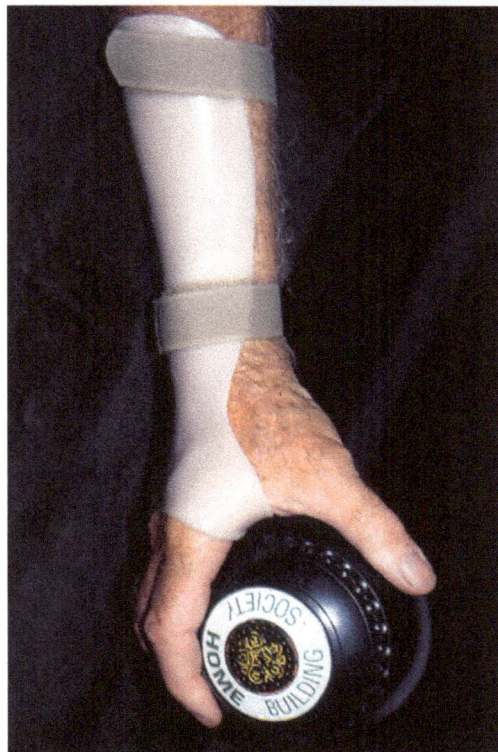

Figure 11: Wrist immobilization orthosis dorsal application. This orthosis meets the patients functional requirements for wrist support (a) whilst maximizing the palmar surface available to contact objects (b).

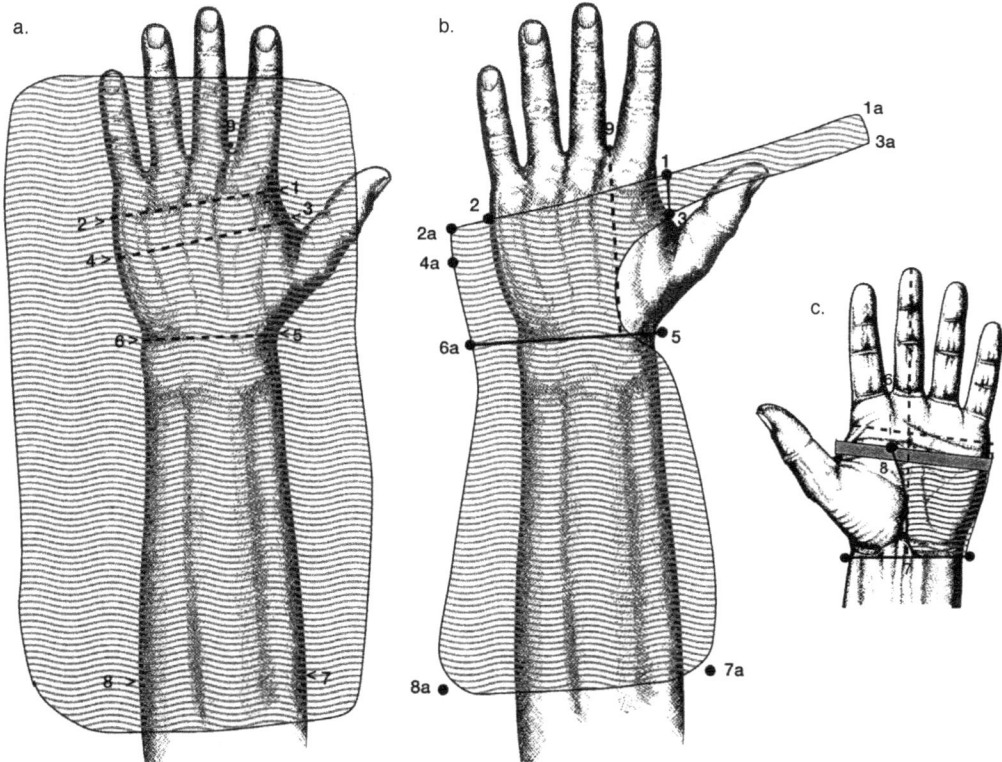

Figure 12: Pattern wrist immobilization orthosis dorsal application. Landmarks are recorded as per (a) with the completed pattern applied to the dorsal surface of application (b). The narrow palmar bar is an extension of the dorsal pattern. The pattern for an extended palmar bar is illustrated in (c).

4. Draw a vertical line from point 9 to intersect the wrist line.

5. Starting at point 2a, draw a line around the forearm through points 4a, 6a, and 8a, curve sharply around to 7a then up to 5. The curve through 7a should be shallow to ensure this aspect of the orthosis does not impede elbow flexion.

6. The line between 5 and 3 touches the vertical line 9 allowing clearance for extensor pollicus longus (EPL) tendon during thumb extension.

7. To incorporate the palmar bar into the dorsal pattern, the distal end of the orthosis is extended through the web space, across the palm of the hand to overlap slightly on the ulnar side of the orthosis. Using a tape, measure the circumference of finger metacarpals just proximal to the MCPs. Extend the MCP and thumb web lines according to the MCP circumferential measurement (2-1a).

8. Cut the pattern out and check for fit on the patient, prior to transferring it to the thermoplastic material.

Fabrication Procedure

1. The arm should be positioned with the elbow supported, the forearm in a vertical position in mid-pronation-supination, and the wrist in the predetermined

position. Allow room for the changing dimensions of the distal ulna by padding out the ulna head prior to fabrication.

2. Remove the thermoplastic material from the heating source. Roll back the distal component from 2a to 1a. The rolled edge decreases shear stress and improves comfort whilst also providing reinforcement.

3. Apply to the patient's hand and secure in place with a bandage. Mould intimately around the wrist, the arches of the hand, and gently flare the proximal and distal ends.

4. Attach three straps, one at the proximal end, one in the vicinity of the wrist and one to the bar at the distal end.

To extend the palmar component, to give greater support to the palmar aspect of the hand, an additional component can be made or incorporated into the dorsal pattern.

Mark the following points as illustrated in Figure 12.

1-2 Medial and lateral aspects of the hand just proximal to the heads of the finger metacarpals.

3-4 Medial and lateral aspects of the wrist at radiocarpal level.

5 The tip of the middle finger.

6 The index and middle finger web.

To shape the pattern:

1. Join points 1 and 2 (MCP line).

2. Join points 3-4 (wrist line).

3. Draw a vertical line from point 5 to intersect the wrist line-point 7.

4. Draw a vertical line from point 6 to intersect the MCP line - point 8 These

lines are used as a guide to determine the location of the thenar crease.

5. Draw a line from 2 to 4 then across the wrist to point 7.

6. The line between 7 and 8 follows the thenar crease.

This component is cut and moulded to the hand with the dorsal component in place. Straps are used to secure it on ulnar and radial aspects. One set of straps can be attached permanently.

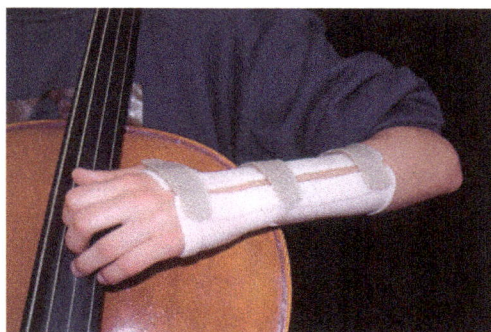

Figure 13: Wrist immobilization orthosis circumferential application. The dorsal opening ensures the transverse arch is completely supported and no radial or ulnar deviation can occur. Finger and thumb motion is not restricted in performance of occupational tasks.

WRIST IMMOBILIZATION ORTHOSIS - CIRCUMFERENTIAL APPLICATION

This orthosis uses the principle of contour to provide rigidity (Figure 13); therefore, thick very rigid thermoplastic material is unsuitable. Climatic and vocational demands will determine the type of material, its thickness and, the degree of perforation. Orfit® Classic or Orfit® Soft 1.6 mm or 2 mm thickness is the preferred thermoplastic material for this type of wrist orthosis. Orfit®Soft is recommended for the novice therapist as the coating makes it easier to handle.

The preference of the author is for the opening to be located along the dorsal aspect of the hand. This ensures there is a complete, well-contoured rigid palmar bar for support, and that radial and ulnar deviation are well controlled. Location of the opening along the ulnar border of the hand allows for easier access; however palmar and ulnar support is less rigid and dependent on securing strap correctly.

Orfit® material is available in pre-cut patterns in three sizes with the opening located on the ulnar side. The following guide is provided for therapists to make their own patterns. Measurements for this orthosis pattern are all taken with a tape measure (see Figure 14).

Procedure To Take A Pattern

For a dorsal opening the hole for the thumb is located two-thirds from one edge of the material.

1-2   (and 3a-4a) Circumference around the heads of the finger MCP joints.
1-3a   (and 2-4a) Length of the orthosis.
1-5   Two-thirds the MCP circumference.
5-2   One third the MCP circumference.
1-1a   and 2-2a The difference in length of the index compared to the little finger metacarpal. Approximately 1-1.5 cm in adults.
5-6   The length from the head of the index finger metacarpal to the head of the thumb metacarpal with the thumb in an adducted position. Approximately

2 cm in adults.
3-4   Circumference of the forearm
3-3a   and 4-4a The difference between the MCP and forearm circumference. This is divided evenly each side.

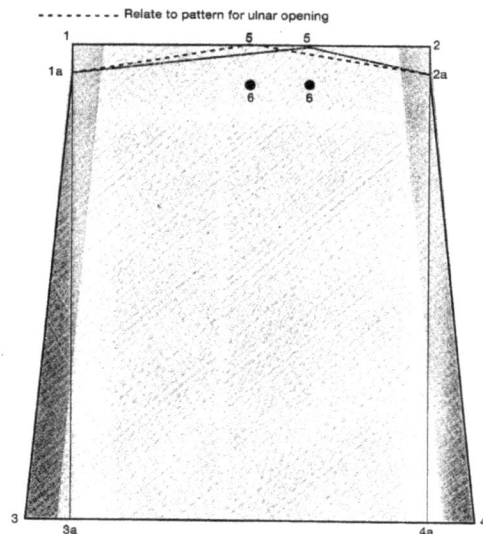

Figure 14: Pattern for wrist immobilization orthosis circumferential application. Pattern dimensions are determined by circumferential and length measurements.

The hole for the thumb is located in the middle of the piece of thermoplastic material when the opening is on the ulnar side.
1-5 The MCP circumference.
5-2 Half the MCP circumference.

When using materials without coating, cover any wound dressings with a thin layer of gauze to prevent removal of dressing when removing the thermoplastic material from the arm. Remove non-stick coating along the length of the orthosis join (shaded in Figure 14) prior to heating materials with coating.

Fabrication Procedure

1. Position the limb in a vertical position and determine the degree of extension required at the wrist. Ensure the thumb is in a position of opposition.

2. Remove the material from the water by the distal ends. Enlarge the hole slightly and place the patient's thumb through it.

3. Wrap the material around the hand and press the distal edges together on the dorsum of the metacarpals.

4. Wrap the proximal ends around the forearm and press together on the dorsum of the forearm. Now the proximal and distal ends are secured, so your hands are free to mould the rest of the orthosis.

5. Join the two edges along the length of the orthosis, ensuring excess material is taken towards the seam on the dorsal surface.

6. Forceful moulding is not required with this material; however, it is necessary to contour around the wrist and palmar arches.

7. When the material is cool, but before it goes completely hard, separate the bond and carefully remove the orthosis from the patient's hand.

8. If the seam on the opening is not of even width along the length of the orthosis, the excess is trimmed.

9. The 3 straps can be secured under each side of the seam trim prior to turning it down on the orthosis to provide reinforcement. Adhere the three pieces of adhesive backed hook Velcro® on one side of orthosis, radial or ulnar depending upon client preference for direction of pull. Heat seam allowance and fold and bond down. Attach the loop Velcro® to the hook and mark on seam allowance the location to adhere the loop Velcro® straps. Dry heat the three locations prior to placing Velcro® with pile facing away from the orthosis under the seam allowance. Heat seam allowance and fold down securing one end of the pile strap.

9. The distal end is also rolled back to provide a rounded edge allowing full motion at the MCP joints. Similarly, the proximal end is heated and folded back on itself.

10. If thumb motion is allowed, the thumb component is heated and a slightly larger hole cut. The edges are rolled back to allow freedom of motion of the thenar muscles. The component in the web space between the thumb and index finger must have a smooth round edge to minimize problems of friction.

WRIST IMMOBILIZATION ORTHOSIS INCORPORATING THUMB IMMOBILIZATION.

If the pathology requires both the wrist and the thumb to be immobilized an additional component may be added to this orthosis. To achieve this, all of the above stages, with the exception of step 10, are completed. A small piece of thermoplastic material is then added. It is slightly larger than the length and circumference of the proximal metacarpal and overlaps the orthosis to bond approximately one centimetre.

The material is positioned around the thumb and the seam cut whilst warm. Prior to the material going hard, the circumference around the proximal phalanx is enlarged slightly to allow for the greater diameter of the IP joint. The heat sealed seam is then re-inforced with an additional piece of material. The distal end is rolled to allow full IP joint motion.

PREFABRICATED ORTHOSES

Prefabricated orthoses have varying capaci-ties for immobilization due to incorporation of reinforcing bars and strapping systems. The majority are made of fabrics that stretch and allow some motion so products need to be selected according to degree of immobili-zation required.

ORTHOSES DESIGNED TO MOBILIZE THE WRIST

Mobilization orthoses fabricated for the wrist either address deficits in passive range of motion (ROM) of the wrist and extrinsic finger muscles, or redirect muscle action to facilitate motion in the presence of paralysis. Orthotic intervention used to mobilize the wrist in the presence of spasticity is discussed in Chapter 8.

ORTHOSES TO ADDRESS DEFICITS IN PASSIVE ROM IN THE WRIST

The requirements for joint motion vary according to the patient's functional and vocational activities. Numerous studies have been undertaken with various types of measuring devices, however the findings of Ryu et al.[19] are most widely used in hand therapy as the norm for functional wrist motions. The authors concluded a minimum of 40° of extension, 40° of flexion, and 40° of combined radial and ulnar deviation, is necessary to perform most activities of daily living. Extension orientated ranges of motion were seen accompanying daily living activities requiring continuous movement. Perineal care required the greatest amounts of wrist flexion.

Mobilizing wrist orthoses apply force to both the radiocarpal and mid carpal joints. Here, application of force perpendicular to the lon-gitudinal axis of the second and third meta-carpals is essential to avoid translational force compressing the joints. Serial progressive and dynamic designs are recommended for adults, with static serial designs recommend-ed for children. Experience suggests that the majority of patients can tolerate mobilizing orthoses through the first 40° in extension and flexion ROM for periods of time up to three hours. However, tolerance time is generally not greater than one hour in ranges greater than 40°.

Serial static orthoses use a wrist immobili-zation (volar) design to address deficits in extension, with the wrist immobilization (dorsal) design for deficits in flexion. These orthoses need to be totally remoulded as range changes. Although the cost is higher, serial static orthoses are generally used to resolve deficits in ROM in young children thus eliminating problems associated with getting appropriate size hinges or issues with traction systems.

Static progressive orthosis generally have a hinge, aligned with the axis of wrist joint motion, to either

- Create the mobilizing force that is applied via the hand-based and forearm components (Figure 15). The commercial hinge transfers the rotational component of the force to the wrist joint thus minimizing any potential compressive forces associated with changing line of pull; or

- Control rotation created by the force from Velcro° or other non-elastic strapping (Figure 16).

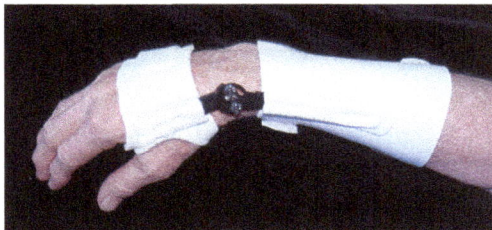

Figure 15: Wrist mobilizing orthoses. The commercial hinge articulation is this orthosis determines axis of rotation with force applied to sustain the wrist at end range using serial progressive principles.

alteration in the arc of motion subsequent to fracture and/or surgery is accommodated.

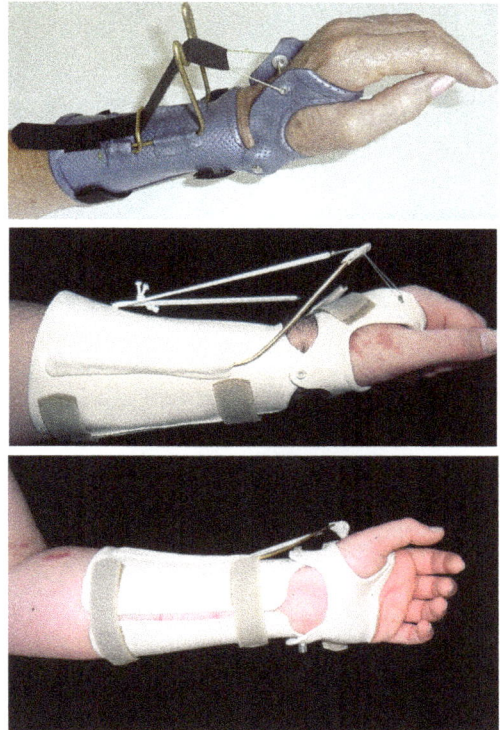

Figure 16: Wrist mobilizing orthosis. Lateral view illustrates hand and forearm components with extensions on the lateral aspect of the wrist to create the screw hinge articulation. Long strong elastic bands apply dynamic force (a) and serial progressive force applied via Velcro® (b) with the outrigger used to increase mechanical advantage to the traction.
(a. Courtesy Michael Fitzgerald)

Dynamic Orthoses use hinges aligned with the axis of wrist joint motion to control rotation created by elastic or Thera-Band® traction (Figure 16). In both type of orthoses hinges prevent the migration of the orthosis components and control deviation of the wrist. Alignment of the axis of the hinge to the axis of flexion/extension of the wrist is essential. Care is taken to ensure that

The hand component must disperse pressure applied to mobilize the wrist, therefore it should be well contoured and support all the finger metacarpals. The pressure is applied to the dorsal and volar surfaces of the hand; therefore the thermoplastic material should disperse it over the length of the metacarpals. Intimate contour and accommodating the transverse and longitudinal arches will help resolve pressure issues. Full motion of the thumb is not essential as this is not a 'functional' orthosis, however care should be taken not to restrict finger MCP joint motion.

Articulated wrist mobilizing orthoses are cost effective, in that modification to the joint angle can be easily undertaken as range of motion improves. Commercial hinges can either create the mobilizing force that is applied via the hand-based and forearm components, or only control rotation generated by another force. Hinges are available from major hand therapy suppliers and have locking devices that can be changed with a small key. The joint is locked at the end of available passive ROM (Figure 15). As tissue responds the end range is gradually increased. Hinges are secured to components moulded around the hand and forearm. If the hinge does not accommodate for the change in dimension from the forearm to the hand causing deviation, modification is necessary to the alignment of the arms of the hinge, or to the area where they will be bonded to the hand or forearm components. Hinges can also be made from screw rivets or by moulding thermoplastic struts within the orthosis design.[3,20,25] They provide a cheaper alternative to connect the hand and forearm components in articulated wrist mobilizing orthoses. Elastic or non-elastic traction is used to provide the mobilizing force.

Wrist Mobilization Orthosis - Articulated

Prior to taking a pattern determine
1. Direction/s of mobilization
2. Type and location of hinge.

3. Requirements for access and thus the location of openings for both hand and forearm components.

Procedure For Taking A Pattern

For forearm component take the following measurements with a tape measure.
1. Circumference of the wrist.
2. Circumference of the proximal forearm.
3. Length from the wrist to two-thirds the length of the forearm.

The hand component pattern is based upon the following measurements.
1. The width is equal to the circumference of the metacarpals.
2. The length is equal to the length of the index finger from the distal palmar crease to the proximal wrist crease. Additional length is added to the medial and lateral aspects of the wrist if using a swivel rivet.
3. Punch a hole for the thumb. The location for the hole is determined by the location of the opening.

Make up pattern and fit to the patient to ensure correct dimensions.

Fabrication Procedure

1. Cut out thermoplastic material for forearm component and heat.
2. Pad out medial and lateral aspects of the wrist to make room to accommodate screws or hinge.
3. Apply the heated material, mindful of the location of the opening of the forearm component.
4. Once thermoplastic material is completely cold mark any excess material

on the volar and dorsal surfaces of the wrist that need to be trimmed so that end range flexion/extension movement is not compromised. Remove and cut off material, noting additional length remains on the medial and lateral borders if rivets are to be used.

5. Reapply forearm component, use adhesive tape to secure in place. Apply a moisturizing cream to area where rivets will be located to prevent hand and forearm materials sticking to each other during fabrication of hand component.

6. Heat the hand thermoplastic material. Roll back the edges of the hole to a size that will accommodate the thumb MCP joint. Do not make this hole too big otherwise you will loose surface area for pressure dispersion. The thumb is placed through the hole and material moulded around the metacarpals and wrist. Good contour is essential.

7. Do not remove until completely cold. Remove then trim excess material on the volar and dorsal surfaces so that end range movement is not compromised. Trim components on the medial and lateral borders to allow for the rivets.

8. To create a swivel joint, a hole slightly larger than the screw rivet is punched into the extensions on the hand component at the axis of joint motion on both radial and ulnar sides. Using the hole as a template, mark the location of the rivet on the forearm component. Secure the rivet by bonding it to the forearm component with a small piece of thermoplastic material. This allows the hand

piece to be removed from over the rivet to increase ease of access to the orthosis.

9. Attach an outrigger if necessary to increase mechanical advantage to the pull of the traction system. The hinge determines the rotation and prevents any compression forces from being directed through the joint so it is not necessary to use a high outrigger. Traction pull does not need to be applied perpendicular to the metacarpal. Outrigger metal 3.2mm thickness is used to ensure strength. The outrigger should be bent to follow alignment along length and width of the finger metacarpals. Bond outrigger to forearm component using additional thermoplastic material.

10. Secure traction, using small hooks to the medial and lateral aspects of the hand and forearm components. Velcro® attached to end of traction can be used for a serial progressive intervention, or thick elastic bands, 10mm wide corded elastic or Orfit Thread in dynamic interventions.

11. Attach the Velcro® straps.

When using a commercial hinge, place hand and forearm thermoplastic components on limb and secure using tape (do not adhere Velcro® until after hinge is bonded). The axis of the hinge is aligned with the axis of the joint and with the arms of the hinge marked on the hand and forearm components. Supplied rivets or an additional piece of thermoplastic material secures the hinge. The joint is positioned at end range and then secured. Attach the Velcro® straps once hinge is secured to hand and forearm components. An outrigger may be used to increase the efficiency of traction application.

The mobilizing force applied by traction must maintain the joint at end range, overcoming the effect of the gravity and the weight of the hand. Forces to mobilize wrist joints are in the vicinity of 500gms. However it is better to err on the lower end of the force spectrum on initial application gradually increasing both force and duration of application according to patient tolerance. Patients should be cautioned that should they develop symptoms of numbness and or tingling in the hand during orthosis wear it should be removed immediately and contact made with the therapist for review.

Currently empirical evidence guides practice in application of mobilizing orthoses for the wrist. The intensity, frequency and duration of application have not been investigated by high-level research studies. Commercially mobilizing orthoses investigated by developers have shown positive outcomes[15] however high quality randomized clinical trials are required to provide unbiased evidence.

ORTHOSES TO ADDRESS DEFICITS IN PASSIVE ROM IN THE WRIST AND FINGERS

Extrinsic flexor/extensor tendon unit tightness can modify the position of both the wrist and finger joints. This problem requires lengthy periods of intervention using mobilizing orthoses. The goal is wrist neutral with mobilizing force applied to the fingers. Only when finger range can accommodate

the wrist in neutral is the mobilization of the wrist is addressed. The principles follow those used when fabricating serial orthoses with multiple remouldings. Gaining finger joint motion, and techniques to achieve this, are discussed in Chapter 6.

TORQUE TRANSMISSION ORTHOSES

In the presence of paralysis without joint contracture orthoses designed using torque transmission principles can redirect active motion of non-paralysed muscles to effect motion in targeted joints. The unique coupling of the wrist and finger musculature in the tenodesis action allows design of orthoses to facilitate grip and pinch function. Where there is paralysis of finger flexor muscles, as is seen following a C6 spinal cord lesion, the action of the wrist extensors is harnessed to approximate fingers to the thumb for pinch. When there is paralysis of wrist and finger extensor muscles in radial nerve palsy, the reverse action is used with wrist flexion effecting finger extension.

The practice of using wrist driven tenodesis orthoses, in acute management of persons with quadriplegia, varies between spinal rehabilitation units. The more permanent tenodesis orthosis is generally manufactured by orthotists. Patient specific components are moulded from high-temperature thermoplastic materials thus requiring a positive-negative plaster mould. Whilst maximizing the potential for wrist movement to facilitate finger thumb approximation for grip during table based activities, the components cover a large proportion of the only sensate area of the hand and impede other functional tasks such as wheelchair mobility and transfers. Continued use of these orthoses following discharge from hospital is quite low. Alternatively, judicious use of orthoses to position the fingers in flexion to create shortening in the finger flexor tendons, combined with appropriate intervention to positioning the thumb in opposition, can result in an effective grasp and release in the long term. Whilst long standing denervation can result in joint contractures, prior to addressing deficits in joint ROM it should be determined that these contractures actually impede and not facilitate, hand function.

Of the peripheral nerve injuries affecting the wrist, the most common, and the most significant due to the impact upon function, is that affecting the radial nerve. Following injury to the radial nerve above the elbow, the characteristic deficit in wrist, finger and thumb extension is evident. The requirement is to position the wrist so that innervated flexor muscles can function effectively. Numerous orthoses are described which use combinations of immobilization of the wrist, with springs, elastic and non-elastic traction to mobilize the fingers. Crochetiere et al.[7] first described an orthosis that used active flexor muscle function to effectively substitute for the paralysed extensor musculature without immobilization or need for springs. As the finger loops are attached directly to the outrigger, accuracy in the alignment of the outrigger is necessary for this orthosis to function effectively. This design was modified by Colditz[6] to increase ease of fabrication for the therapist. A static line supports the finger loops, suspended by an outrigger that redirects the line of pull along the dorsum of the hand. Less precision is required in the manufacture of the outrigger with adjustment being in the lengths of the static lines for each finger. The author's experience with a design based upon the Granger orthosis (Figure 17) suggests an easier manufacturing procedure.

The patient should gently grasp a cylindrical shaped object so that the wrist is in 20°-30° extension, MCPs 45° flexion and rest of the joints flexed. A rolled crepe bandage is good; however a tool handle specific to the patient's trade is also appropriate. Take a piece of 3.2 mm brass welding rod or outrigger wire 50 cm in length.

The outrigger traverses the lateral aspects of the forearm, is angled into extension at the wrist, and then traverses across the middle of the proximal phalanges following the descending angle of the heads of the metacarpals. To bend the outrigger refer to Figure 18.

1-2 Length of forearm component to the wrist, angle the rod at the wrist into 20°-30° extension.

2-3 Wrist to middle of the proximal phalanx allowing approximately 1 cm clearance to the top of the finger. This point is at 90° perpendicular to the middle of the proximal phalanx.

3-4 The width of the hand across the proximal phalanges plus 0.5 cm clearance on medial and lateral sides.

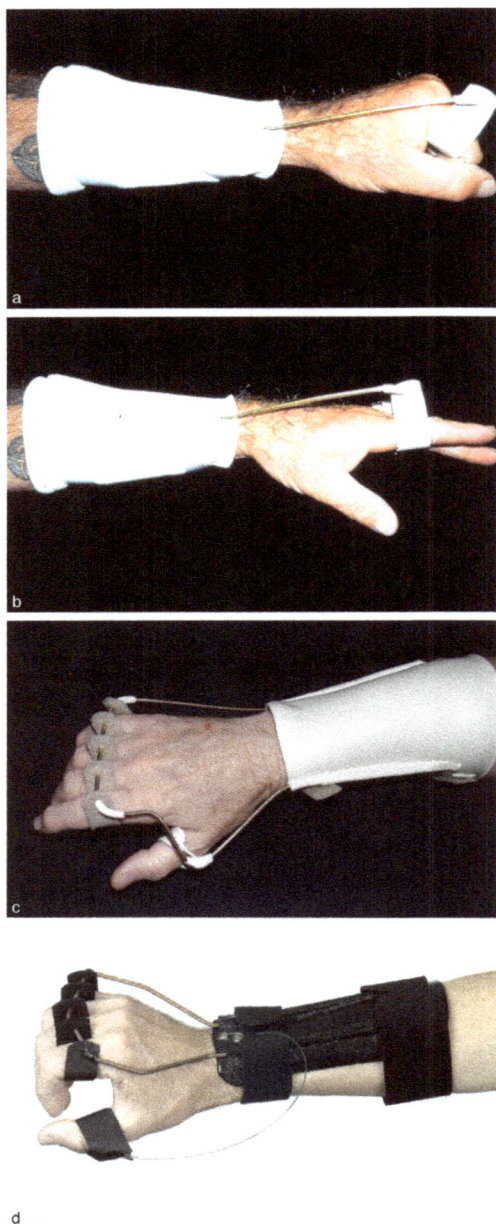

Figure 17: Torque Transmission Radial Nerve Palsy Orthosis. An outrigger secured to a long forearm base redirects wrist and finger action so that wrist extension is associated with active finger flexion (a), and finger and thumb MCP extension with active wrist flexion (b). Thumb extension is aided by a modified outrigger (c) or a spring wire loop (d). (d. courtesy Helen Fitzgerald)

This component must also be angled to accommodate the decreasing lengths of the metacarpals. To accommodate the changing transverse arch of the hand the metacarpal component is secured in a vice and then the finger component rotated medially.

4-5   1 cm distal to the top of the proximal phalanx of the little finger to the axis of the wrist

5-6   Length of forearm component.

Finger loops are measured with a tape measure allowing 1.5 cm above the dorsum of the finger on both sides. Holes are punched for insertion of the outrigger 0.5 cm from the edge. Finger loops are made from narrow Velcro® or very thin leather. If the hand is to be used in water Velcro® loops are recommended.

The pattern for the forearm component, to which the outrigger is attached, requires a series of length and circumferential measurements.

1.   Length from just proximal to the ulna head to two thirds the length of the forearm. Mark these two points to locate the next two circumferential measurements.

2.   Circumference of wrist just proximal to the ulna head.

3.   Circumference of proximal forearm.

Attach the finger loops to the outrigger and check lengths prior to bonding the outrigger to the forearm component. Ensure alignment along the lateral aspects of the wrist and the

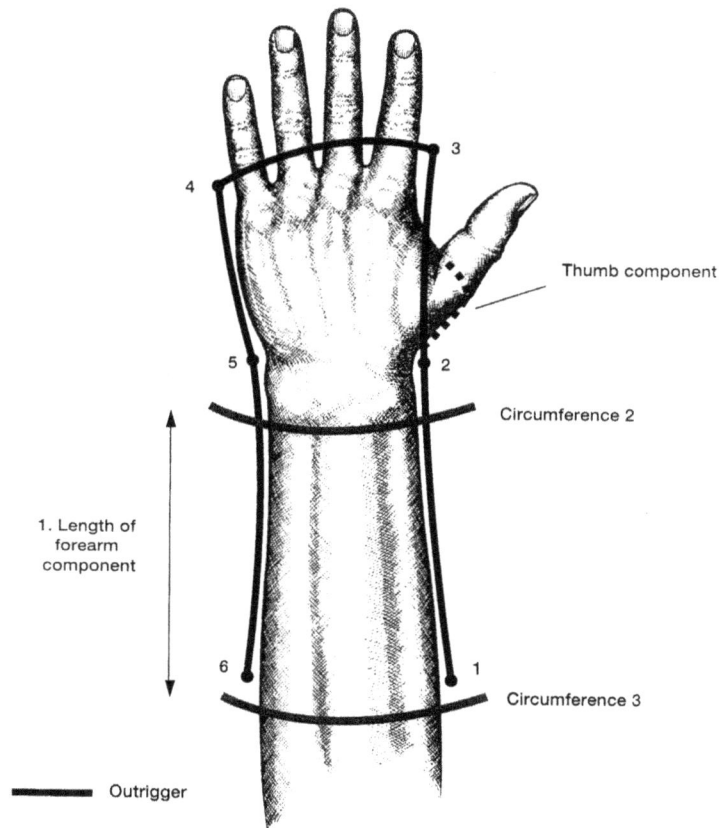

Figure 18: Pattern for the radial nerve orthosis outrigger torque transmission orthosis. Thick brass welding rod is shaped according to the pattern illustrated. If extension abduction of the thumb is also required the outrigger follows the broken line along the thumb metacarpal.

hand. The bond should allow the outrigger to be pulled out so that finger loop length may be adjusted and replaced if necessary. Attach the Velcro® straps at the proximal and distal ends of the forearm component.

This orthosis requires a period of supervised therapy to ensure that the patient has an understanding of how to achieve efficient finger opening and closing. It is worn during the day to achieve functional goals with an orthosis to immobilize the wrist at night.

Many persons with radial nerve palsy can use abductor pollicus brevis to abduct the thumb sufficient for functional grip. However if greater thumb extension is required the outrigger is modified to follow the line of the thumb metacarpal to the MCP joint with the thumb in slight extension. A loop around the thumb is attached to the outrigger with an elastic band so that extension is assisted when the wrist is flexed (Figure 17c). Alternatively a spring wire can provide the mobilizing extension force (Figure 17d). It is secured to the dorsum of the orthosis, and then follows the alignment of the thumb metacarpal to position a loop around the proximal phalanx of the thumb.

ORTHOSES DESIGNED TO RESTRICT MOTION IN THE WRIST

Orthoses that restrict motion in the wrist are used for two groups of patients. The first group have sustained injuries to the carpals or distal radius and require limited movement to facilitate the healing of tissues. The second group are those persons with permanent disabilities, such as rheumatoid arthritis or cerebral palsy, where the wrist requires some form of support but not rigid immobilization. Recovery of, or sustaining functional movement of the wrist, is the primary objective of orthotic intervention for both groups. In selecting orthoses to restrict motion in the wrist the therapist has a very large choice of prefabricated orthoses or the option to use customised orthoses.

Numerous designs are described in the literature to restrict wrist motion in either flexion extension, or radial and ulnar deviation. This is achieved by a hand and forearm component articulated by metal hinges or flexible thermoplastic tube.[3] These orthoses are manufactured using the hand and forearm components described in the previous section.

PREFABRICATED WRIST ORTHOSES

The hardness and rigidity of thermoplastic materials have often led to complications and diminished acceptance of these materials for fabrication of wrist orthoses for persons with rheumatoid arthritis or other permanent disability. Prefabricated wrist orthoses have established a niche in the market due to their accessibility in pharmacies and easy application by medical practitioners and therapists who require no knowledge of orthotic fabrication. With many styles, materials, sizes, and features, application can minimize the time and expense of orthotic intervention. Studies investigating various brands suggest they can reduce pain and improve functional use of the hand. [5,11,13,21,24,28]

The majority of these orthoses are made of elastic-based materials, reinforced on the volar surface with thermoplastic or metal, and secured by Velcro® tabs. However, universal sizing to a 'normal shaped' hand often results in inadequate support due to poor fit, inadequate length, and impingement of motion of the thumb and MCP joints of the fingers.[11,12] In addition, the difference in flexibility between the orthosis material and reinforcing bar will always allow movement between these two components, and between the hand and the orthosis. Taking the time to fit the appropriate size and modify reinforcing inserts to accommodate the shape of the patient's hand, are essential to ensure adequate support with restriction of motion limited to the wrist.

CUSTOM MADE ORTHOSES

Customized orthoses have advantages over prefabricated orthoses in accommodating the unique dimensions of the hand and the specific requirements of the pathology. Those persons who prefer orthoses with softer flexible material, who have significant deformities require customized orthoses. Flexible materials used for customized orthoses can accommodate bony architecture but do not sustain any shape on concave surfaces. Therefore, contour can only be achieved by design, and the manner in which components are sewn or held in place by reinforcement.

Commercially available custom-made orthoses have advantages over therapist-manufactured orthoses because of the expertise and equipment of the manufacturer. It allows for more choices in design, selection of materials and leads to a more professional finished product. Measurement and prescription details are available from the manufacturers.

CONCLUSION

Wrist stability and mobility are critical factors in the successful use of the upper limb in a wide variety of functional and vocational activities. Subsequent to disease or injury affecting the wrist, these essential assets may be lost with significant consequences to function. Orthotic intervention is an extremely valuable therapeutic tool in the management of wrist dysfunction. Multiple designs and materials are used to immobilize,

restrict or mobilize tissues according to the involved pathology and the occupational performance objectives of the patient.

REFERENCES

1. Adams J, Burridge J, Mullee M, et al. The clinical effectiveness of static resting splints in early rheumatoid arthritis: a randomized controlled trial. Rheumatology. 2008;47(10): 1548–53.

2. Berger RA, Garcia-Elias M. General anatomy of the wrist. In An K, Berger R, Cooney WP editors. Biomechanics of the Wrist Joint. New York:Springer-Verlag. 1991. p. 1–22.

3. Bora FW, Culp RW, Osterman AL, Skirven T. A flexible wrist splint. Journal of Hand Surgery. 1989;14A: 574–575.

4. Bulthaup S, Cipriani DJ, Thomas JJ. An electromyography study of wrist extension orthoses and upper-extremity function. American Journal of Occupational Therapy. 1999;53: 434–440.

5. Callinan NJ, Mathiowetz V. Soft verses hard resting hand splints in rheumatoid arthritis: Pain relief, preference and compliance. American Journal of Occupational Therapy. 1995;50:347–353.

6. Colditz JC. Splinting for radial nerve palsy. Journal of Hand Surgery. 1987;1:18–23.

7. Crotchetiere W, Granger CV, Ireland J. The 'Granger' orthosis for radial nerve palsy. Orthotics and Prosthetics. 1975;27:27–31.

8. De Boer IG, Peeters AJ, Ronday, HK, et al. The usage of functional wrist orthoses in patients with rheumatoid arthritis. Disability and Rehabilitation. 2008;30(4):286–295.

9. Egan M, Brosseau L, Farmer M, et al. Splints and Orthosis for treating rheumatoid arthritis. The Cochrane Collaboration. John Wiley and Sons. 2010 Issue 7.

10. Grenier ML, Chinchalkar S, Pipicelli J. Static progressive orthosis for patients with limited radial and/

or ulnar deviation: An innovative orthotic design. Journal of Hand Therapy. 2012; 5–8.

11. Haskett S, Backman C, Porter B, et al. A crossover trial of custom-made and commercially available wrist splints in adults with inflammatory arthritis. Arthritis Rheumatology. 2004;51(5): 792–799.

12. Henshaw JL, Satren JW, Wrightsman JA. The semi flexible wrist splint. Journal of Hand Therapy. 1989;2: 35–40.

13. Kjeken I, Møller G, Kvien TK. Use of commercially produced elastic wrist orthoses in chronic arthritis: A controlled study. Arthritis Care and Research. 1995;8:108–113.

14. May-Lisowski TL, King PM. Effect of wearing a static wrist orthosis on shoulder movement during feeding. American Journal Occupational Therapy. 2008;62:438–445.

15. McGrath MS, Ulrich SD, Bonutti P, et al. Evaluation of static progressive stretch for the treatment of wrist stiffness. Journal of Hand Surgery. 2008;33A: 1498–1504.

16. Mell AG, Friedman MA, Hughes RE, Carpenter JE. Shoulder muscle activity increases with wrist splint use during a simulated upper-extremity work task. American Journal of Occupational Therapy. 2006;60:320–326.

17. Moritomo H, Apergis EP, Herzberg G, et al. IFSSH committee report of wrist biomechanics committee: biomechanics of the so-called dart-throwing motion of the wrist. Journal of Hand Surgery. 2007;32A: 1447–53.

18. Patterson RM, Williams L, Andersen CR, et al. Carpal kinematics during simulated active and passive motion of the wrist. Journal of Hand Surgery. 2009;32A:1013–1019.

19. Ryu J, Palmer AK, Cooney WP. Wrist joint motion. In An KN, Berger RA, Cooney WP editors. Biomechanics of the Wrist Joint. New York:Springer-Verlag. 1991, p. 37–60.

20. Schwartz D. Thermoplastic hinges: eliminating the need for rivets in mobilization orthoses. Journal of Hand Therapy. 2012;25(3): 335–40.

21. Stern EB, Ytterberg SR, Krug HE, et al. Immediate and short-term effects of three commercial wrist extensor orthoses on grip strength and function in patients with rheumatoid arthritis. Arthritis Care Research. 1996;9(1): 42–50.

22. Steultjens EMJ, Bouter LLM, Dekker JJ, et al. Occupational therapy for rheumatoid arthritis. The Cochrane database of systematic reviews. 2004;1:CD003114. 26

23. Steultjens EMJ, Dekker J, Bouter LM. Evidence of the efficacy of occupational therapy in different conditions: an overview of systematic reviews. Clinical Rehabilitation. 2005;19: 247–54.

24. Stewart D, Mass F. Splint suitability: A comparison of four splints. Australian Journal of Occupational Therapy. 1990;37: 15–24.

25. Sueoka SS, Detemple K. Static-progressive splinting in under 25 minutes and 25 dollars. Journal of Hand Therapy. 2010;24(3): 280–6.

26. Tubiana R. Architecture and functions of the hand. In Tubiana R editor. The Hand Vol 1. WB Saunders:Philadelphia; 1981; p. 25.

27. Valdes K, Marik T. A systematic review of conservative interventions for osteoarthritis of the hand. Journal of Hand Therapy. 2009;(4), 334–50.

28. Veehof MM, Taal E, Heijnsdijk-Rouwenhorst LM, van de Laar MA. Efficacy of wrist working splints in patients with rheumatoid arthritis: a randomized controlled study. Arthritis Rheumatism. 2008;15;59(12):1698–704.

6

ORTHOSES/SPLINTS TO ADDRESS THE FINGERS

INTRODUCTION

The fingers with their varying orientation and degrees of mobility provide the hand with an incredibly versatile tool to gain information through the sensory innervation of the skin and to transmit force in grasp and pinch. Stability and mobility of the fingers are required for the hand to achieve its unique functional requirements.

Fingers are vulnerable to injury and to the effects of diseases of the musculoskeletal system. Whilst often considered relatively minor, injuries to a finger can impact upon the whole hand and therefore functional performance of the individual. Orthotic intervention is used to provide joint stability and protection of injured or repaired structures; however in the majority of cases, it is used to restore mobility. Regaining motion in finger joints is the focus of the majority of research studies into casting and orthotic interventions for the hand. The theoretical basis of intervention/s and the outcomes of mobilizing studies are discussed in Chapter 1 from a clinical reasoning perspective. This chapter describes the orthoses and fabrication techniques used to maximize functional potential of diseased or injured fingers.

ANATOMY

Successful application of an orthosis to the hand demands a sound knowledge of anatomy and kinesiology. The unique arrangements of the structural components of finger bones and joints, combined with the interconnections between intrinsic and extrinsic musculature, allow adaptation of shape with variance in force transmission for the many demands normal function requires. The finger carpometacarpal (CMC) joints are plane synovial joints, where the second through fifth metacarpals articulate with the distal carpal row. The comparative stability of the index and middle finger CMC joints, and mobility of the ring and little finger CMC joints can be understood by noting the anatomical relationships of the CMC articulations, and their associated ligamentous and tendinous supports. The shape of the articulations between the carpals and metacarpals determines the mobility of the finger CMC joints. Index and middle finger articulations are highly congruent with minimal movement possible, while flatter more shallow articulations of the ring and little fingers allow greater mobility. The index and middle finger metacarpals act like a rigid central pillar to support the movement of the more mobile adjacent fingers and thumb. CMC joint flexion motion is negligible in the index and middle fingers, 8-10 degrees in the ring finger and 15°-30° in the little finger.[1] The range of movement available at the finger CMC joints is most readily observable at the metacarpal heads on full finger flexion.

The finger CMC joints are supported by the dorsal and palmar carpometacarpal ligaments with additional dynamic stabilization afforded via the insertions of the wrist muscles on the metacarpals. The CMC joints contribute to the palmar arch system together with the thumb. The proximal transverse arch is a relatively fixed arch at the level of the CMC joints. The distal transverse arch and longitudinal arches are relatively mobile arches, with mobility greatest at the little and ring fingers and the thumb. The relative mobility of the little and ring finger CMC joints facilitates cupping and flattening of the hand, and opposition to the thumb (see Figures 1 and 2 Chapter 5, pages 111-112).

The longitudinal axis of the second metacarpal and radius align at rest, with some degrees of deviation at other metacarpals. Deviation of the proximal phalanges on the metacarpals is evident in ulnar deviation in the index and middle fingers, and radial deviation in the little finger. The progressive decrease in length of the finger metacarpals means the metacarpophalangeal (MCP) joints together form an oblique angle to the longitudinal axis of the forearm. The dynamic structures of the hand, i.e. the transverse and longitudinal arches, are associated with the two oblique angles created by the changing length and mobility of the finger metacarpals. This dual obliquity must be evident in all orthoses addressing finger metacarpals.

The articulations of the fingers are designed to function in the direction of flexion. The capsule is reinforced with strong collateral ligaments, a volar plate and tendons that traverse the joints. The MCP joints are ball and socket joints allowing active motion in flexion and extension, abduction and adduction, and passive rotation. The shapes of the metacarpal heads, combined with slightly longer radial, as compared to ulnar, collateral ligaments, allows rotational motion during flexion.

The orientation of the longitudinal axis of the fingers varies from extension to flexion. Fess[14] determined that convergence of this axis changed from an area at the base of the thumb for individual finger flexion to the radial distal half of the forearm in simultaneous flexion of all fingers (Figure 1). Variation between the orientations of the finger axis in extension as compared to flexion was greater in the index and little fingers. The wrist position did not influence convergence. Thus care is required to correctly orientate the direction of force in traction used to mobilize a finger, or fingers, into flexion.

The anatomical arrangement of the capsular structures of the MCP joints determines the safe position for immobilization. The collateral ligaments are located eccentrically with respect to the centre of rotation of the joint. Thus the distance from origin to insertion of the collateral ligaments progressively increases during joint flexion reaching a plateau after 45°.[18] Immobilizing MCP joints in greater than 45° flexion will maintain length in the collateral ligaments, minimizing potential for stiffness and contracture in extension commonly seen in many pathologic conditions.[3, 15] The tension of the ligaments in MCP flexion will restrict abduction

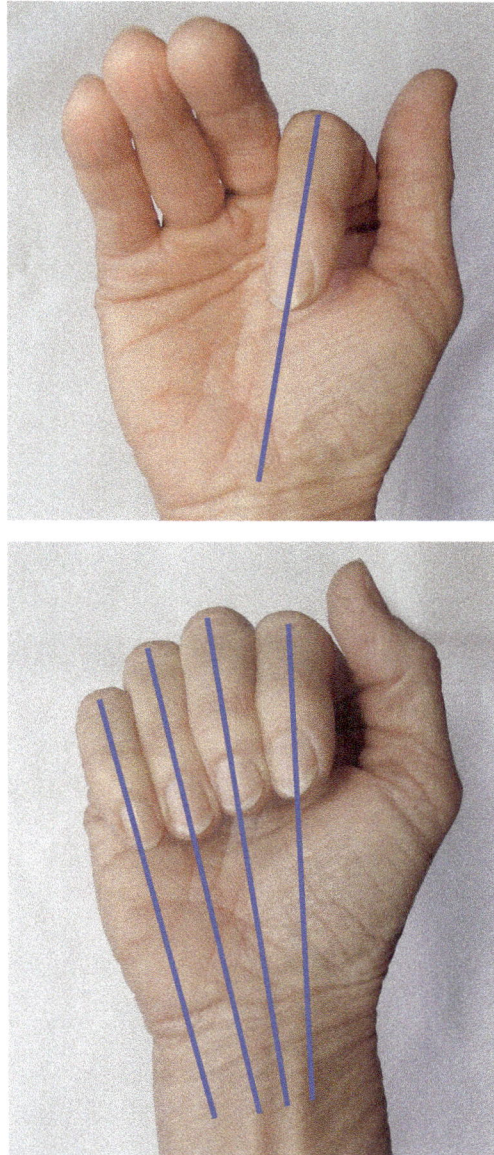

Figure 1: The difference in orientation of the longitudinal axis of the fingers is noted between individual finger flexion and simultaneous finger flexion.

movements at these joints.

The IP joints are trochlear, allowing only flexion and extension movement. Hyperextension in the DIP is usual. The capsule of the IP joints is reinforced by the extensor mechanism, the collateral ligaments and the volar plate. Fibres of the proper collateral ligament, which arise dorsal to the axis of the joint thus have an eccentric origin, and become taut as they pass over the flare of the condyle in flexion greater than 60°. Fibres that arise volar to the joint axis, the accessory collateral ligament-volar plate system, are taut in terminal extension.[4] In the presence of oedema, or collagen rearrangement associated with immobilization, the capsular structure will tighten further, limiting full extension and full flexion.

The oblique retinacular ligament (ORL), which arises from the volar aspect of the distal third of proximal phalanx, crosses the lateral side of the PIP joint to insert on the distal half of the middle phalanx with fibres intermingling with the distal extensor tendon.[21] These fibres influence motion of the IP joints. Greater resistance to DIP flexion with the PIP in extension as compared to flexion is suggestive of abnormal tightness of the ORL. The possibility of contracture in this structure requires consideration in protocols to mobilize the IP joints of the fingers.

Immobilization of joints is commonly used to allow healing of bone and surrounding soft tissue structures. Immobilization positions need to consider the impact of the pathology on the arrangement of capsular, ligamentous and musculotendinous structures.

It is beyond the scope of this anatomical review to describe the complex interconnections between the extrinsic wrist and finger muscles, and the intrinsic finger muscles during motion of the digits. Digital motion is influenced by wrist position with interdependence of muscle action across the three finger joints. For this reason prior to designing an orthosis to immobilize, mobilize, or restrict any finger joint motion careful anatomical analysis is required to determine the implications to both proximal and distal joints, and to adjacent digits. The interconnections between the tendons of the extrinsic muscles, extensor digitorum communis (EDC) and flexor digitorum profundus (FDP), influence the manner in which orthoses are fabricated to address injuries to these tendons. Interconnections between the EDC tendons, through the junctura on the dorsum of the hand, allow transmission of tension between tendons of adjacent fingers. FDP is one muscle with four tendon units, perhaps with some independence in the index finger. Therefore, protection of one FDP or EDC tendon following tendon repair impacts upon motion of the tendons of adjacent digits.

Complex interconnections between the intrinsic and extrinsic musculature through the extensor digital expansion are designed to extend the IP joints. The length relationships of the tendinous fibres are very precise as they cross the MCP, PIP and DIP joints. Therefore swelling, altered bone length, and or adhesions to surrounding tissue can markedly effect digital movement. With movement of the PIP and DIP joints interconnected orthotic solutions must consider how movement deficits or immobilization of one joint could impact or potentially facilitate greater movement at another. Extension of the IP joints occurs without significant force while PIP and DIP flexion is powered by the strong extrinsic flexors FDP and FDS. Differentiating between deficits in extensibility of the intrinsic verses extrinsic musculature is vital to ensure orthoses target the relevant tissues.

Deformities seen in fingers following paralysis of muscles arising from damage at the spinal cord, brachial plexus or peripheral nerve, or from joint instability or tendon disruption, are determined by length, tension, and function in residual muscles. Preventing contracture in positions of deformity, and augmenting residual muscle action to gain functional use in areas of paralysis can be achieved by appropriately designed and fabricated orthoses.

In their path from the forearm to their insertions distally, the tendons are constrained by retinacular ligaments on the volar and dorsal surfaces of the wrist. A series of pulleys distal to the MCP joints also maintain the finger and thumb flexors close to the phalanges. Retinacular and pulleys are often sites of inflammation. Immobilization or restriction of tendon motion by orthoses can be used to facilitate healing.

Skin on the palmar surface of the fingers and hand has two primary functions. The first is that of a sensory organ, due to the enormous number of sensory receptors present. The second function is to resist and disperse the very large mechanical forces applied during performance of functional tasks. Volar skin ridges, the adherence of skin to underlying fascia, and the location of fat pads between the digital flexion creases, all contribute to increasing friction and pressure dispersion. Orthotic design should therefore maximize the area on the palmar surface of the fingers and hand available for both sensory and mechanical functions.

Dorsal skin is very mobile with loose connections to underlying tissues. This extensibility is essential to allow movement as the fingers go from extension to flexion. However, thin epidermis and minimal connective tissue elements in the dermis increase the risk of injury should pressure be applied. Nails add support to the pulp and precision to grip. Dynamic orthoses commonly apply hooks and Velcro® to the nail as a means of securing a force applied to the finger. Application of force to the proximal end is essential to prevent disruption of the nail bed, or modification of nail contour, secondary to sustained pressure.

Clinical experience would suggest that deficits in passive motion in flexion of the MCP, extension of the PIP, and flexion of the DIP joints present the greatest therapy challenges in restoring function in the finger ray. These problems can be traced back to the effect of muscle action combined with swelling and contracture of capsular and ligamentous structures.

Therapists are encouraged to consider the intimate relationships between finger and wrist anatomy as detailed in Chapter 5, as many finger orthoses incorporate the wrist. In addition pathology often has implications for orthotic interventions affecting both wrist and fingers.

ORTHOSES TO IMMOBILIZE THE FINGERS

Immobilization of the fingers can be undertaken for a specific joint or several joints within the one digit. The impact of immobilization on proximal and distal joints, and other digits within the hand must be considered when designing orthoses and adjunctive therapy programs.

ORTHOSES TO IMMOBILIZE THE METACARPALS

Specific immobilization of the metacarpals is required following injury and surgery to facilitate healing or functional use of the hand. The extent of orthotic intervention is determined by location of the injury and which metacarpal/s are involved. When planning orthotic intervention therapists should consider:

1. The number of metacarpals to be immobilized and how this can be achieved.

2. The extent of proximal and distal immobilization, particularly proximal phalanges, and the wrist in the case of ring and little fingers.

3. The position of immobilization of the MCP joints protecting capsular structures in the context of pathology.

4. The potential impact on distal finger movement, particularly rotation and or deviation and whether this needs to be addressed.

ORTHOSES TO IMMOBILIZE CMC AND MCP JOINTS WRIST BASED

Immobilization of the fingers incorporating the wrist may be required following stable metacarpal fractures, where the orthosis immobilizes the joints above and below the fracture - MCP joints and the wrist. Immobilization of the wrist is of particular relevance where the fracture is located in the proximal third of the metacarpal, and in the more mobile less stable little and ring fingers. The wrist is immobilized following little finger metacarpal fractures to prevent the potentially deforming forces of the wrist tendons that insert at the base of the 5th metacarpal.

The orthosis is similar to that described in chapter 5 for a circumferential wrist immobilization orthoses, but extended to include the MCP joints (Figure 2). The location of the opening, whether radial or ulnar, is determined by which metacarpal is to be immobilized. For little and ring fingers, the seam is located dorsally, and for index and middle fingers, the opening is on the ulnar side. The wrist is immobilized in comfortable extension, with the MCP joints in greater than 45 degrees flexion to maintain the length of capsular structures. The wrist-based orthoses may be used in combination with 'buddy taping' to prevent rotation of the finger fracture.

ORTHOSES TO IMMOBILIZE MCP JOINT/S HAND BASED

The immobilization of the MCP joint in a hand based orthosis is indicated in ligament injuries, stable fractures of the index and

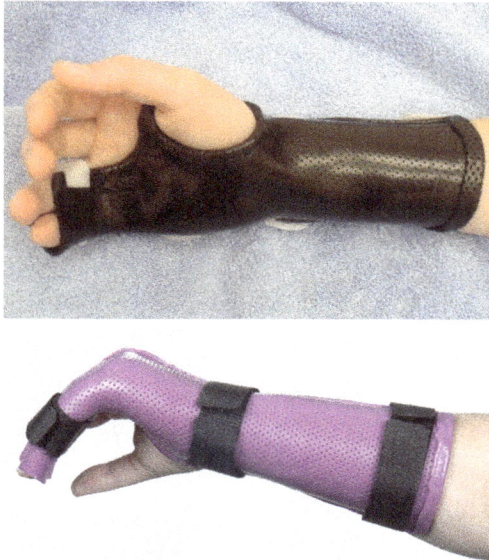

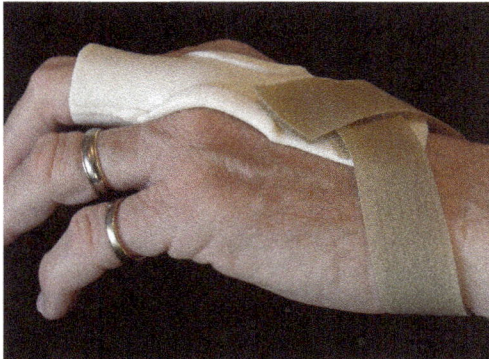

Figure 2. MCP immobilization orthosis wrist based. Mobility of the ring and little finger metacarpals require immobilization of CMC joint and MCP joints (a) with need to immobilize distal joints determined by pathology (b). (b courtesy Michael Fitzgerald).

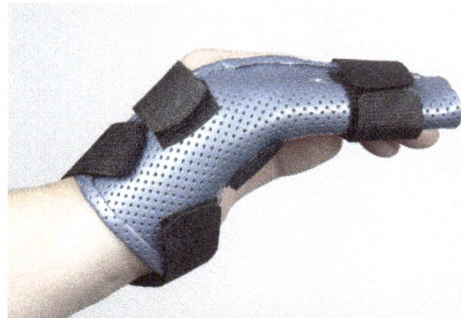

Figure 3. MCP Immobilization Orthoses. The design is circumferential around the proximal phalanx extending along length of metacarpal on dorsal surface to control flexor tendon movement. Contouring the thermoplastic material through the narrow region of the MCP joints provides strength to the design.

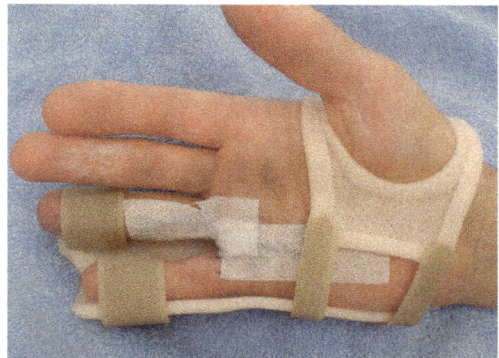

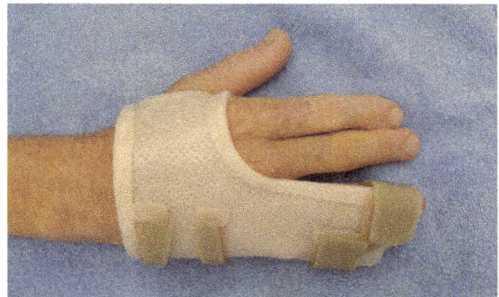

Figure 4. MCP, PIP and DIP immobilization orthoses. (a) Circumferential design for the ring and little fingers will maximize degree of immobilization for a proximal phalanx fracture. (b and c) Immobilizing finger joints in extension post surgical release of Dupuytren's contracture facilitating wound healing. (a. Courtesy Helen Fitzgerald)

middle metacarpals, or where control of tendon movement is required (Figure 3 and 4a). The degree of joint immobilization will be determined by pathology with con-

sideration as to consequences of prolonged immobilization in a position likely to cause collateral ligament shortening. Immobilization of the MCP joint in extension while per-

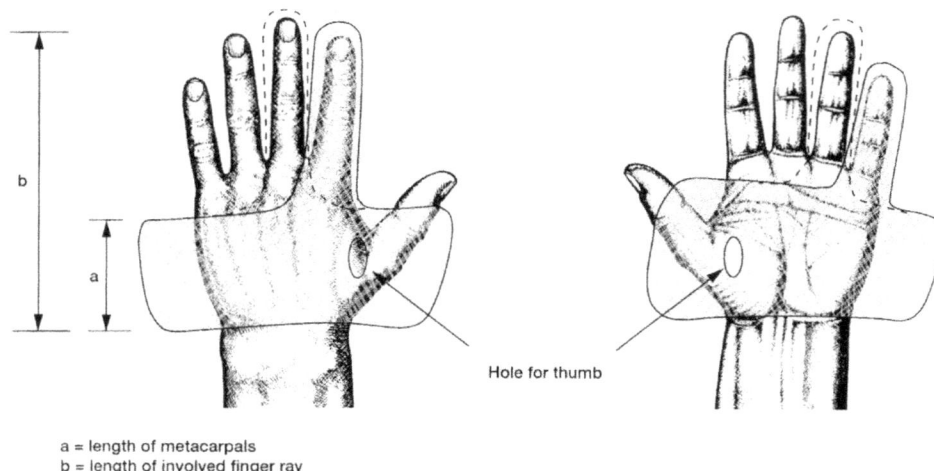

a = length of metacarpals
b = length of involved finger ray

Figure 5. Pattern for finger immobilization orthosis hand based. A precise pattern is not required when orthoses are manufactured from plastic based materials. Variations for volar and dorsal views are illustrated. Multiple fingers may be included.

mitting unrestricted motion at the PIP joints is used in conservative management of trigger finger.[8] Limiting finger flexion and excursion of the thickened and inflamed flexor tendon through the tendon sheath and pulleys minimizes triggering. The orthosis traverses the length of metacarpal on either dorsal or volar surfaces, with a circumferential finger component that permits full PIP joint flexion.

ORTHOSES TO IMMOBILIZE MCP AND IP JOINTS HAND BASED

Orthoses that are designed to immobilize one or more fingers from the volar or dorsal surface are very similar in design (Figure 4). Materials with stretch are used; therefore, precise patterns are not required. The width is the circumference of the hand. The length is determined by length of the metacarpals with extension to include the length of the involved finger ray/s (Figure 5). The piece

of material used is always slightly larger than required to allow for rolled edges. Rolled edges reinforce the narrow component over the MCP joint adding strength in the finger component by use of contour. A hole is punched to create access for the thumb.

The position of immobilization of the MCP and PIP joints can vary from full extension, as post Dupuytren's release, to varying degrees of flexion at the MCP and IP joints depending upon pathology of involved tissues. Dorsal application is recommended in the presence of palmar wounds to allow better air circulation around the wound and to allow active and passive flexion exercises without need for removal of the orthosis (Figure 4b and c). The same pattern can be used for volar application.

ORTHOSES TO IMMOBILIZE THE PIP JOINT

PIP joint immobilization may be required following injury and repair to the soft tissues at the level of PIP joint. The resultant flexed position of the PIP joint is commonly described as a Boutonniere deformity. Any contracture must be resolved by other forms of orthotic fabrication prior to immobilization of the joint. Cylindrical orthoses for the PIP joint are not successful in immobilizing the joint for two reasons. Firstly, the length of the proximal phalanx around which thermoplastic material can be placed is limited, owing to webbing of the skin between digits. Proximal length is therefore limited, approximately half the length of the phalanx, resulting in poor mechanical advantage. Secondly, the soft tissues on the volar surface can be compressed on attempted flexion. Therefore, to achieve sufficient stabilization of the orthosis on the proximal phalanx, a volar component must be added to extend the orthosis proximally (Figure 6).

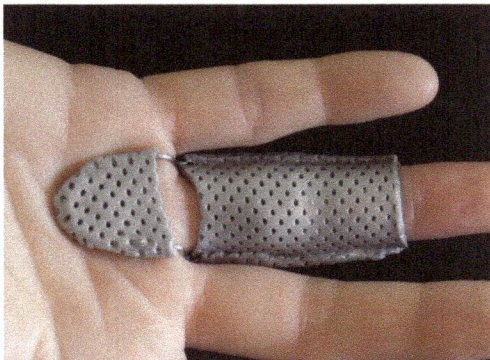

Figure 6. PIP immobilization orthosis. Effective immobilization of the PIP joint is achieved with addition of a volar component over the proximal end of the phalanx. Range of motion of the DIP joint should not be compromised. This is a good design to facilitate active DIP flexion exercises.

Fabrication Procedure

A cylindrical orthosis is made with the joint maintained in 0° extension.

1. A piece of 1.6 mm thickness micro perforated thermoplastic material is used. The length is determined by the distance between the webspace and the DIP joint. The seam is placed on the lateral aspect of the finger so that it is secured when the base is bonded on. This seam is cut while material is hot to achieve a smooth contoured bond.

2. A piece of 1.6 mm outrigger wire or stainless steel welding rod (15 cm in length) is used. Form a U shape in the centre by bending around a small round object adjusting the width to that of the finger. It is then placed over the proximal end of the phalanx and bent to accommodate the differing lengths identified in Figure 7:

    1-2 Distal palmar crease to proximal digital crease. Note the lengths on the ulnar and radial sides will differ according to finger webbing.

    2-3 Palmar surface to midway between dorsal and palmar aspects of the finger

    3-4 Length to just proximal to the DIP joint.

A small piece of thermoplastic material is then moulded over the proximal end. The two components are assembled using a thin bond along the length of the metal rod. The therapist should ensure that full motion of the DIP joint is possible. Flexion of the MCP joint is restricted to approximately 60°. The patient is taught to put on and remove the orthosis whilst the finger is resting on a flat surface so no flexion of the joint occurs.

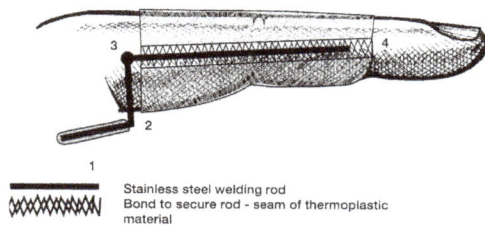

Figure 7: PIP immobilization orthosis pattern. This orthosis has good mechanical advantage.

Stainless steel welding rod
Bond to secure rod - seam of thermoplastic material

ORTHOSES TO IMMOBILIZE THE DIP JOINT

The immobilization of the DIP joint is required following a dorsal fracture of the phalanx distal to the insertion of EDC into the phalanx, or rupture of the EDC tendon close to it's insertion. This is commonly described as a Mallet deformity. There is insufficient evidence from comparisons tested within randomised trials to establish the relative effectiveness of different finger splints/orthoses used for treating mallet finger injury.[17] The critical position for an orthosis used to immobilize the DIP to allow healing of this injury is up to 15° hyperextension of the distal phalanx, while not limiting movement of the PIP joint. No pressure should be applied by the orthosis to the skin on the dorsum of distal phalanx proximal to the nail.[20] Figure 8 illustrates three orthoses designed to immobilize the distal phalanx. The cylindrical thimble style orthosis provides good positioning and does not require strapping however, must be altered as the size of the finger changes. Less alteration is required to the designs with lateral openings as the straps and openings along the side of the finger allow these orthoses to be tightened as the swelling resolves. Strapping should be kept to a minimum with adhesive tape often preferred. A small extension to the orthosis can be interlocked with the DIP immobilization orthosis to restrict extension of the PIP to -40°. This will relax the lateral bands during the first 4-6 weeks, prevent hyperextension and thereby reduce tension on the terminal tendon.[13]

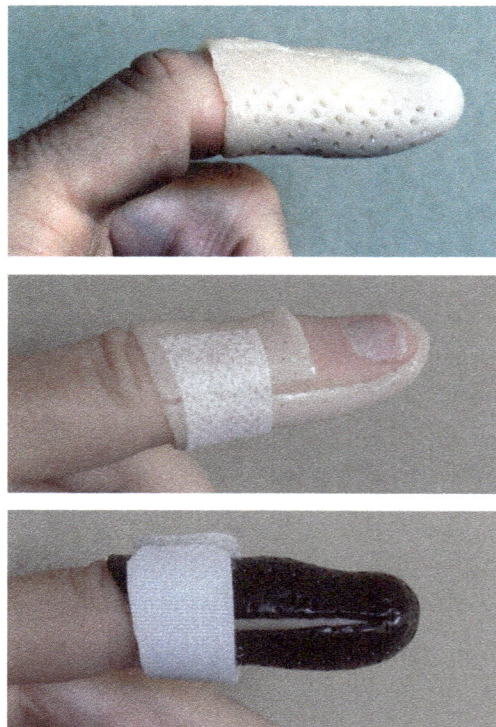

Figure 8: DIP immobilization orthoses. A cylindrical design (a) provides excellent immobilization when the size of the finger does not fluctuate. Designs with lateral openings maintain the finger in the required position whilst allowing adjustment via strap or tape as oedema resolves (b and c).

Fabrication Procedure
Circumferential Design

1. A piece of 1.6 mm thermoplastic material the length of the finger distal to the PIP joint and approximately the circumference of the finger is required.
2. Heat the material and place around the finger. Place the bond along the dorsal surface. This bond is cut flush with the skin while the material is still warm.
3. Position the finger in an extended position by a sling of Thera-Band® (Figure 9) whilst applying gentle pressure to position the material around the middle phalanx. Pressure is not applied over the dorsum of the distal phalanx.
4. Remove orthosis from the finger while it is sustained against a firm surface in an extended position. Secure seam with an additional thin strip of thermoplastic material.
5. Ensure PIP joint flexion is not restricted. Cut off excess material and very slightly flare the volar surface at the proximal end.

Open Design (single lateral opening)

Modify placement of the bond of heated material to either the radial or ulnar surface of the digit. Cut flush with the skin while the material is still warm and mould as described in circumferential design. On removing from the finger, split the bond and cut out the dorsal section distal to the DIP joint crease exposing the fingernail. Slightly flare the area along the opening. A small piece of adhesive backed hook Velcro® is then bonded directly to the thermoplastic material to secure strap for the orthosis. Alternatively tape can be

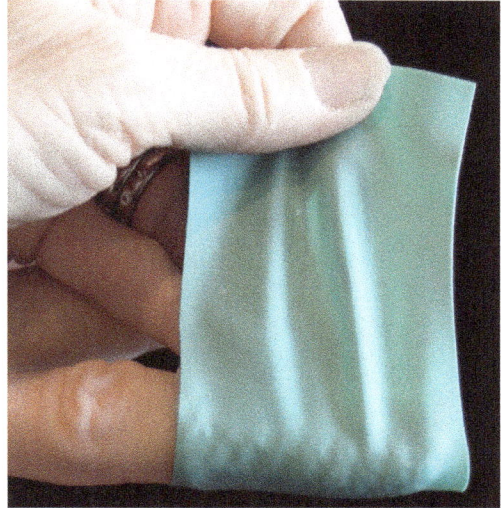

Figure 9: Gentle traction on Theraband® provides hyperextension positioning of the distal phalanx with excellent contour to the volar surface of the orthosis.

used to secure closing if lower profile orthosis is required.

Dorsal-Volar Design (bilateral openings)

This design is useful when there is significant swelling in the digit or when regular review of the orthotic fit is not possible.

1. Cut a piece of 1.6 mm thermoplastic material at least twice the length of the finger distal to the PIP joint and two thirds the circumference of the finger in width (approximately 10cm x 4cm).
2. Heat material and place on the volar surface just distal to the PIP joint and then over dorsal surface of the finger, bonding material along the sides of the finger. This bond is cut flush with the skin while material is still warm.
3. Apply required force to position the DIP joint in hyperextension while material cools.

4. Remove from the finger, split the bonds and trim along the openings ensuring PIP joint flexion is not impeded.

5. A single circumferential strap is then bonded directly to the thermoplastic material, securing the dorsal and volar components of the orthosis.

Although these orthoses may look simple, they require great care to achieve the hyperextended position whilst ensuring the orthoses are snug but not tight on the finger. Orthoses must be modified to accommodate changes in finger dimension in order to maintain the extended position. They are generally worn 24 hours per day for six to eight weeks and therefore should be comfortable and robust enough for everyday use.[19] The critical issue is to educate the client to ensure good skin hygiene, and to maintain the DIP joint in hyperextension at all times particularly when putting on and taking off the orthosis.

ORTHOSES TO MOBILIZE JOINTS OF THE FINGERS

Mobilization orthoses fabricated for the fingers address deficits in passive range of motion (ROM). Deficits in extension limit opening of the hand for grasp, while deficits in flexion limit manipulation of objects, power of grasp, as well as opposition for pinch. Where there are deficits in both extension and flexion within the one digit, priorities must be set to regain that ROM of greatest functional significance to the patient. The expected functional outcome will determine time spent in mobilizing orthoses. For example, in the stiff hand, gaining flexion to approximately 70° at the PIP joints has precedence over gaining the last 30° of extension. Acknowledging that the ideal is to treat both deficits, but being realistic that there are a limited number of hours available for orthotic intervention, a 2:1 ratio of flexion:extension may be adopted. Information from various assessments, described in Chapter 2, will determine the type of orthotic intervention.

ORTHOSES TO MOBILIZE MULTIPLE FINGER JOINTS - EXTENSION DEFICITS

Various designs are used to address all fingers in the presence of extension deficits associated with flexor tendon unit tightness. Serial progressive designs are generally used as the low force for extended periods of time between changes in position allow adaptation and growth in muscle and tendon tissues. Fabrication requires careful attention to both the wrist and finger positions. Whilst the wrist hand immobilization orthosis (Chapter 5 Figure 5, page 116) is commonly used, an orthosis that has a dorsal forearm component and volar finger component not only increases ease of fabrication, but can distribute force more effectively through orthotic components as opposed to straps (Figure 10). For the novice therapist, it is often easier to complete fabrication of the wrist and forearm components prior to moulding the finger component to apply gentle tension to the fingers to gain greater extension.

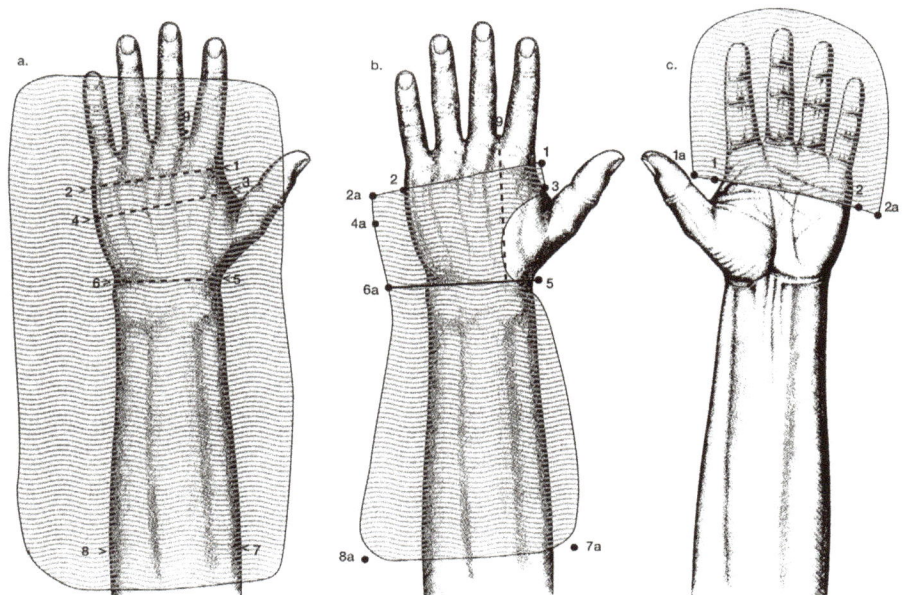

Figure 11: Pattern for wrist and finger extension orthosis.

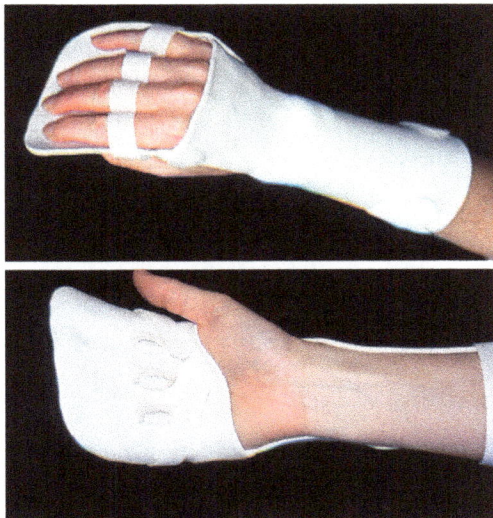

Figure 10a: Wrist and finger extension mobilizing orthosis. This design is used to address extrinsic flexor tendon tightness or extension deficits in the joints of multiple fingers. An extension force is applied to the palmar surface of the fingers (a). Finger position is maintained by finger loops, threaded through a 'D' ring on the volar surface (b). Loops are lengthened to gain access to the orthosis then secured flush with each digit.

Procedure To Take A Pattern

1. The length of the orthosis from wrist to proximal end is two-thirds the length of the forearm. This roughly equates to the length of the hand. Measure length using a tape and mark with a small dot.

2. Position the wrist at an angle close to neutral and allow the fingers and thumb to remain flexed. Lay pattern material over the dorsum of the hand and mark the following points illustrated in Figure 11a.

   1-2 Medial and lateral aspects of the hand just proximal to the heads of the finger metacarpals.

   3-4 Medial and lateral aspects of the hand at the thumb web level.

   5-6 Medial and lateral aspects of the wrist at mid carpal level.

   7-8 Medial and lateral aspects of the forearm at the length previously determined.

151

Allowance is added to support the side of the little finger (2a). The width of the orthosis should be half the circumference at the forearm and wrist. This can be determined by wrapping the pattern material around, and marking the desired width at the forearm and wrist. These width points are indicated on the diagram as 6a, 8a, etc.

The volar finger component extends from the heads of metacarpals to the tips of the fingers. Place the pattern material under the client's fingers with the wrist in some flexion so that the fingers can be extended. Mark the medial and lateral aspects of the hand just proximal to the heads of the finger metacarpals as illustrated in Figure 11.c. The finger component should be slightly longer than the fingers.

To shape the pattern refer to Figure 11.b:
1. Join points 1 and 2 (MCP line).
2. Join points 3-4 (thumb line).
3. Join points 5-6 (wrist line).
4. Draw a vertical line from point 9 to intersect the wrist line.
5. Starting at point 2a draw a line around the forearm through points 4a, 6a and 8a, curve sharply around to 7a then up to 5. The curve through 7a should be shallow to ensure this aspect of the orthosis does not impede elbow flexion.
6. The line between 5 and 3 touches the vertical line 9 allowing clearance for thumb tendons.
7. Points 1 and 3 are joined.
8. Cut the two pattern pieces out. When fitted to the hand the proximal edge of the palmar component is aligned to the thumb line of the dorsal component.

Check for fit on the patient, prior to transferring it to the thermoplastic material.

Fabrication Procedure

Prior to fabricating this orthosis it is important to determine the angle at which the wrist and the MCP joints are to be immobilized.

1. The arm should be positioned with the elbow supported, and the wrist in the predetermined position. Do not be concerned with the finger position when moulding the forearm component. Pad out the ulna head using a small piece of exercise putty.
2. Remove the forearm component from the heating source and apply to the patient's hand and secure it in place. Mould intimately around the wrist, the arches of the hand, and gently flare the proximal and distal ends, and around the thumb.
3. When the forearm component is completely cold, the palmar component is attached. The wrist is flexed so that full extension can be achieved at the fingers. The wrist component remains in place on the dorsum of the hand. The palmar component is positioned under the fingers with the sides turned up to bond onto the dorsal component on the sides of the index and little finger metacarpal heads.
4. Once the bonds are secure, the palmar component is moulded to position the fingers in the degrees of MCP flexion previously determined. IP joints are held in extension to prevent flexion.

5. Remove from the hand and bond the two components together using a heat gun. A strap is attached at the proximal end of the forearm, and if necessary over the proximal phalanx of the fingers to prevent flexion.

To increase the extension of the fingers, only the palmar component needs to be modified till the neutral position of the IP joints of fingers is achieved. Then the MCP joint position is gradually extended in combination with the wrist.

Securing each finger by a loop threaded through the palmar component will ensure position is maintained. A small slit is made between the fingers. The strap is threaded through the hole, through a securing loop or 'D' Ring on the volar surface and then back through the same slit. Thus one strap secures all fingers. The sides of the orthosis should not be higher than the fingers so that the strap sits flush with the dorsum of the index and little fingers.

ORTHOSES TO MOBILIZE MULTIPLE FINGER JOINTS - FLEXION DEFICITS

Extrinsic extensor tendon unit tightness can be addressed using composite flexion force directed to all three-finger joints. The orthosis may include the wrist using a circumferential wrist immobilization design with the goal of achieving neutral position. A soft fabric or leather strap is anchored via Velcro® to the dorsum of the distal end of the orthosis in alignment with the finger/s involved. It then traverses the dorsum of

the finger and is directed back into the palm under a pulley, and anchored to the orthosis (Figure 12). Anatomical differences in both length and potential joint mobility make it difficult to address the extensibility of all four fingers using a single strap. Individual finger straps are recommended. The patient is educated how and when to adjust straps as passive flexion increases. Tolerance to this type of mobilization is generally limited to several intervals per day.

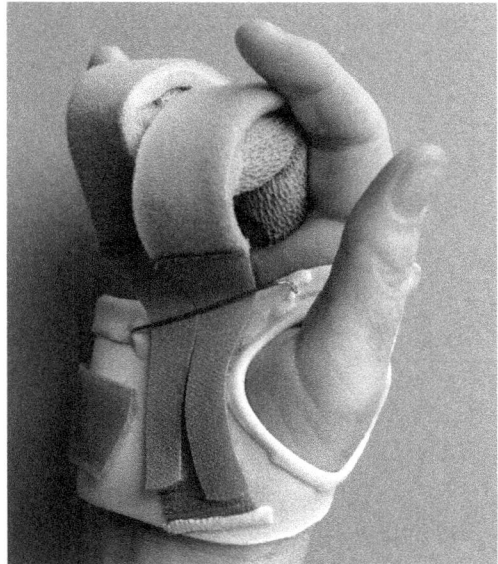

Figure 12: Finger flexion mobilizing orthosis.
This design is used to address multiple finger joint flexion deficits in the joints of multiple fingers. Traction applied to each finger accommodates movement differences in each digit.

When all joints of the finger have similar deficits in passive joint flexion, an orthosis designed to effect motion at all three joints may be used. However if the mobility of successive joints is not similar, the line of pull of the mobilizing traction should be directed specifically to each joint. Traction applied at one point on the digit to mobilize multiple joints will always mobilize the joint with the greater movement, and therefore least stiffness, first. Hand based orthoses may be used for a single finger with forearm based orthoses recommended where multiple fingers are to be mobilized. Forces can be applied to multiple joints of the same digit using separate outriggers with static and/or dynamic traction systems. Figure 13 illustrates two examples. Close monitoring is required to maintain correct line of pull and force of traction. Patients can be educated to monitor alignment and advance the tension as tissues respond with increased range of motion.

MOBILIZING ORTHOSES FOR MCP JOINTS

In designing serial progressive and dynamic orthoses to address active and passive ROM deficits in the finger joints, consideration must be given to the length of the base. Orthoses that include the wrist provide secure anchorage, a larger area for pressure dispersion, and potential for use of multiple outriggers and longer traction. However these advantages must be weighed against immobilization of proximal joints, and patient tolerance issues that are associated with larger orthoses. Orthoses traversing the wrist are used for multiple digit problems, where ROM deficits pertain to extrinsic musculotendinous adhesions, and when deficits in both flexion and extension are to be addressed within the one orthosis. Hand-

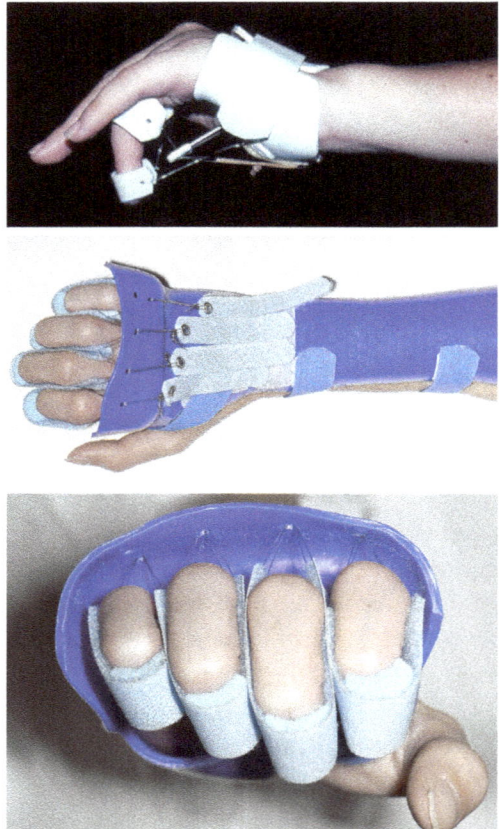

Figure 13: MCP, PIP and DIP Flexion Mobilizing Orthosis. Analysis of tissue/s contributing to passive ROM deficits determines direction of mobilizing force impacting on multiple joints. (a) Individual loops and outriggers are necessary to direct a perpendicular force when joint motion is not equal in all joints of a single finger. (b & c). Coupling finger loops that impact IP joints in combination with non elastic traction to impact MCP joint motion addresses muscle tendon unit length across multiple joints (Courtesy Helen Fitzgerald).

based designs are generally used for single digit or single joint problems.

Orthoses require regular review so that the direction of force remains at the correct angle, and where dynamic traction is used that elastic band tension is not diminished by material fatigue. After initial fabrication the patient should be seen within 2 to 3 days to determine the response of tissues to the force applied, and then on a regular basis thereafter.

Due to its capsular and ligamentous arrangement the MCP joint will generally contract in extension. Contracture of this joint is often associated with paralysis of intrinsic musculature, inappropriate immobilization subsequent to wrist casting or the presence of significant pain when the hand is immobilized. Resolution of contracture tends to be aided by functional use of the hand after approximately 45° flexion. Flexion contracture of the MCP joints is seen, but generally associated with conditions that impact upon other joints and structures in the hand.

Wrist immobilization orthoses (Figure 13 and 14 in Chapter 5, page 125) form the base of finger mobilizing orthoses that require a long base to secure an outrigger and traction. The circumferential design is most commonly used as a base for orthosis addressing deficits in MCP flexion, whilst the dorsal design with an extended palmar component is used for deficits in MCP extension (Figure 11 and 12 in Chapter 5). To fabricate the orthosis the base component is made in the usual manner. If the outrigger is likely to traverse the same location as the straps, temporarily secure orthosis using tape while marking outrigger position. The outrigger is bonded to the base prior to straps being attached. In the presence of flexion deficits in the index MCP joint, the thumb is positioned in a more extended position to allow room for the outrigger. The outrigger must accommodate the unique angle of pull for each digit. The pull should always be at 90° to the longitudinal axis of the proximal phalanx. For passive range of motion deficits serial progressive and dynamic mobilizing orthoses (Figure 14) use a low-profile outrigger attached using principles of advantageous application of mobilizing force as discussed in Chapter 2. Figure 5 in Chapter 3 (page 78) illustrates various outrigger and traction options.

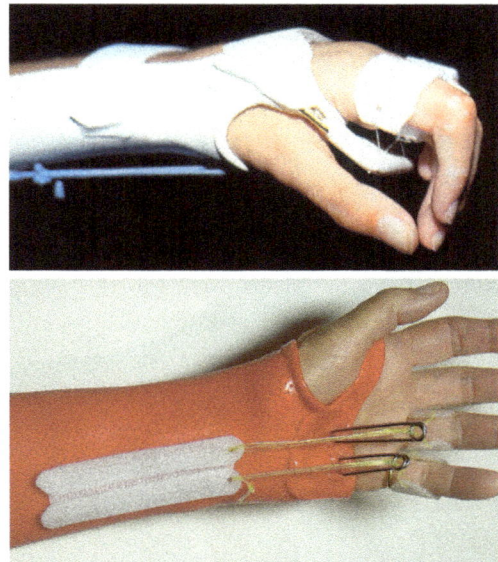

Figure 14: MCP Flexion Mobilizing Orthoses. Regaining passive flexion motion in the MCP joints via elastic traction (a) or inelastic traction (b).

For active range of motion deficits, where mobilizing orthoses are used to facilitate movement through a predetermined range, dynamic orthoses are used. A common example is the flexion/extension deficits and ulnar deviation of the MCP joints, seen in rheumatoid arthritis pre and post reconstructive surgery. The profile of the outrigger is generally higher, with long elastic bands providing dynamic force, to allow for movement against the traction unit (Figure 15). The procedure to create the dynamic traction system to facilitate active motion is described in Chapter 3.

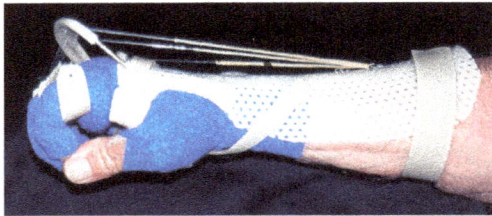

Figure 15: MCP extension mobilizing orthosis (active motion post arthroplasty surgery). A dorsal wrist immobilization orthosis with an extended palmar bar forms the basis of this orthosis.

In the case of single digit MCP movement deficits hand based orthoses use a circumferential design, not involving the thumb. Consideration is given to the location of the outrigger in determining the position of the opening and the straps.

MOBILIZATION FOR THE PIP JOINT

The design of orthoses to mobilize the PIP joint is determined firstly by the number of digits involved. Single digit deficits are generally addressed using casting or finger based orthoses, whilst hand and forearm based orthoses with traction components can address multiple digits and deficits in multiple directions.

Finger Based Interventions

Serial casting is recommended for resolution of PIP joint flexion contractures where there is significant pain or chronic inflammation, when contractures are long standing, or to maximize total end range time (TERT) and compliance. Plaster casting involves gentle positioning of the contracted tissue near the end of its elastic limit for 24 hours per day, that is maximal TERT (Figure 16). Bell[2] states "no force greater than that which would be used to extend the tissue is applied". Duration of casting depends on chronicity of the pathology–the longer duration of contracture the longer the duration between casts. Authors along with experienced clinicians would recommend casting acute injuries for 3-5 days with greater duration up to seven days for more chronic contractures.[11, 16]

On removal of the cast active and passive movements through the available range of motion are undertaken to prevent complications of prolonged immobilization. A new cast is then applied in the new lengthened position. Four or five casts are applied, with casting ceasing when the desired passive ROM is reached or when other forms of mobilizing orthoses can be used. While there may be some loss of flexion on immediate removal of casts, this is generally resolved within a short time using the greater power of the finger flexors.

For information regarding qualities and procedures for use of Plaster of Paris, and other synthetic plaster options, refer to Chapter 3.

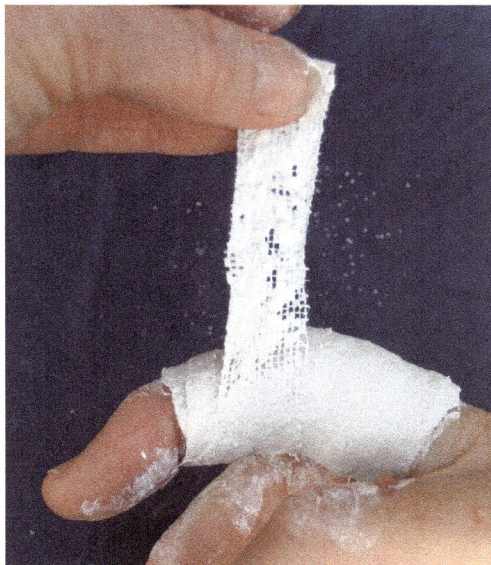

Figure 16: Spiral wrapping of narrow plaster bandage around the finger provides a neat but strong cast.

Finger Casting Fabrication Procedure

1. Very small amounts of cotton wool can be used to minimize shear between skin and plaster over the dorsum of the PIP joint. Alternatively a single layer of wax (as used in the wax bath) can be painted strategically over the PIP joint. As the plaster is setting the heat melts the wax that impregnates the plaster bandage creating a smooth area.

2. Small plaster bandage strips, 2 cm in width and between 20-25 cm in length, are rolled into small bandages. Prepare a minimum of two per finger.

3. Neat smooth edges are achieved on the proximal and distal ends of the cast by turning 5 mm over to form a small hem on the plaster bandage.

4. The finger is positioned and the plaster dipped into luke warm water and then applied to the finger without tension (Figure 16). A complete wrap is made around the proximal end prior to over-lapping by half as it is wrapped distally around the digit. Inclusion of the DIP joint will be determined by pathology. Two applications of plaster bandage are all that is necessary.

5. To position the finger the therapist holds the MCP and the distal phalanx over the nail and gently extends the finger until the plaster becomes warm and sets firmly. Slight traction may also be applied by the patient resting their finger in a cradle of Thera-Band® (Figure 9).

6. Smooth all edges and surfaces of the cast. Talcum powder rubbed into damp plaster gives a smooth surface.

7. The plaster can be removed by soaking in water. Should pain and discomfort arise the patient should be instructed to soak the plaster off.

On occasions when dealing with very small fingers it is necessary to modify the casting technique. To increase mechanical advantage, or prevent forces hyperextending the DIP joint, the casting technique is modified to im-mobilize the DIP joint first. Once plaster to this joint is rigid a second layer of plaster can be applied over DIP cast extending past PIP joint using the longer lever to gain extension torque at the PIP joint.

If active motion is not able to sustain gains in range of motion other forms of static orthoses should be considered post casting. Application during non-functional times of the day is recommended.

Capner orthosis is the common name for the PIP extension orthosis where the mobilizing force is generated by spring wire.[6] Custom-made orthoses ensure better fit and comfort as the springs can be exactly aligned to the PIP joint axis (Figure 17). This is essential to the resolution of forces and biomechanical efficiency of the orthosis. Prefabricated designs available from hand therapy suppliers are recommended over choosing not to provide a mobilizing intervention due to inability to overcome the challenges of orthotic fabrication. Thin non-perforated material is used for the moulded components of this orthosis. Thermoplastic components have advantages over soft tape. The moulded thermoplastic ensures intimate contact with changing dimensions of the finger, particularly in the vicinity of the PIP joint that is often enlarged. It also ensures that the longitudinal alignment of the springs is maintained over the narrower distal phalanx, thereby minimizing rotation and preventing the patient adjusting the force applied.

PIP Extension Orthosis (Capner) Fabrication Procedure

Two fabrication procedures are described here. The first uses two separate springs that can be premade, or purchased ready made from hand therapy material suppliers. For novice therapists having ready made springs can increase efficiency by avoiding some of the pitfalls of spring winding during fabrication. The second uses one piece of spring wire bent to the patient's dimensions incorporating the two spring coils. Small pliers are used to bend the wire and wax crayons to mark it. In both designs the dimensions of

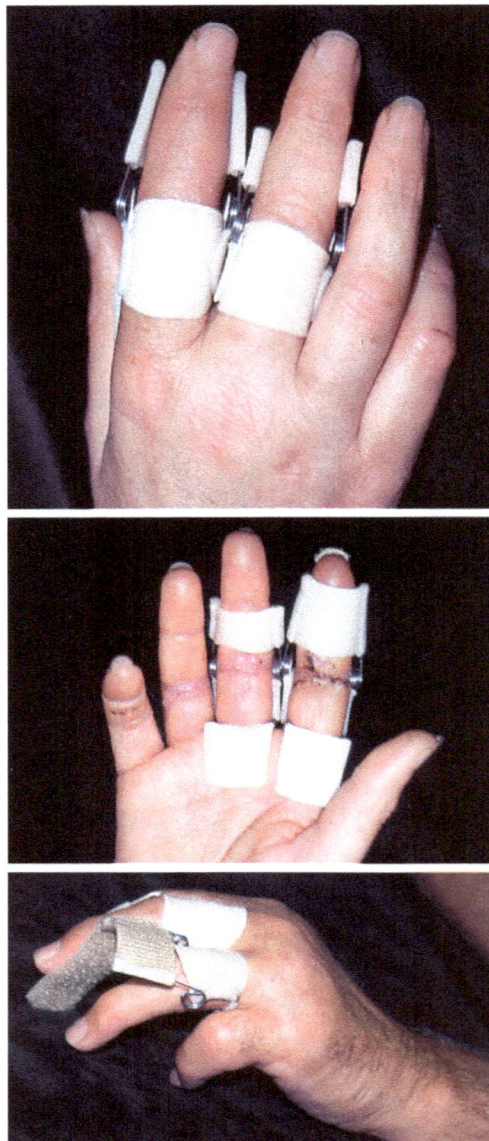

Figure 17: PIP extension mobilization orthoses (Capner). (a & b) Pressure to extend the PIP joint is applied by a thermoplastic sling. (c) The application of a Velcro ® strap, as opposed to a moulded thermoplastic component, allows easier access and more adjustment to the force applied by the spring.

the wire and thermoplastic components are the same (Figure 18), the difference relates to wire bending procedure. When bending wires note:

- The web-spaces provide a guide to the width of the finger.
- The distance from the distal palmar crease to webspace will vary on ulnar and radial aspects of each finger.
- The distance from the webspace to the PIP joint will vary on ulnar and radial aspects of each finger. The lengths are usually even for the middle finger, with the greatest variation being at the little finger.
- Centre of both springs are parallel and aligned to axis of the joint. This is critical to ensure axis of spring corresponds to axis of joint.
- Coils in wire must be wound in the same direction as the spring curve of the wire.
- Proficiency in making springs requires practice.
- For safety the ends of spring wire are curved over and buried in thermoplastic material components.

For two-wire fabrication procedure start with a piece of spring wire (gauge 12), length 15 cm. Two tight complete coils of equal diameter are located one-third from the end. A simple jig (available from hand therapy suppliers) is used to make springs winding in the direction of the coil of the wire. Place wire in the slot of the jig and wind spring in the direction of the wire curve two and a half times. One wire is wound clockwise and the other in a counter clockwise direction. The spring coils should be tight and parallel with the arms horizontal for appropriate end range of force.

The spring is positioned at the axis of the PIP joint with the spring arm distal and then bent according to the lengths illustrated in Figure 18.

1-2 Length from PIP joint to the web of the digit.

2-3 Height midway between dorsal and palmar aspects of the finger and the palmar surface.

3-4 Length from the finger web to proximal palmar crease.

1-5 Length from PIP joint to just proximal to the DIP joint. This length may be longer if the orthosis traverses this joint. It is important to remember that the torque at the PIP joint will differ depending on where the force is applied on the middle phalanx or distal phalanx.

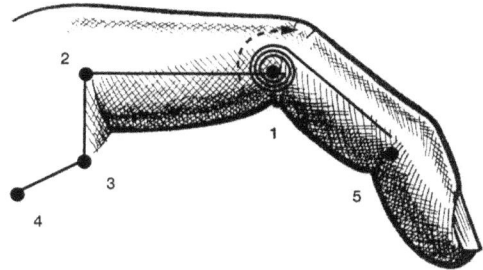

Figure 18: PIP extension mobilization orthosis pattern. Wire spring aligned to the axis of the joint with balance aligned to accommodate finger dimensions.

1. The end of both wires is bent across the palm at the proximal end before being cut close to the bend to ensure the sharp end faces away from the patient's skin.

2. The dorsal hood is made from a piece of 1.6 mm thermoplastic material moulded over the dorsal aspect of the proximal phalanx.

3. The springs are aligned to the PIP joint and the position marked on dorsal hood. The edge of the material is reheated and folded over securing the springs.

4. The small piece of thermoplastic material is moulded over the wires to form the palmar component and to maintain the finger width.

5. The orthosis is then fitted to the finger and the final loop moulded to the volar surface of the middle phalanx, or middle and distal phalanges. Align the distal arm of the springs and mark the location on the thermoplastic material. Reheat the edges and fold the thermoplastic material over the wire. This design is used to address deficits in extension of the PIP joint less than 45°.

6. Place a small piece of thermoplastic to cover the wire between finger web spaces to increase comfort.

For deficits greater than 45° the thermoplastic material is placed over the dorsum of the finger to secure the spring arms. A Velcro® loop is then attached to this piece of thermoplastic material allowing access as well as allowing the patient to adjust the force applied (Figure 17c).

The second procedure uses a single piece of (gauge 12) spring wire, length 30cm.

1. The wire is gently bent at it's mid-point to create a 'shallow 'V' or 'U' shape.

2. Pliers are used to straighten the tails of the wire, by sliding outwards from the centre point of the 'V' towards the ends of the wire whilst applying a gentle force in the opposite direction to the resting curve of the wire.

3. The centre of the 'V' is paced on the palmar aspect of the hand, at the level of the distal palmar crease and in the centre of the finger.

4. Mark on the wire the width of the finger then bend the wire 90° at the two marks, with the tails pointing distally towards the finger.

6. The proximal edge is positioned on the distal palmar crease. Mark wire just distal to the web spaces (measurement 4-3).

7. Bend the wire 90° at the two marks, so that it passes between the fingers to the dorsal aspect of the hand.

8. A small piece of thermoplastic material is heated and folded over palmar component of the wire, cut, shaped and moulded to contour the metacarpal head.

9. The wire tails are marked at half the height of the finger (measurement 2-3), and bent 90° so that they run along the longitudinal axis of the finger.

10. A mark is made half a coil (3mm) distal to the PIP joint axis, identified by locating the volar PIP joint crease. The marks on each tail should be exactly parallel.

11. Place wire in jig with the mark at the front of the slot. Place jig handle over base; hold wire firmly while turning the handle towards the palmar aspect of the finger to create the two tight parallel coils. An extra half turn may be necessary to complete coil. Remove spring and place second tail in jig, ensuring correct orientation prior to winding second coil.

12. Mark the wire tails to finger length required (measurement 1-5) then cut. Bend distal end over to help anchor the distal thermoplastic component.
13. Cut and mould the dorsal hood over the proximal phalanx, gently flaring the edges for comfort. Secure to wire maintaining spring alignment.
14. Cut and mould a thin rectangle of thermoplastic to create the palmar component under the middle phalanx and secure to wire.

Moleskin, Velcro® or filament tape may be used instead of thermoplastic materials in this design.[7]

To determine the force applied by the spring in this orthosis a Haldex® gauge and finger goniometer are required. Stabilize proximal component of orthosis. Apply force to the distal volar cuff using the Haldex® gauge to bend the component to the degree of the patient's PIP flexion contracture as measured by the goniometer. The Haldex® gauge is measuring resistance, in other words the opposing force being generated by the spring. Adjusting the resting angle of the spring will modify the force generated by deformation.

Hand Based Mobilization Orthoses

In order to apply an effective force to mobilize the PIP joint in a hand based orthosis it is essential that the proximal phalanx be immobilized to prevent the reactive force moving the proximal phalanx within the confines of the orthosis. This is best achieved by volar and dorsal components effectively sandwiching the proximal phalanx as illustrated in

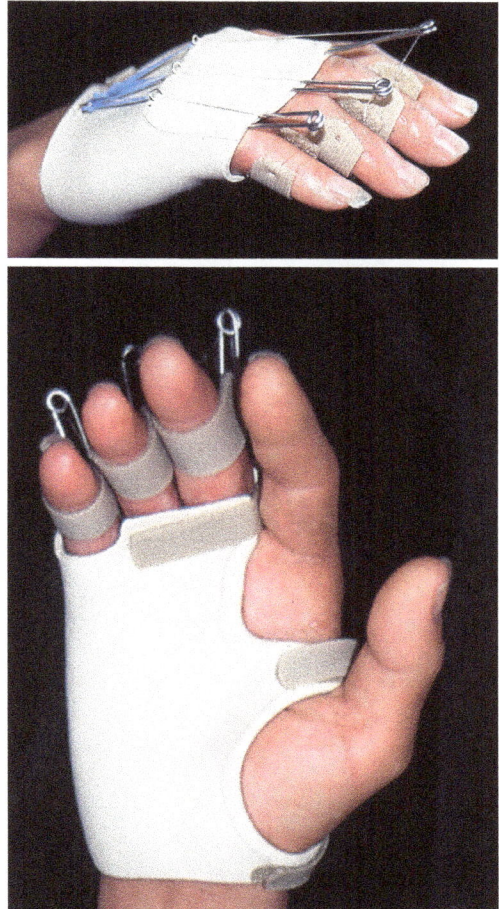

Figure 19: PIP extension mobilizing orthosis. Dynamic traction is applied via a series of low profile outriggers to three fingers with differing deficits in ROM. Volar view illustrates blocking of the proximal phalanges to eliminate reactive forces.

Figure 19. Effective mobilization of the PIP joint into flexion is often best achieved by immobilization of the MCP joints in extension as illustrated in Figure 20. The patterns used for these orthoses start from the same base as those used to immobilize the finger (Figure 5). Ensure you adjust length of the pattern for the finger component to accommodate

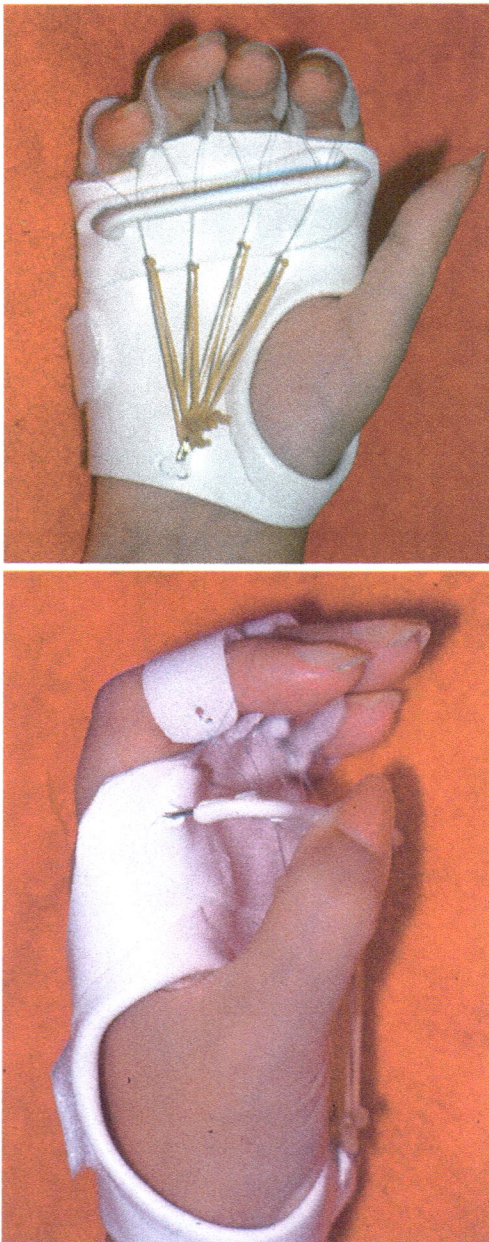

Figure 20: PIP flexion mobilizing orthosis. Similar deficits in passive ROM in flexion of PIP joints are addressed limiting motion at the MCP joints and directing traction force via a single outrigger.

increased dorsal length as the MCP is flexed. The location of the outrigger is considered in positioning the opening and the straps. A single outrigger may be appropriate if all joints have similar deficits in motion however individual outriggers (as illustrated in Figure 19) allows for easy adjustment to ensure line of pull of the traction remains a perpendicular to the middle phalanx of each digit.

While a single outrigger can be used, van Veldhoven[23] describes a rotating swing fabricated with the axis of movement at the level of the PIP joint. This ensures the correct angle of pull into flexion is maintained throughout mobilization without need for adjustment. A flexible strap is suspended perpendicularly over the swing with traction attached to the swing and orthosis base.

ORTHOSIS DESIGNS TO MOBILIZE THE DIP JOINT

Deficits in motion of the DIP joint are not uncommon with lack of flexion having the greatest impact upon function. Joint and capsular injuries may require some form of mobilizing orthosis, where as pathologies involving tendon adhesions, particularly those that restrict distal and volar movement of the lateral bands of the dorsal apparatus, are better addressed by restrictive orthoses.[10, 11] An orthosis that restricts flexion motion at the MCP or PIP will enable strong active FDP force to be directed to the DIP. Holding the joint in slight flexion with small orthosis on the dorsum of the DIP joint can enhance the effectiveness of FDP action at the DIP joint.

A finger-based orthosis (Figure 21) can effectively apply a mobilizing force to the DIP joint. Immobilization of the PIP joint means all the torque is directed to the DIP joint. The base to this orthosis is that used to immobilize the PIP joint described in Figure 6. A small outrigger made from a safety pin directs the correct line of pull to a hook secured over the palmar component. Tolerance to wearing DIP flexion orthoses is generally not greater than one hour. Therefore, repeated applications are recommended to maximize end range time. This orthosis is also an effective means to direct active force of FDP to the distal phalanx once some degrees of passive ROM have been achieved.

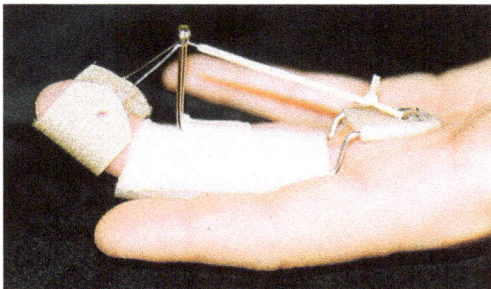

Figure 21: DIP Flexion mobilizing orthosis, finger based. Traction applied to the DIP joint requires good immobilization of the PIP joint. A safety pin forms the outrigger and a dress hook anchorage for the traction.

Prefabricated Dynamic Finger Orthoses

Numerous prefabricated dynamic finger orthoses are available from hand therapy suppliers. Their advantage is that no orthotic fabrication skills are required and the cost of time for fabrication and application is minimal. The disadvantage of these orthoses is that the location of the axis of the orthosis often does not match the axis of joint, with other components not matching the size of the finger. However, for therapists without the skill or resources to fabricate mobilizing finger orthoses, prefabricated orthoses can be used to fulfil therapeutic objectives for increasing range of motion.

ORTHOSES TO RESTRICT MOTION IN FINGER JOINTS

Orthoses designed to restrict motion in a finger are used to protect healing structures, particularly ligaments and tendons, to redirect active motion of non-paralysed muscles to effect motion in targeted joints, or to redirect active effort to effect motion in stiff distal joints. When restricting finger joints to facilitate healing the surface of application dictates the motion to be limited. Dorsal application will limit extension, volar application flexion, and medial or lateral application will restrict deviation.

ORTHOSES TO FACILITATE HEALING

There are many protocols for the postoperative rehabilitation of finger flexor and extensor tendons repairs. The reader is encouraged to source review articles for more detailed information on management protocols following flexor and extensor tendon repairs.[7,12,13] Within each protocol a form of restrictive orthosis is used with the specific angles of joint position varying.

Finger Extension Restriction Orthosis (Finger Flexor Tendon Repairs)

A dorsal hand orthosis is used to restrict

the range of extension of the fingers, whilst allowing either passive, active, or active and passive digital motion into flexion (Figure 22). Protocols vary with the wrist immobilized between 20°- 30° flexion, the MCP joints between 30°- 50° flexion, with the position the IP joints are allowed to achieve dependent on the level of tendon injury and whether protection of end range DIP extension is desired.[13] Differing positions relate to potential to modify tension force of the lumbrical muscle on FDP and ability to achieve differential excursion of the FDP and FDS tendons. A moulded palmar component is recommended when fabricating the orthosis to support the transverse arch and decrease potential for flexion to occur at either the wrist or the MCP joints.

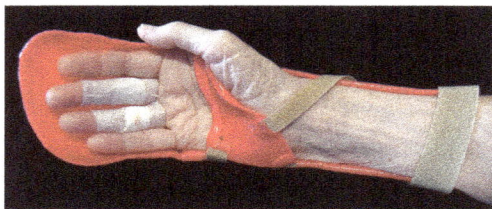

Figure 22: Finger extension restriction orthosis. The basic component of all protocols for management of finger flexor tendon repairs is an orthosis that immobilizes the wrist and blocks MCP joint extension.

Procedure To Take A Pattern

1. Position the patient's hand in safe position. In the presence of flexor tendon repairs it is advisable to support the wrist in flexion and between neutral and 10° ulnar deviation, with the fingers and thumb completely relaxed. Place the pattern material over the dorsum of the hand.

2. The length of the orthosis from wrist to proximal end is generally two-thirds the length of the forearm. This roughly equates to the length of the hand. Measure and mark with a small dot.

Mark the following points as illustrated in Figure 23.

1-2 Medial and lateral aspects of the hand just proximal to the heads of the finger metacarpals.

3-4 Medial and lateral aspects of the wrist at mid carpal level.

5-6 Medial and lateral aspects of the forearm at the length previously determined.

7   Length of the middle finger.

8   Between the index and middle finger web.

The width of the orthosis should be half the circumference at the forearm and wrist. This can be determined by wrapping the pattern material around, and marking the desired width at the forearm, wrist and MCP joints. These width points are indicated on the diagram as 1a, 2a, 3a etc.

To shape the pattern

1. Join points 1 and 2 (MCP line) and 3-4 (wrist line).

2. Draw a vertical line from point 8 to intersect the wrist line. This line is used as a guide to allow movement of the thumb.

3. Starting at point 7 draw a line connecting 2a, 4a, and 6a, curve sharply around to 5a then up to 3. The curve though 5a should be shallow to ensure this aspect of the orthosis does not impede elbow flexion. The line between 3 and 1a

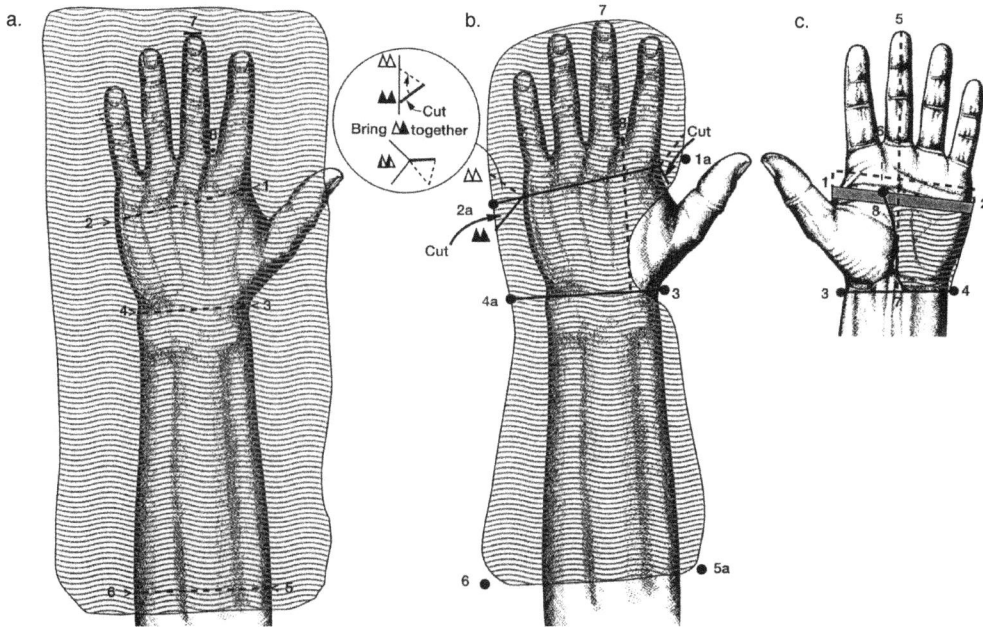

Figure 23: Finger extension restriction orthosis pattern.

allows for movement of the thumb in extension.

4. Cut the pattern out. Cut the material on the medial and lateral aspects of the MCP joints (as illustrated in the circle in Figure 23 b) to reposition the dorsal finger component into flexion. Check for fit on the client, ensuring the forearm is maintained in a pronated position, prior to transferring it to the thermoplastic material. Ensure the extensor action of extensor pollicus longus is not compromised by the orthosis distal to its exit from the extensor retinaculum.

A separate palmar component is used to contact the palmar surface of the hand for support of the arches and dispersion of pressure. Mark the following points with reference to Figure 23 c.

1-2 Medial and lateral aspects of the hand just proximal to the heads of the finger metacarpals.

3-4 Wrist at mid carpal level.

5 Tip of the middle finger.

6 Between the index and middle finger web.

To shape the pattern

1. Join points 1 and 2 (MCP line).

2. Join points 3-4 (wrist line).

3. Draw a vertical line from point 5 to intersect the wrist line-point 7.

4. Draw a vertical line from point 6 to intersect the MCP line - point 8. These lines are used as a guide to determine the location of the thenar crease.

5. Draw a line from 2 to 4 then across the wrist to point 7.

6. The line between 7 and 8 follows the thenar crease.

165

This component is cut and moulded to the hand with the dorsal orthosis in place. Straps are used to secure it on ulnar and radial aspects. Hook Velcro® is attached to the palmar component with pile Velcro® attached to the dorsal component. The ulnar strap can be attached permanently to both orthosis components to act as a hinge for ease of access.

Flexion Restriction Orthosis (Extensor Tendon Repairs)

Various protocols are used following repair of extensor tendons repaired in zones V – VII. Immobilization protocols require a volar wrist hand immobilization orthosis, as illustrated in Figures 5 and 7 in Chapter 5, with wrist and finger joints immobilized in extension. Other protocols use dynamic extension traction to maintain the finger MCP joints in a 0° extended position while allowing approximately 30-35° of flexion motion for the index and middle digits and 40-45° of motion for the ring and small digits.[12] The orthosis has a dorsal forearm component that positions the wrist in an extended position, while the palmar component restricts flexion to predetermined angles.

The pattern is the same as that used for the static serial hand orthosis (Figure 10 and 11). During the pattern taking and fabrication procedure the fingers must be supported in extension at all times.

1. The dorsal forearm component is moulded first with the patient supporting the fingers.

2 The straps are then applied to the forearm component so that they can secure this part of the orthosis to the forearm while the finger component is made.

3. The palmar component is heated, positioned on the hand and bonded on the medial and lateral surfaces of the dorsal component. MCP joint flexion is adjusted to the predetermined angle initially around 30°.

4. The outrigger is bent to accommodate the fingers suspended in a zero position at the MCP joints.

The patient is required to actively flex to the palmar component and let the traction return the fingers to a zero position. Gradually over the period of six weeks the orthosis is modified to allow increased MCP, PIP and DIP joint flexion.

Hand and Finger Based Orthoses to Restrict Finger Motion

Hand based orthoses that restrict motion of the finger joints are used for management of isolated digit injuries or as a means of controlling motion during specific exercise protocols. Orthoses that block extension are commonly used for certain fracture dislocations of the PIP joints, and following repair to the volar plate or digital nerves (Figure 24). The pattern for fabrication is illustrated in Figure 5. The amount of restriction in motion at each of the finger joints is determined by the pathology.

Restricting hyperextension or medial or lateral deviation of the PIP joint can be achieved with a small orthosis (Figure 25). This design does not impede other

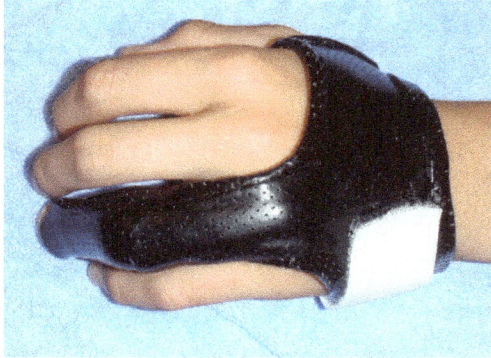

Figure 24a: Dorsal Extension Restriction Splints. The pathology will determine the degree of restriction at the MCP, PIP and DIP joints. A position of MCP flexion with IP extension is used for digital nerve repairs (a) while flexion of both MCP and PIP joints is often required following volar plate injuries (b).

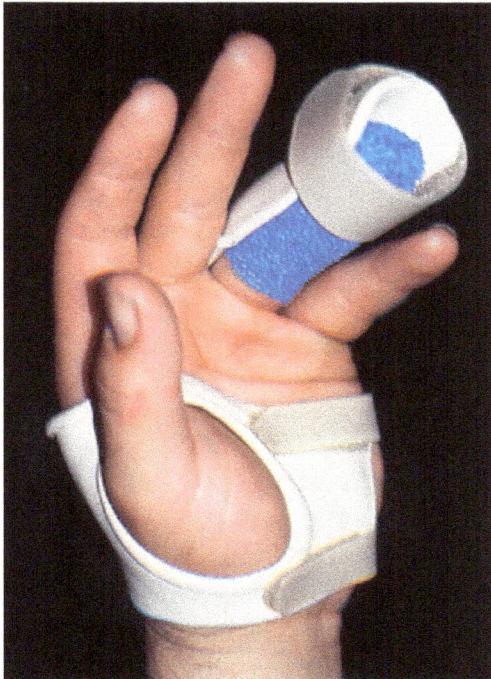

Figure 24b

functions of the PIP joint. The orthosis used to resolve both deformities requires a piece of thin thermoplastic material cut according

to Figure 26. Orfit 1.6mm non-perforated material is recommended for this orthosis. The tendency for Aquaplast to shrink slightly when cooling can lead to constriction of the finger if care is not taken during moulding.

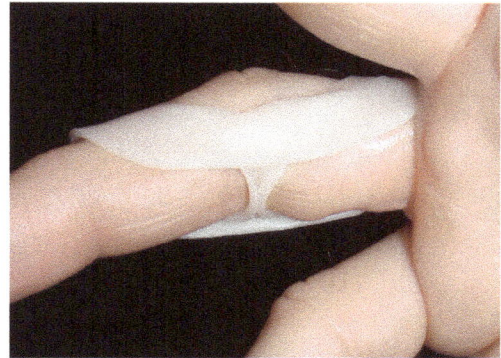

Figure 25: PIP Extension Restriction Orthosis. Hyper extension deformity secondary to a volar plate injury at the PIP joint is managed by an orthosis that restricts PIP joint hyperextension without compromise to other joint function.

Length is determined by distance from the webspace to the DIP joint, with the width at least half the circumference of the finger. Two large holes are punched.

1. Hand cream is applied to the slightly flexed finger to ensure the material slides on easily.

2. On removing material from the heating source slightly stretch the holes. Place the finger through the holes and move the material down the finger being careful not to overstretch it.

3. The sides are folded volarly and well contoured against the side of the digit.

4. This orthosis is removed from the finger when the material is *completely cold*. The edges are then trimmed to ensure

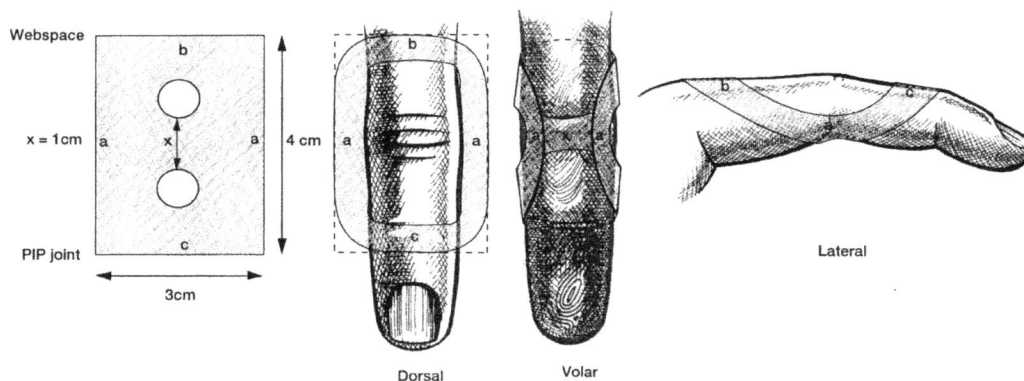

Figure 26: Pattern PIP Extension Restriction Orthosis.

no material extends beyond the volar surface of the finger.

5. If necessary the volar bar is rolled to decrease its width across the PIP joint, as flexion should not be compromised.

For persons with a permanent deformity a more acceptable solution is the use of custom made ring orthoses. These are manufactured in silver and can be ordered from the Silver Ring Splint Company (USA) or manufactured to specification by jewellers.

Restriction of medial and lateral motion of the MCP and PIP joints, whilst still allowing flexion extension, is achieved by coupling the involved finger to its non-involved neighbour by what is commonly described as a 'Buddy Tape'. The non-injured finger can provide both support and passive motion during functional movements of the fingers. The length discrepancy of ulnar digits requires the loops for each finger to be offset otherwise flexion of the digits is compromised. Bowers[5] cautions that there is a risk of undesirable rotational forces occurring in the injured finger

forced to track in tandem with its neighbour. Where this risk is present orthoses should be specifically directed to the involved joint.

Buddy tapes can be manufactured from Velcro®. The simplest design requires a length of Velcro® equal to the circumference of the involved fingers plus 2.5 cm (Figure 27). Narrow Velcro® is recommended. A small hole is cut 0.5 cm from one end. With the pile side towards the inside, the end is threaded through the hole and looped around the adjacent finger. Hook Velcro® sewn to the dorsal aspect secures the loop. Alternatively a small piece of hook Velcro® is sewn to a longer length of pile Velcro®. Both textured surfaces are orientated in the same direction so that the pile can attach to the hook as it is brought around the finger. The little finger generally requires the loops to be offset to accommodate different positions of the phalanges. In the presence of oedema, when a Lycra® fingerstall would be an appropriate intervention for the injury, multiple digit fingerstalls can be used to effectively buddy the involved digit.

MCP Ulnar Deviation Orthoses

The deviation of the fingers in an ulnar direction presents a fabrication challenge to the very experienced therapist. Correction of the deformity can be achieved in a volar wrist hand immobilization orthosis however it is during performance of functional tasks that limitations become evident. Experience suggests the customised low-profile orthosis, first described by Rennie[21] is effective in select cases where patients identify specific functional problems. For the orthosis to achieve its objectives, the advantages in positioning the fingers for function must outweigh the impediment of thermoplastic material in the hand. Many prefabricated styles are available but tend to be bulky.

RESTRICTIVE ORTHOSES TO FACILITATE ACTIVE RANGE OF MOTION

Selective restriction of finger joints to promote active mobilization of proximal or distal joints can address issues including joint stiffness and tendon adhesion. Both extrinsic and intrinsic hand muscles have influence over more than one joint. By blocking motion at proximal or distal joints the muscle tendon unit crosses, all the force of contraction can be directed to the targeted joint/tissues. These orthoses can be worn for completion of specific active ROM exercises, as well as for periods of functional activity, to promote ROM of targeted joints and excursion of affected tendons. Similar principles are applied when using non-removable plaster of

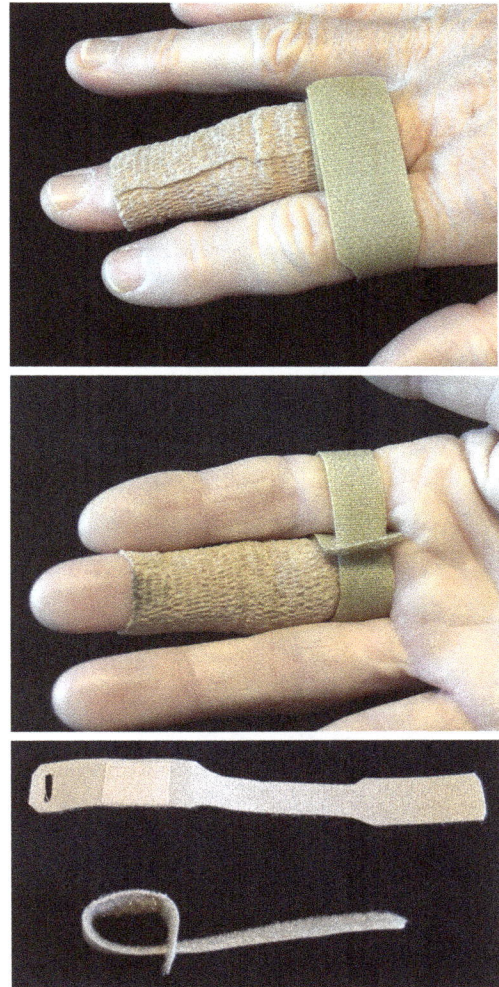

Figure 27: 'Buddy Tape' Splints.
A 'Buddy' tape configuration made of a single piece of Velcro¨ is appropriate when adjacent fingers are the same length. 'Buddy' tape for the little finger generally requires two loops that are then stitched together.

Paris casts to selectively immobilize proximal joints in an ideal position while constraining distal joints to optimize active motion over a longer period of time.[10]

169

Orthoses may restrict the MCP joint to mobilize the PIP joint, or restrict the PIP joint to mobilize the DIP joint. In some instances it may be necessary to include the wrist (positioned in slight extension) to facilitate the most efficient transmission of flexion force to the targeted joint.

The hand based orthosis, similar in design to that illustrated in Figure 20 positions the MCP joint in extension, allowing the active flexion force to be directed to the stiff PIP joint. The pattern and fabrication of this orthoses is the same as those used to immobilize the MCP joint. The orthosis illustrated in Figure 6 positions the PIP joint in extension; directing the flexion force to mobilize the DIP joint, addressing issues such as capsular tightness, oblique retinacular ligament tightness, and diminished FDP tendon glide. The critical issue with these 'exercise' orthoses is length of wear and repetition of the exercises during wear time.

ORTHOSES TO FACILITATE FUNCTIONAL MUSCLE ACTION (TORQUE TRANSMISSION)

Where damage to the median and or ulnar nerve has occurred within the vicinity of the wrist, extrinsic muscle action predominates in the fingers resulting in deformities that are exacerbated by resisted motion of the fingers. Paralysis of the interossei and lumbricals, results in flexion of the DIP and PIP joints with extension at the MCP joints, described as an intrinsic minus position. This impacts upon grasp due to the inability to extend the IP joints limiting the size of objects grasped. To overcome this deformity restriction of

extension of the MCP joints allows the full action of FDP and FDS to effect IP flexion, and EDC to extend the IP joints through its interconnections in the extensor hood (Figure 28). Clinical experience suggests that patients discard many orthoses designed to address this deformity, as the deficits associated with their use are greater than the benefits. When the patient identifies an occupational task where finger function would be enhance by restricting extension a simple orthosis is recommended.

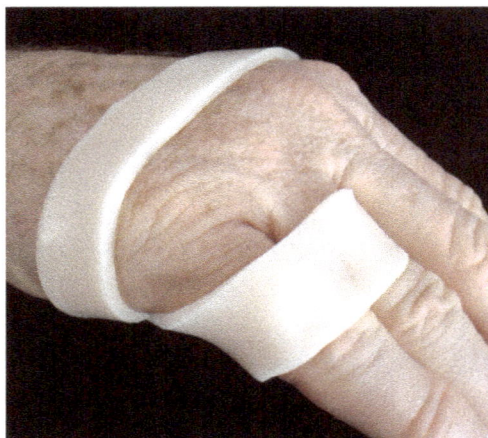

Figure 28: Torque Transmission Orthosis. Blocking hyperextension at the MCP joint will facilitate functional extension of the IP joints by transmitting extensor torque from the MCP to the PIP joints.

The orthosis requires anchorage to the palm of the hand. An additional piece of material is moulded across the dorsum of the involved fingers to prevent extension of the MCP joints. Ideally, the orthosis components should be thin, however, if too thin they will move and rotate on the hand creating discomfort.

This orthosis is manufactured from two pieces of thermoplastic material. To prevent rotation of the orthosis on the hand, the material that traverses the dorsum is slightly wider than the component across the palm. Width of the material is determined by the size of the hand. The length equals the circumference of the hand.

1. Material is intimately moulded to contours of the hand just proximal to the heads of the metacarpals. The join is placed on the ulnar aspect of the hand and heat cut to ensure a smooth bond.
2. The fingers are then positioned in flexion at the MCP joints. A second piece of material is adhered to the palmar bar on the ulnar aspect of the hand over the seam, taken over the dorsum of the fingers and then adhered back to the palmar bar on the radial aspect. Contour is especially important over the dorsum of the fingers.
3. When only the ring and little fingers are involved, the piece of material through the webspace of the middle and ring fingers should not create pressure or cause friction with movement.
4. All edges are gently flared to avoid pressure.

ORTHOSES TO OPTIMIZE FUNCTION

In situations where paralysis or injury impairs ability to grasp and position objects in the hand an orthoses may be used. These orthoses are generally performance specific, in that they secure an object such as a pen or eating utensil, positioning a digit for effective access to technology and communication devices, or secure hand on a control so that proximal

limb function can be used to achieved the functional objective. Creative solutions require therapist and patient to work together to achieve functional outcomes.

CONCLUSION

Function of the hand is dependent upon movement and stability of the fingers for fine dexterity in addition to transmission of force in object and tool manipulation. Mobility is perhaps the major focus of orthotic intervention for the fingers, preventing loss of motion in the acute phases of healing and regaining motion in the presence of contracture. To achieve desirable outcomes, orthotic design must consider the pathology, the anatomy and the kinesiology of the hand, in addition to applying sound biomechanical principles. The patient's unique functional demands and future occupational tasks will also direct the course of therapy and determine participation in the orthotic programme.

References

1. Ahmad S, Plancher KD. Carpometacarpal dislocations of the fingers. Operative Techniques in Sports Medicine. 1996;4: 257–267.
2. Bell J. Serial casting. In Fess EE, Philips CA. Hand Splinting: Principles and Methods. 2nd ed. St Louis: Mosby; 1987. p. 454.
3. Boscheinen-Morrin J, Conolly WB. The Hand: Fundamentals of Therapy. 3rd edn. Kent: Butterworth Heinemann; 2001.
4. Bowers WH. The anatomy of the interphalangeal joints.

In Bowers WH editor. The Interphalangeal Joints. Edinburgh:Churchill Livingstone; 1987. p. 1–20.

5. Bowers WH. Injuries and complications of injuries to the capsular structure of the interphalangeal joints. In Bowers WH editor. The Interphalangeal Joints. Edinburgh:Churchill Livingstone; 1987. p. 56–76.

6. Capner N. Lively splints. Physiotherapy. 1967;53: 371–374.

7. Chesney A, Chauhan A, Kattan A, et al. Systematic review of flexor tendon rehabilitation protocols in zone II of the hand. Plastic Reconstructive Surgery. 2011;127: 1583–92.

8. Colbourn J, Heath N, Manary S, Pacifico D. Effectiveness of splinting for the treatment of trigger finger. Journal of Hand Therapy. 2008;21: 336–43.

9. Colditz JC. Spring-wire extension splinting of the proximal interphalangeal joint. In Hunter JM, Makin EJ, Callahan AD editors. Rehabilitation of the Hand: Surgery and Therapy. 4th ed: St Louis: Mosby; 1995. p. 1617–1629.

10. Colditz JC. Therapists' management of the stiff hand. In Skirven TM, Callahan AD, Osterman AL, Schneider LH, Hunter JM editors. Rehabilitation of the Hand and Upper Extremity. 5th ed: St Louis: Mosby; 2002. p. 1021–1049.

11. Colditz J. Plaster of Paris: the forgotten hand splinting material. Journal of Hand Therapy. 2002;15: 144–57.

12. Evans RB. Clinical management of extensor tendon injuries: the therapist's perspective. In Skirven TM, Osterman AL, Fedorczyk, Amadio PC, eds. Rehabilitation of the Hand and Upper Extremity. 6th ed. Elsevier. 2011, p. 521-554.

13. Evans RB. Managing the injured tendon: current concepts. Journal of Hand Therapy. 2012;25(2): 173–89.

14. Fess E. Convergence points of normal fingers in individual flexion and simultaneous flexion. Journal of Hand Therapy. 1989;2: 12–19.

15. Fess EE, Gettle KS, Philips CA, Janson JR. Hand and Upper Extremity Splinting: Principles and Methods, 3rd edn. St Louis:CV Mosby. 2005.

16. Flowers KR, LaStayo P. Effect of total end range time on improving passive range of motion. Journal of Hand Therapy. 1994;7: 150–7. Reprinted in January 2012.

17. Handoll HG, Vaghela MV. Interventions for treating mallet finger injuries. Cochrane Database of Systematic Reviews. John Wiley and Sons Ltd. 2008.

18. Minami A, Kai-Kan A, Cooney W et al. Ligament stability of the MCP joint: a biomechanical Study. Journal of Hand Surgery. 1985;12A: 548-260.

19. O'Brien LJ, Bailey MJ. Single blind, prospective, randomized controlled trial comparing dorsal aluminum and custom thermoplastic splints to stack splint for acute mallet finger. Archives of Physical Medicine Rehabilitation. 2011;92(2): 191-8.

20. Rayan G, Mullins P. Skin necrosis complicating mallet finger splinting and vascularity of the distal interphalangeal joint overlying skin. Journal of Hand Surgery. 1987;12A: 548–550.

21. Rennie HJ. Evaluation of the effectiveness of a metacarpophalangeal ulnar deviation orthosis. Journal of Hand therapy. 1996;9: 371-377.

22. Tubiana R, Thomine JM, Mackin E. Examination of the Hand and Wrist, 2nd ednigure. London: Martin Dunitz. 1996.

23. Van Veldhoven G. The proximal interphalangeal joint swing traction splint. Journal of Hand Therapy. 1995; 5: 265–268.

7

ORTHOSES/SPLINTS TO ADDRESS THE THUMB

INTRODUCTION

The position, orientation and motion of the thumb afford the human hand unique opportunities for function. Stability is essential for force transmission to objects during grip and pinch, whilst mobility is necessary to orientate the pulp of the thumb to the pulp of the fingers for fine object manipulation. Mobility may be sacrificed to achieve stability in functional use of the hand. Disruption of the joint surfaces, and or the ligamentous arrangement, is commonly associated with rheumatoid and osteoarthritis. Altered muscle function is associated with paralysis or spasticity secondary to either peripheral or central nervous system dysfunction. Both joint and muscle integrity have a profound impact upon the thumb's contribution to function of the hand.

Orthotic intervention may be used to provide stability to the thumb in the presence of subluxation, to reduce mechanical stress that may be causing joint instability and disorganization, and or to reduce pain and inflammation. Orthoses may also be used to position the thumb for function, such that it can provide an effective opposition post in the presence of muscle imbalance, or to prevent

173

maceration of the skin seen in severe cases of neurological dysfunction. An understanding of the musculoskeletal forces contributing to deformity in all three thumb joints is essential to designing orthoses to decrease pain, and increase hand strength and function.

The literature specific to a presenting pathology will provide clinicians with information on the efficacy of various orthotic interventions for the thumb. Literature on rheumatoid and osteoarthritis, pathologies where orthotic intervention is common, suggests positive outcomes in the use of orthoses to decrease pain, increase grip strength and improve hand function with no clear consensus on the 'best orthosis or protocol'.[1,3,10,11,15] With a myriad of client centered factors that influence choice of intervention and diversity of reasons orthoses are prescribed, findings from systematic reviews and research studies are used as tools to aid clinical reasoning when making decisions with the patients regarding orthotic choices.[4,12,13,14,16]

ANATOMY

An understanding of the anatomy and biomechanics of the thumb provides a foundation to understanding it's pathophysiology and dysfunction. The complexity of the subject is beyond this review, however therapists are encouraged to seek this knowledge prior to orthotic fabrication. The carpometacarpal (CMC) joint of the thumb is a complex joint with minimal stability offered by the biconcave-convex or reciprocal saddle joint. Multiple ligaments reinforce the capsule and interplay with intrinsic and extrinsic muscle action to achieve stability, to prevent translation of the metacarpal during loading, as well as facilitating the desired orientation of thumb pulp for function. To achieve opposition, the thumb must first abduct to position the metacarpal on the part of the articular surface of the trapezium where rotation occurs. As can be seen from close observation of the orientation of the thumbnail, the movements of flexion/extension, and a small range of abduction/adduction, occur without rotation of the metacarpal. Without rotation of the metacarpal, orientation of the thumb pad to the pad of the fingertips is not possible. Motor units act as dynamic stabilizers of the thumb with movement at the CMC joint a result of the combined action of the thumb intrinsic and extrinsic muscles and the constraining influence of the ligaments.

The compressive forces transmitted through the joint in occupational tasks are believed to be one reason osteoarthritis of the CMC joint, is relatively common. Alterations in CMC joint contact forces may occur after joint injury, disease effecting cartilage or bone integrity, changes in neuromuscular balance affecting the thumb, and contact stresses influenced by changes in forces transmitted by differential positioning of the thumb metacarpophalangeal (MCP) and interphalangeal (IP) joints.[6] Therefore when applying forces to correct or position or re-establish 'normal' relationships of tissues via an orthosis, therapists need to understand pathological processes and consider implications of orthotic forces for immobilization, mobilization, or restriction to all thumb joints.

The condyloid shape of the MCP joint, surrounded by strong collateral ligaments and the volar plate sesamoid bone complex, allows motion in flexion/extension with passive deviation. The collateral ligament of the MCP joint of the thumb has two components one of which is always taut giving the joint stability in full range of motion. The greater length of the ulnar collateral ligament allows some passive radial rotation essential in opposition. This ligament is more commonly injured than the radial ligament. Intrinsic muscles, abductor pollicis brevis (APB), adductor pollicis (AP), flexor pollicus brevis (FPB), and extensor pollicis brevis (EPB), provide dynamic stability to the joint during pinch and grasp activities. The normal range of motion is quite variable in this joint.

The IP joint is a trochlear articulation. The ligamentous capsular structures are reinforced by flexor pollicus longus (FPL), and extensor pollicus longus (EPL) tendons. Joint stability is more important than mobility. Hyperextension is common.

The MCP joint capsular and ligamentous arrangements are reinforced by the fibrous aponeurotic formation in the thumb index web space. This attaches to bone, tendon sheath and skin. Contracture of this and other structures spanning the web space is very common with oedema in the hand following trauma, or from immobilization secondary to muscle dysfunction.

Intrinsic muscles control the position of the thumb during function. These muscles are arranged in a fan shape around the metacarpal. The median nerve innervated muscles are responsible for movements of abduction and rotation while the ulnar nerve innervated muscles produce adduction and flexion towards the fingers for grip and pinch. The radial nerve innervated extrinsic abductor and extensor muscles position the thumb away from the palm in preparation for grip and pinch. Orthotic fabrication has an important role in sustaining functional use of the thumb in the presence of paralysis of one or more of these nerves. Recognition of the pathomechanics of injury and disease as it affects all thumb joints facilitates the consideration of appropriate orthotic treatment particularly as stability and mobility of one joint has implications to proximal and distal joints.

ORTHOSES TO IMMOBILIZE THE THUMB

Orthoses may be required for the thumb in isolation or in combination with the wrist or the rest of the hand. Perhaps the most critical issue in design and fabrication of all thumb orthoses is the position in which the CMC joint is immobilized. This has implications to the maintenance of the web space and rotation of the metacarpal to meet the functional requirements of the patient for grip and pinch.

A variety of orthotic designs are used to immobilize the thumb. In deciding which is the most appropriate design the two key issues for consideration are:

1. The pathology and the degree of immobilization required. Orthoses may address specific joint structures, or include more than one joint and the wrist if there is extensive pathology involving multiple joints or extrinsic muscle tendon units. It is not unusual that more extensive immobilization is undertaken in acute phases of healing, or inflammatory joint disease, with reduction in size of the orthosis as greater mobility is allowed.

2. The patient's functional requirements. Function determines the forces that are transmitted through the thumb, and the requirement for skin friction and sensory input for objects and tool manipulation.

IP JOINT IMMOBILIZATION ORTHOSES

Due to the nature of tissues in the thumb, a circumferential orthosis provides a more rigid means of immobilization following injury (Figure 1). Cylindrical orthoses can be easily applied and removed, thereby avoiding problems with straps or tapes getting wet or needing to be replaced. However, sensory input to the pulp of the thumb is important for function and therefore modification of design will be necessary if grip and pinch are essential functional requirements.[2] Orthoses designed to correct a hyperextension

deformity or lateral instability to facilitate pinch require the palmar surface to be cut down to maximize the area of pulp available for pinch. Thermoplastic material is slippery and therefore prevents good purchase for pinch.

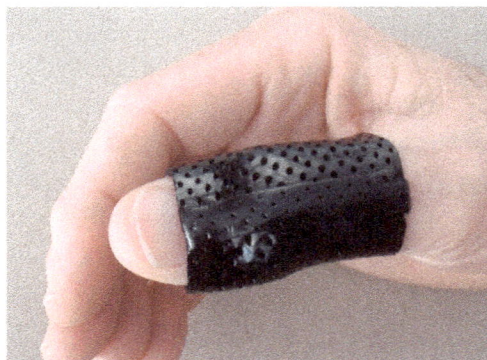

Figure 1: Thumb IP Immobilization Orthosis.
The circumferential design has advantages for joint immobilization and dispersion of pressure, however limits the area available for sensory input during pinch.

When moulding thermoplastic materials for cylindrical orthoses therapists should be mindful of the oval shape of the IP joint, with tissues more proximal tending to be smaller in circumference. Splitting the seam over the proximal phalanx will improve access, but necessitate strap closure.

MCP JOINT IMMOBILIZATION ORTHOSIS

When pathology is specific to the MCP joint, a decision has to be made as to the degree at which the orthosis will immobilize the metacarpal. Complete immobilization of the thumb metacarpal can only be achieved if the CMC joint is also immobilized, thereby preventing any rotation. An orthosis that protects structures around the MCP joint whilst still allowing rotation is designed to transmit much of the radial stress associated with pinch through the orthosis. Final stages of healing following ulnar collateral ligament injury of the MCP joint or arthritis are diagnoses commonly immobilized in this manner (Figure 2).

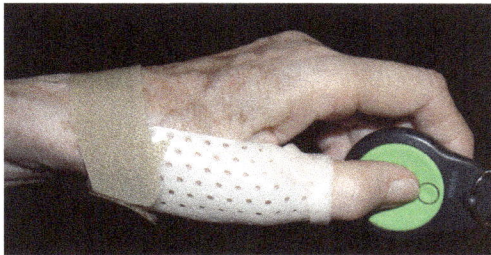

Figure 2: Thumb MCP joint immobilization orthosis. Stability for the thumb MCP joint is achieved without compromise to function of the thumb.

Procedure to Take a Pattern

The easiest way to make this pattern is to wrap the plastic pattern material directly onto the hand with the distal edge just proximal to the IP joint. The pattern material should be approximately 15 cm square depending upon the size of the hand. Mark the following points referring to Figure 3.

1. Wrap the pattern material around the thumb and thenar eminence as indicated.
2. On the volar ulnar aspect, mark the circumference of the proximal phalanx from IP joint proximal to the web at the MCP joint.
3. Mark the proximal end at the radial styloid at the wrist.
4. On the volar surface, outline the thenar eminence from MCP joint level to the wrist.
5. On the dorsal surface, outline the thumb through the middle of the web space to the wrist.

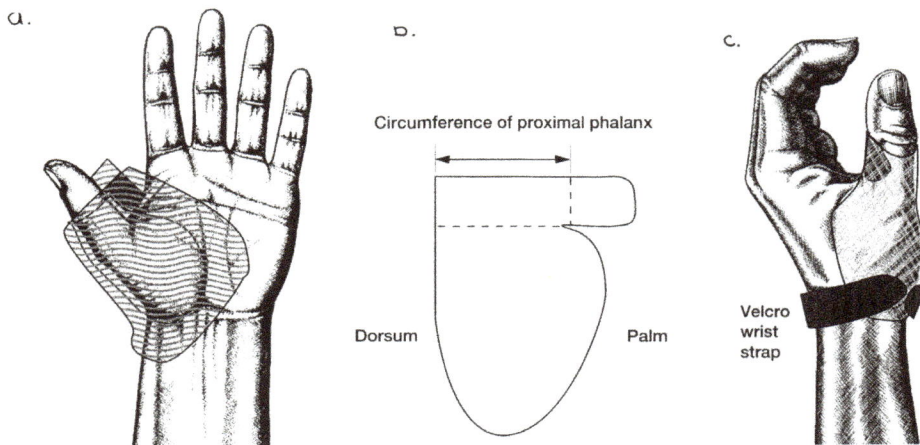

a.

b.

c.

Circumference of proximal phalanx

Dorsum

Palm

Velcro wrist strap

Figure 3: Thumb MCP joint immobilization orthosis pattern. Placement of pattern material is illustrated in a, the shape of the completed pattern in b and radial view of completed orthosis in c.

6. A small extension is added to the circumference of the thumb to form a bond. The pattern should resemble the diagram in Figure 3.

7. Cut out the pattern. Check for fit on the patient prior to transferring it to the thermoplastic material. Materials that have good mouldability are recommended for this orthosis.

Fabrication Procedure

1. Position the arm on the table with the thumb in the required position. If there is a large difference between the circumference of the IP joint and the circumference of the phalanx, place some exercise putty around the proximal phalanx of the thumb.

2. Position the heated thermoplastic material on the thumb as for the pattern, overlapping the area to be bonded. Mould the material ensuring the thenar eminence is well supported.

3. Slightly flare the proximal end ensuring it does not impede wrist motion.

4. When the material is cold, check the freedom of IP motion. Mark any modifications required. Unseal the bond and remove.

5. Carefully reheat the two bond surfaces and reseal. Smooth the bond on the inside surface too. Make any modifications required.

6. Attach the Velcro® strap.

THUMB MCP AND CMC IMMOBILIZATION ORTHOSES

Two designs for orthoses that immobilize the first metacarpal in relation to the finger metacarpals are discussed. Both immobilize the MCP and CMC joints whilst supporting the transverse arch of the hand. The design that provides circumferential contact around the length of the metacarpal provides considerable stability and most efficient immobilization (Figure 4). It is, therefore, used when the greatest stability is required as in the case of trauma, arthritis, and neurological conditions with spasticity of adductor pollicus muscle. The spiral design maintains the thumb position in relation to the fingers whilst maximizing the area of the palm available for sensory input and object contact (Figure 6). This design is commonly used to facilitate functional pinch grip in the presence of paralysis. In peripheral nerve and spinal cord injuries the forces transmitted through the thumb are not so great, therefore, this design is used more for positional control.

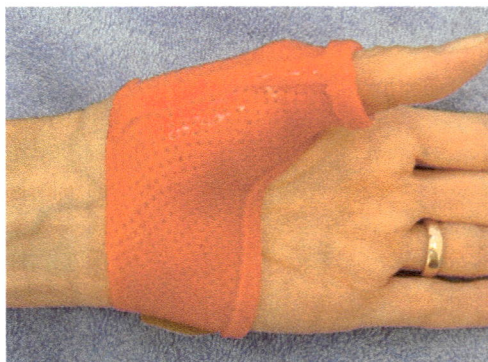

Figure 4 Thumb MCP CMC immobilization orthosis hand based. A hand based thumb orthosis effectively immobilises the thumb metacarpal and proximal phalanx in relation the finger metacarpals. Wrist and thumb IP joint function is unrestricted.

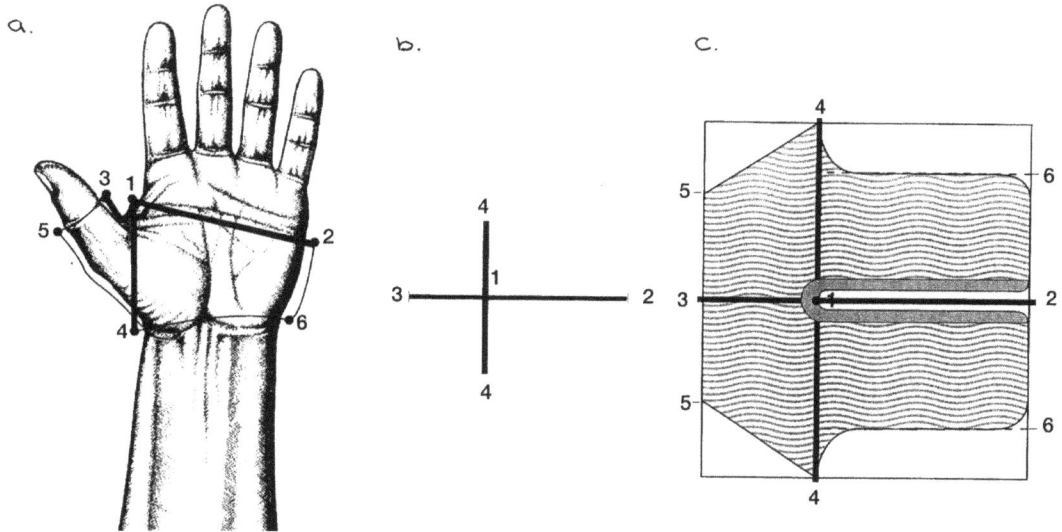

Figure 5 Thumb MCP CMC immobilization orthosis hand based pattern. The location of key markers are illustrated in a, the linear measurements taken from point 1 are translated into a cross as in b which is the basis of the completed pattern in c.

THUMB MCP AND CMC IMMOBILIZATION ORTHOSIS - HAND BASED

Procedure to Take a Pattern

You will need four measurements (see Figure 5). All measurements are taken from point 1 at the level of the distal palmar crease of the index metacarpal.

1. Width of the hand just proximal to the MCP joints.
2. Length of the thumb web - from point 1 to the IP joint crease of the thumb.
3. Depth of hand through the thenar eminence.
4. Circumference of the thumb at the IP joint plus 2 cm.

The dorsal and volar parts of this pattern are the same. In the centre of the pattern material, mark point 1 and draw a vertical and horizontal line through it. Mark the following points (see Figure 5).

1-2 Width of the hand (a).
1-3 Length of the thumb web (b).
1-4 Depth of the thumb through the thenar eminence (c).

From points 1, 2, 3 and 4 square across the vertical and horizontal lines then mark in the following points.

2-6 Length of fifth metacarpal proximal to the distal palmar crease plus 1 cm.
3-5 Half the circumference of the thumb plus 1 cm.

179

Fabrication Procedure

1. To shape the pattern, draw a horizontal line from point 6 to intersect line 1-4. Curve corners where indicated.

2. Join points 4-5 with a diagonal line.

3. Cut out pattern slashing down vertical line 1-2. Transfer to a highly drapable thermoplastic material.

4. To mould this orthosis, the thumb is placed in a position of opposition. If there is a large difference between the circumference of the IP joint and the circumference of the phalanx, place some exercise putty around the proximal phalanx of the thumb.

5. Remove heated material from the water, and then roll the edge the complete length of 1-2 away from the palm of the hand.

6. Place material on the patient's hand with length 1-3 through the thumb web space.

7. Wrap the hand components across the metacarpals, proximal to the distal palmar crease, to slightly overlap and bond on the ulnar dorsal aspect of the little finger.

8. Wrap the components around the thumb pressing together into a flat seam the length 4-5.

9. Quickly mould the orthosis ensuring correct position prior to cutting the bond 4-5 flush with the skin. This bond must be cut while the material is still warm.

10. Mould orthosis ensuring good contour through the palm and on the dorsum of the hand.

11. When cold, unseal the bond on the ulnar aspect and remove from the patient's hand. Trim the ulnar components.

12. Add an extra strip of material to reinforce the seam 4-5.

13. Roll the distal end of the thumb to allow clearance for IP joint motion. Roll the component across the dorsal aspect of the hand so that wrist motion is not impaired.

14. Attach Velcro® straps with adhesive-backed hook on the dorsum of orthosis.

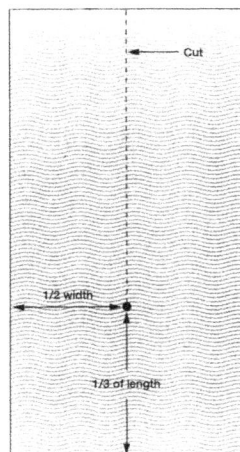

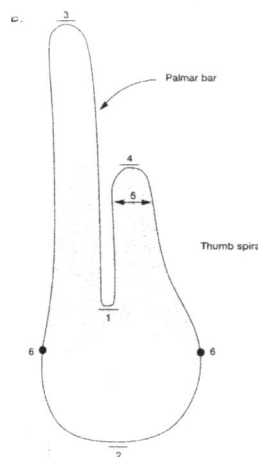

Figure 7: Thumb CMC MCP immobilization orthosis spiral design pattern. The pattern material is wrapped around the hand. Markers determine the shape of final pattern b.

THUMB MCP AND CMC IMMOBILIZATION ORTHOSIS SPIRAL DESIGN

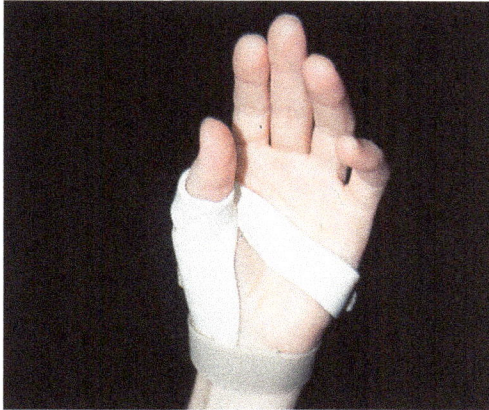

Figure 6: Thumb CMC MCP immobilization orthosis spiral design. This orthosis immobilizes the thumb CMC and MCP joints with minimal impact to the palmar surface of the hand.

Procedure to Take a Pattern

Take a piece of pattern material approximately 25 cm x 15 cm.

1. Mark point 1 at half the width and two-thirds the length of pattern. Cut the pattern through the length to this point as shown in Figure 7.
2. Place point 1 over the dorsum of the MCP joint and mark the wrist crease at the base of the thumb - point 2.
3. Wrap the palmar piece through the web space across the palm and mark the length on the dorsal aspect of the ring finger.
4. Take the thumb piece and spiral around to encircle the proximal phalanx of the thumb. Mark this length.
5. Width of the thumb spiral is determined by the length of the proximal phalanx on the volar aspect of the thumb.
6. To determine the width of the thenar component, mark the thenar crease on the volar surface at MCP joint level and the middle of the web space on the dorsum of the hand.
7. Cut out the pattern. Check fit on the patient prior to transferring to thermoplastic material. Thermoplastic materials that have good mouldability are required for this orthosis. The thickness of material will determine the strength offered by the orthosis - 1.6 mm for very young children to 3 mm for adults.

Fabrication Procedure

1. To mould this orthosis the thumb is placed in a position of opposition. Heat then cut out pattern.

2. Apply the material to the hand orientating along the length of the metacarpal and the markers as identified in the pattern. Secure with a bandage if necessary. Ensure the thumb is in an appropriate position and the palmar bar is well contoured. Unless immobilization of the IP joint is required thermoplastic material should not impede movement.

3. The straps are attached with adhesive backed Velcro®. An extra wrap of the strap around the wrist will increase anchorage of the orthosis.

THUMB MCP, CMC AND WRIST IMMOBILIZATION ORTHOSIS

Movement of the wrist and associated movement of the carpals impact upon pathology of the thumb. Post reconstructive surgery or complex injuries of the CMC joint orthoses are required to immobilize the wrist as well as the thumb. To completely immobilize the thumb in relation to the rest of the hand, it is necessary to include the index and middle finger metacarpals and the wrist. This is best achieved by a circumferential wrist immobilization orthosis with an extension to immobilize the CMC, MCP and, if necessary, the IP joint of the thumb. It is suggested that immobilization of wrist and thumb can

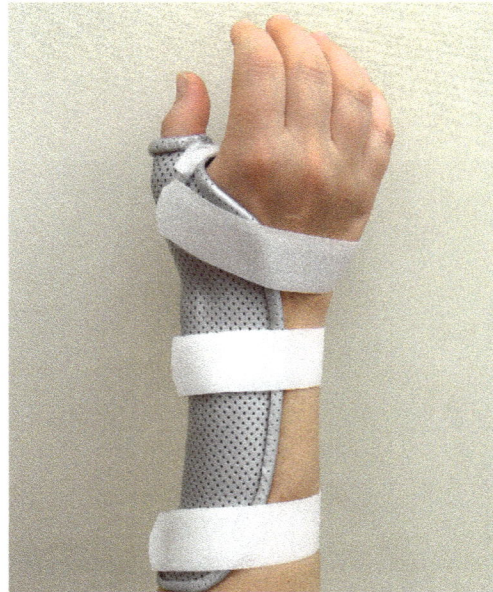

Figure 8: Thumb MCP CMC Wrist immobilization orthosis. the thumb is positioned so that opposition to the index and middle fingers is easily achieved.

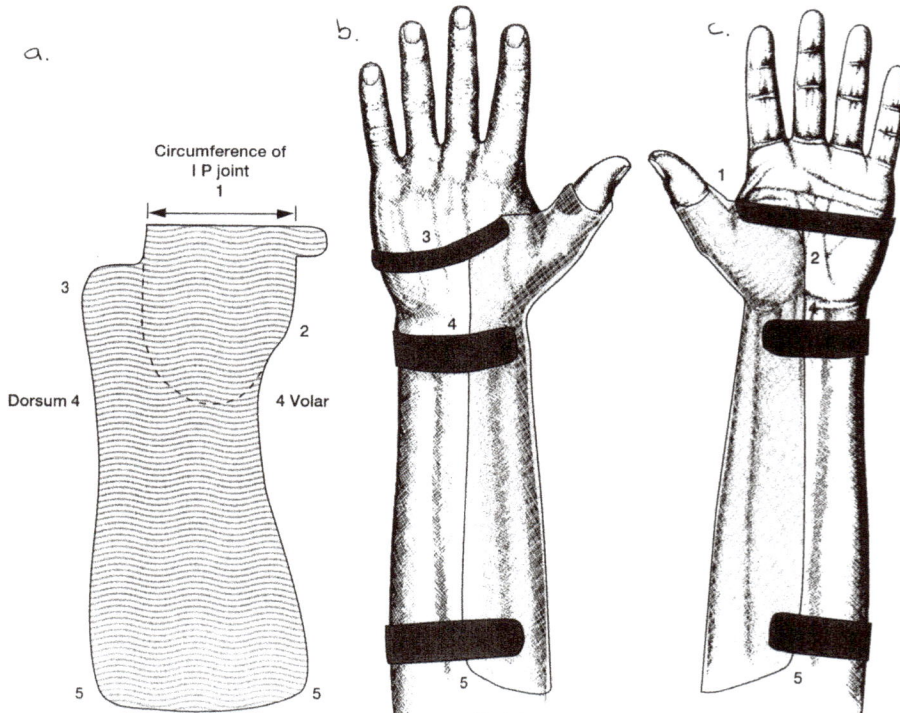

Figure 9: Thumb MCP CMC and wrist immobilization orthosis pattern. The pattern is illustrated in (a), with dorsal (b) and volar (c) views of the completed orthosis with straps in situ.

relieve the pressure on the palmar side of the CMC joint, the area most susceptible to degenerative changes.[7, 8] A description of the pattern and procedures for fabrication are found in Chapter 5, page 125-6.

Where thumb joint stability is not a concern, but pathology requires immobilization of the thumb and wrist, a radially based orthosis can be used (Figure 8). Tenosynovitis of the EPL and APL tendons (DeQuervain's tenosynovitis) is an example of pathology requiring this type of orthosis. Eliminating thermoplastic material on the ulnar surface allows greater mobility of the ulnar metacarpals and less impedance to sensation in functional grasp. This has an advantage to the patient who is required to undertake writing or table based activities.

Procedure to Take a Pattern

The easiest way to make this pattern is to wrap the pattern material around the thumb and forearm so that the distal end is just proximal to the IP joint. The pattern material should be approximately 25 cm x 15 cm depending upon the size of the hand.

Mark the following points (Figure 9).

1. The circumference of the proximal phalanx from IP joint proximal to the web at the MCP joint.
2. Outline the thenar eminence on the volar surface from MCP joint level to the wrist.
3. On the dorsum, the middle finger metacarpal at the level of the thumb MCP joint.
4. The wrist on volar and dorsal surfaces in line with middle finger metacarpal

so that width of the orthosis is half the circumference at the wrist.

5. Two-thirds the length of the forearm and the radial half of the circumference.
6. A small extension is added to the circumference of the thumb to form a bond. Connect marks on the thumb with those on the forearm so that the pattern resembles the diagram in Figure 9.
7. Check fit on patient and mark modifications. Adjust pattern prior to transfer to thermoplastic material.

Fabrication Procedure

1. Position the thumb. Place some putty around the proximal phalanx of the thumb if there is a large difference between the circumference of the IP joint and the circumference of the phalanx.
2. Position the heated thermoplastic on the thumb and forearm as for the pattern overlapping the bonded area. Mould the material ensuring the thenar eminence and wrist are well contoured.
3. When the material is cold check the freedom of IP joint motion. Mark any modifications required. Unseal the bond and remove.
4. Carefully reheat the two bond surfaces and reseal. Smooth the bond on the inside surface too. Modify areas marked.
5. Velcro® straps are applied to the proximal end and at the wrist. A narrow strap is applied around the hand.

Place the adhesive hook Velcro® in the desired position to mark the correct location of loop Velcro®.

ORTHOSES DESIGNED TO MOBILIZE THE THUMB

Deficits in mobility of the thumb have a significant impact upon function of the hand. Minimizing potential for contracture of the webspace by sustaining the length of the skin, fascia, AP and other intrinsic muscles is a major consideration in all orthoses that impact the thumb. Serial orthoses are used to gain range of motion in the web space while dynamic orthoses tend to be used to address deficits in the MCP and IP joints.

MOBILIZING ORTHOSES FOR THE CMC JOINT

Pathology effecting mobility of the CMC joint of the thumb, capsular and ligamentous structures, fascia and skin tissues on the palmar or dorsal surfaces of the hand, as well as intrinsic and extrinsic muscles will impact upon the web space between the first and second metacarpals. The multifaceted nature of this contracture challenges therapists to direct effective forces to achieve end range in all these tissues. Mobility is influenced by the degree of abduction or extension, and flexion of the thumb and index MCP joints. All orthoses designed to increase motion of thumb joints compromise function during the period of wear.

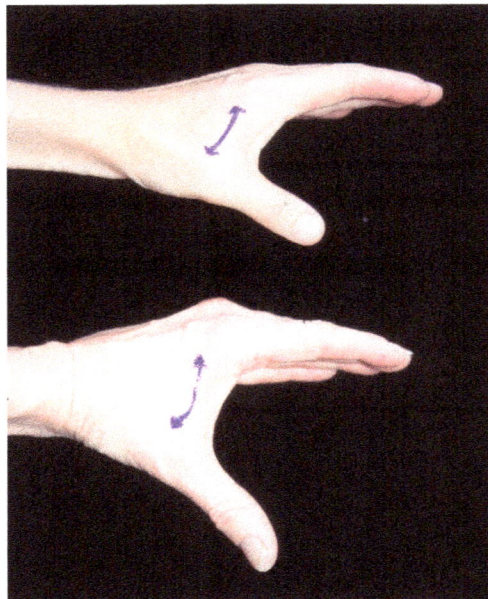

Figure 10: Normal thumb index finger spans.
Normal span can vary greatly. To effectively mobilize the region, forces have to be applied to the metacarpal proximal to the MCP joint. The arrows indicate the appropriate location to avoid stress to the MCP joint capsular structures.

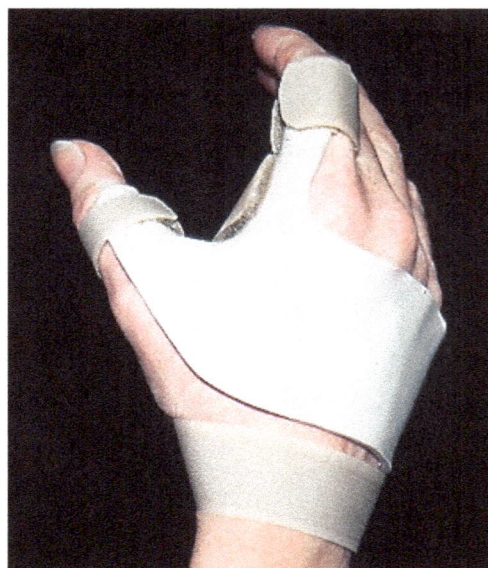

Figure 11: Thumb CMC mobilizing orthosis hand based. Dorsal radial view of the orthosis. Strap location is critical to achieve good anchorage and prevent distal migration.

Serial orthoses are the most effective means of addressing range of motion deficits in the web space as intimate moulding increases the area of the first and second metacarpals over which force is applied. Long standing contractures may require a series of orthoses. Time between remoulding to change position will depend upon the compliance of tissues and their response to force. Once range of motion has plateaued, orthotic intervention can cease if the patient is able to maintain the range by patterns of functional use. If function will not maintain gains, the last orthosis may continue to be worn at night.

In one of the few randomised controlled clinical trials on this region Harvey and colleagues[5] studied a diverse sample of persons with established webspace contractures secondary to stroke, acquired brain injury and cervical spinal cord injury. Using a standardised torque outcome measure they failed to find any change in passive range of motion when serial progressive orthoses were worn for 8 hours per night over a 12-week period. The authors suggested reasons for the failure to find an effect might have related to the diagnosis of participants, or the fact that orthoses did not administer a sufficiently large torque for sufficient time. With no accurate means of measuring torque applied to the thumb metacarpal via serial progressive orthoses therapists must rely on clinical judgement to determine intensity, frequency and duration of torque being applied. These findings suggest further research is required in relation to prevention of webspace contractures for clients with neurological pathology with determination of effective parameters for orthotic interventions.

Mechanically it is often difficult to apply an effective force to mobilize the thumb metacarpal as there is little surface area on which force can be applied proximal to the MCP joint,[2] while at the same time stabilizing the orthosis on the hand so that it does not migrate. An orthosis designed to increase passive range of motion in extension or abduction of the CMC joint must apply the force to both the thumb and index metacarpals and not the proximal phalanx (Figure 11). In the non injured hand, the web tissues extend past both the index and thumb MCP joints, therefore these joints must be included if length is to be gained. Web space length is quite variable as indicated in Figure 10. Fear of shortening the collateral ligament of the index MCP joint,[9] by maintaining it in an extended position in a mobilizing thumb orthosis is without basis unless the orthosis is on 24 hours per day and active and passive movements of the joint are not undertaken. Effectiveness of this orthosis is achieved by:

- Identifying location and direction of forces required to effectively mobilize the joint while effectively stabilizing the orthosis.
- Application of force to the thumb metacarpal without stress to the ulnar collateral ligament of the MCP joint.
- Extending the orthosis to the distal end of the proximal phalanx of both the index finger and thumb provides greater mechanical advantage and potential torque.
- Anchoring of the orthosis around the wrist to prevent distal migration and sustain appropriate forces.
- Selecting appropriate thermoplastic material that provides good contour,

and that can withstand pressure applied during fabrication and numerous remouldings.

Extended periods of wear at night or during times when functional use of the hand is not required.

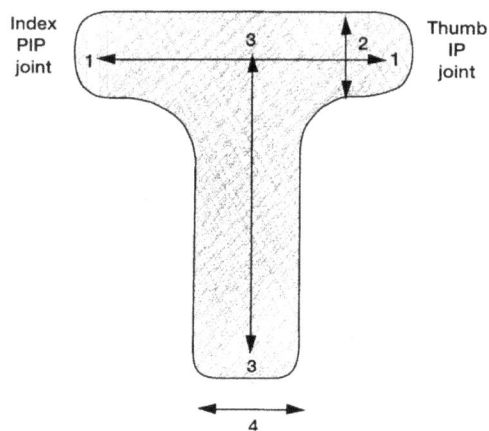

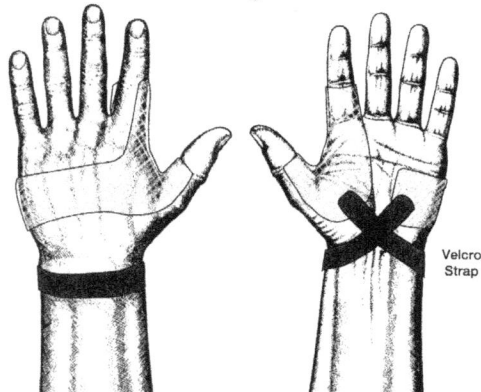

Figure 12: Thumb CMC mobilizing orthosis hand based pattern. This serial static design uses measurements of the hand to shape pattern (a). Dorsal (b) and volar (c) views of the completed orthosis illustrate one style of strapping.

Procedure to Take a Pattern

A piece of thermoplastic pattern material is cut roughly in a very thick 'T' shape and positioned through the web space and across the dorsum of the hand (see Figure 12).

1. The length of the horizontal of the 'T' is the length of the web space from the index finger PIP joint to the thumb IP joint.

2. The width of the horizontal of the 'T' is approximately two thirds the circumference of the thumb MCP joint.

3. The length of the vertical of the 'T' is determined by the distance from the volar surface of the thenar crease across the dorsum of the hand to the volar surface of the ring finger metacarpal.

4. The width of the vertical of the 'T' is the length of little finger metacarpal proximal to the distal palmar crease.

Fabrication Procedure

1. The thermoplastic material is cut roughly to these dimensions, heated then applied to the thumb and index finger webspace before wrapping section around across dorsum of the hand. Ensure there is excellent contour through the thumb index web space. Pressure to abduct or extend the thumb (depending upon the objective) should be applied proximal to the MCP joints of the thumb and index finger.

2. Once the material is cold, excess material is cut and edges smoothed.

3. The strapping must be spiralled around the wrist to prevent distal migration.

For those patients who require greater anchorage, or for postoperative patients where straps could compromise venous and

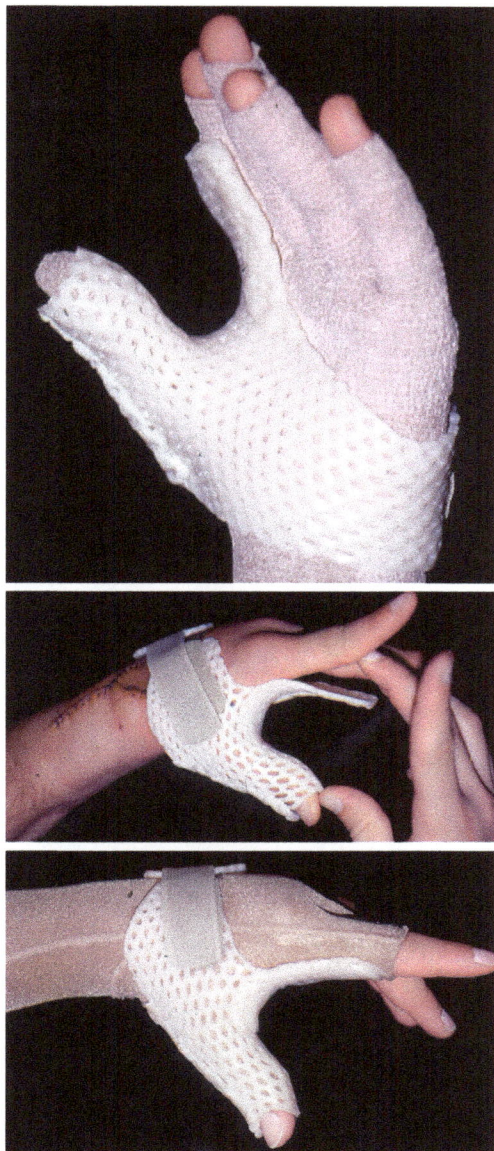

Figure 13: Thumb MCP CMC mobilizing orthosis hand based. Serial static principles are used to mobilize the webspace following surgical release. As the orthosis is worn over a surgical wound with dressings secured by Coban (a), and subsequently a Lycra® pressure garment (c), maxi perforated thermoplastic material was chosen.

lymphatic drainage, the thumb MCP CMC Joint Immobilization Orthosis is modified (Figure 13). The orthosis is fabricated in the usual way, and then an additional piece of thermoplastic material is added to extend the web space to the length of the proximal phalanx of the index finger.

THUMB MCP AND IP JOINTS MOBILIZING ORTHOSES

Hand based orthoses are recommended to address deficits in joint motion at the MCP and IP joints of the thumb (Figures 14-16). Care needs to be taken to ensure rotational force is applied perpendicular to the longitudinal axis of the thumb metacarpal to ensure no stress is applied to the collateral ligaments. The same principle is used when applying traction to the IP joint. Deficits in extension of the MCP joint are often closely associated with contracture of the web space, therefore, it may be necessary to combine gentle force to both the web space and proximal phalanx.

The base orthosis to address a contracture of the MCP joint is the same irrespective of the deficit. Therefore, the orthosis must have components that traverse the palm and the dorsum of the hand both for stability of the metacarpal and anchorage of the traction. A thumb MCP and CMC joint immobilization pattern is recommended. It is cut down to allow either IP or MCP motion. The procedure to determine the shape and location of the outrigger is described in Chapter 3.

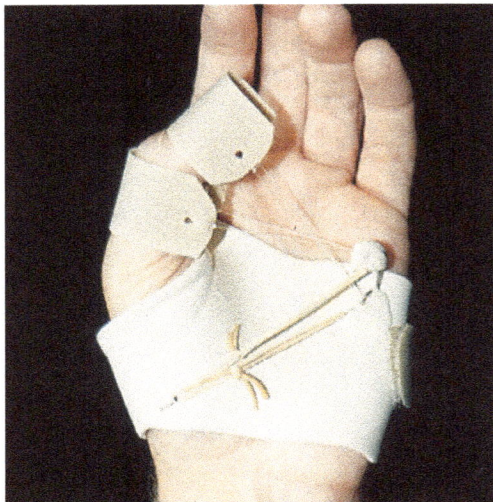

Figure 14: Thumb MCP and IP joints flexion mobilization orthosis. The deficit in thumb flexion is addressed by application of separate forces to mobilize the MCP and the IP joints.

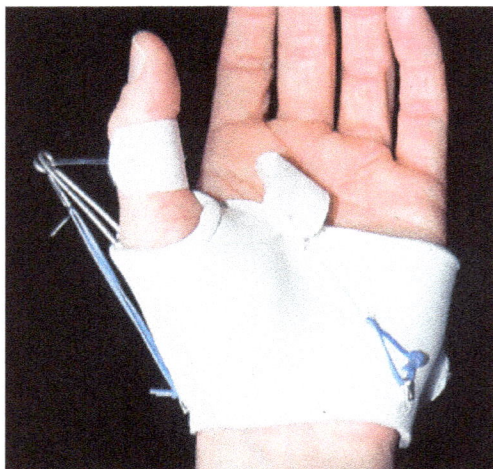

Figure 15: Thumb MCP extension mobilizing orthosis. Dynamic traction can be applied in the thumb to specifically address one joint using an outrigger, as is the case in extension. A loop over the distal phalanx will address several joints in the direction of flexion to the palm. Wearing regime will determine the time the tissues spend at end range in each direction.

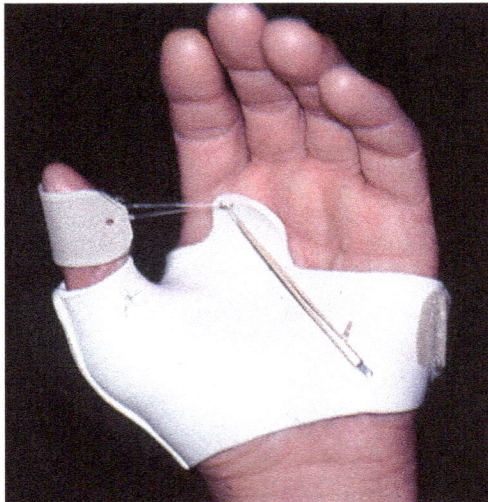

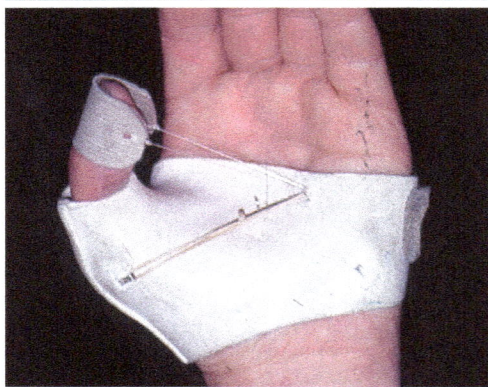

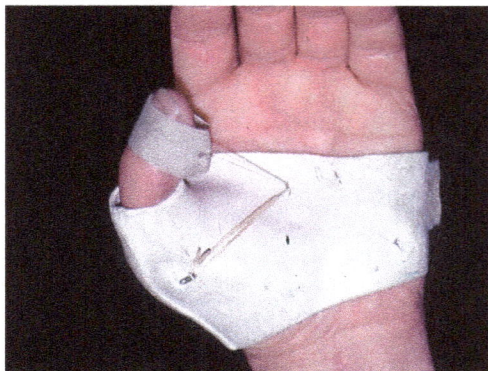

Figure 16: Thumb IP joint flexion mobilization orthosis. This series illustrates the change in anchorage required to ensure the direction of pull by the traction remains at 90° to the longitudinal axis of the distal phalanx as greater range is gained in the IP joint.

If the ROM deficit is due to thumb extensor muscle tendon tightness impacting upon several joints, then traction applied to the distal phalanx in the direction of the longitudinal axis of the thumb will rotate the thumb. Where there is little flexion a loop over the nail will apply traction. As greater flexion is gained, securing the traction loop to the nail may be achieved by use of Fabrifoam®, or adhesion of hook Velcro® to the nail.

ORTHOSES TO RESTRICT MOTION IN THE THUMB

Orthoses that restrict motion in the thumb are used to either gain stability in the thumb for performance of functional tasks or to protect structures during healing.

RESTRICTION DURING WOUND HEALING

There are many protocols described for the management of tendon repairs. From an orthotic perspective, FPL is protected from full extension (Figure 17) whilst EPL is protected from full flexion (Figure 18). Further information regarding protocols can be found in hand rehabilitation publications.

Determination of the position of restriction in orthoses that limit movement following repair of extrinsic thumb tendons is undertaken in consultation with the hand surgeon. Generally for restriction of extension thermo-

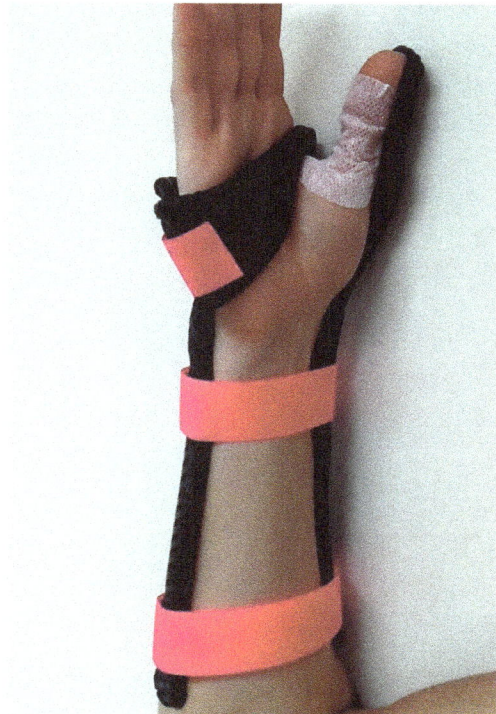

Figure 17: Thumb Flexor Tendon Repair Orthosis. Restriction of thumb extension is achieved when the thermoplastic material is placed on the dorsal surface of the wrist and thumb a. Passive flexion of the IP and MCP joint should not be impeded by thermoplastic material on the volar surface b. (a. Courtesy Ceri Pulhman)

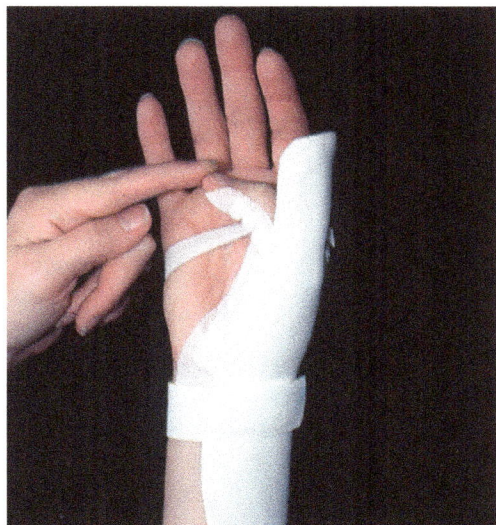

plastic material is position on the dorsoradial surface of the thumb, for restriction of flexion the dorsal component extends from the MCP joint proximal whilst the volar component extends from the MCP distal. Wrist is positioned in greater extension and thumb flexion blocked

Procedure To Take A Pattern

The thumb is supported by the patient in a neutral position of extension/abduction. The pattern material should be approximately 25 cm x 15 cm depending upon the size of the hand. The pattern material is placed along the radial aspect of the hand and the following points marked. Refer to Figure 19a.

1. Tip of the thumb.
2. Half the circumference of the MCP joint on the medial and lateral aspects of the thumb. Add 1 cm - 2 cm to each side depending upon size of the hand.
3. Half the circumference of the wrist on

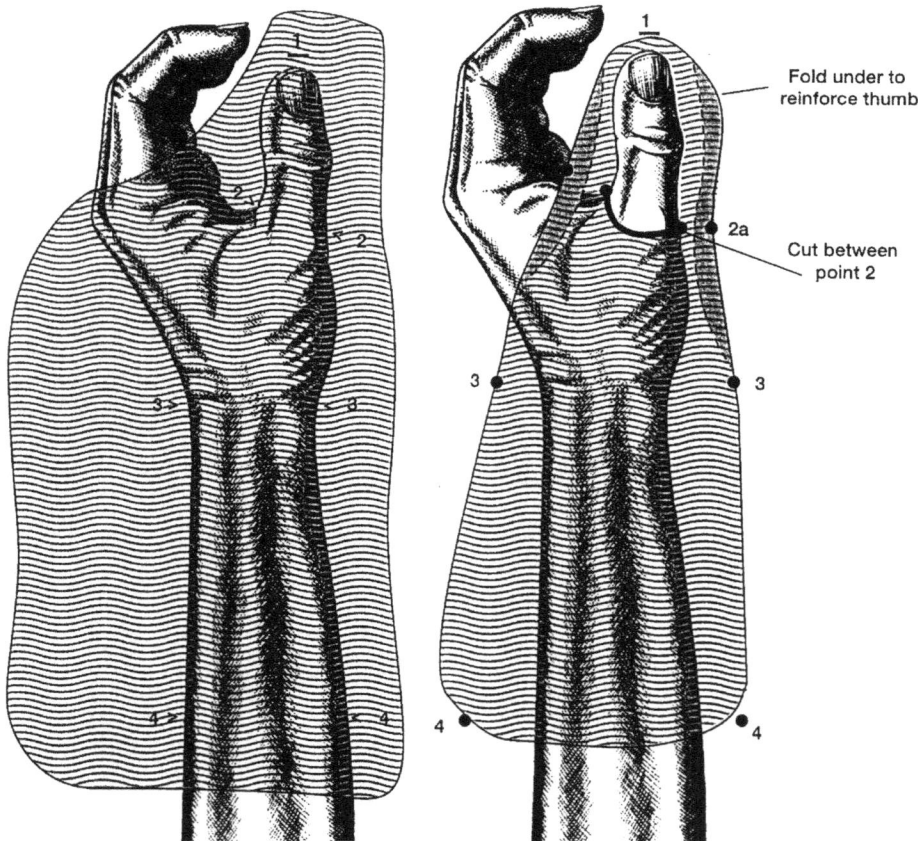

Figure 18: Pattern for thumb restriction orthosis wrist and hand based. To restrict extension or flexion of the thumb following tendon repair requires pattern landmarks identified in a. To restrict thumb flexion it is placed through a hole at the level of the MCP joint as illustrated in b.

volar and dorsal surfaces in line with middle finger metacarpal.

4. The point at two-thirds the length of the forearm and half the circumference on the volar and dorsal surfaces.

(If designing an orthosis to restrict flexion cut between points 2 so that the thumb may be threaded through the hole. The components on the side of the thumb are folded volarly to reinforce the thumb component). Check fit on patient and mark modifications. Adjust pattern prior to transferring to thermoplastic material.

Fabrication Procedure

1. Position the thumb and wrist with the required degrees of extension.
2. Apply heated thermoplastic, ensuring good contour.
3. Attach the Velcro® straps.

To restrict extension of the thumb the orthosis is applied to the dorsal radial surface of the thumb, wrist and forearm. The wrist is positioned in neutral and slight ulnar deviation, the CMC joint in neutral, the MCP and IP joints at 0° or according to the degree of extension allowed in the thumb joints. It is important that the passive flexion of all thumb joints is not restricted.

When restricting flexion heat thermoplastic material, create hole and roll back edges. Be careful not to make this hole bigger than the MCP joint circumference. The heated thermoplastic is placed on the thumb, volar to phalanges and dorsal over metacarpal and wrist. If mobilizing traction is to be used attach the outrigger prior to applying straps.

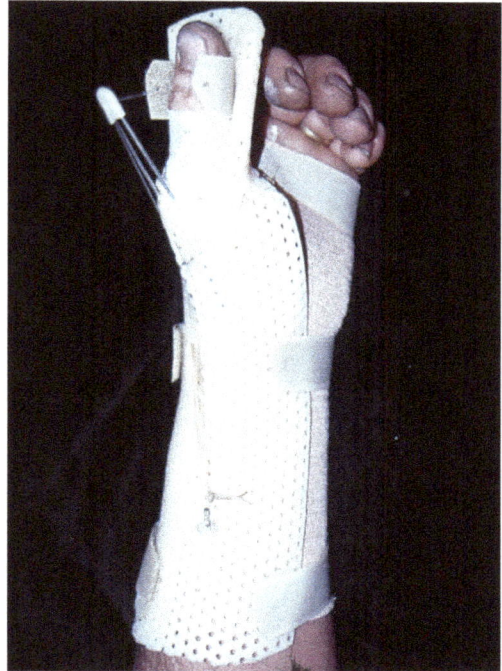

Figure 19: Orthosis EPL Tendon Repair. Following repair to EPL tendon restriction of flexion is achieved by the volar aspect of the orthosis distal to the MCP joint, whilst dynamic traction extends to thumb away from the volar block to facilitate tendon glide.

RESTRICTION FOR FUNCTION

The nature of the skin through the web space often means poor tolerance to the use of hard thermoplastic materials to position the thumb. Total immobilization of the thumb may also limit functional choices for hand use. Soft fabrics are incorporated into custom made and prefabricated orthoses used to address the functional limitations of the thumb. In order to have an influence in controlling the thumb position the fabric must have potential to resist the deforming forces created in the thumb during use.

PREFABRICATED THUMB ORTHOSES

There are a number of brands of prefabricated thumb splints/orthoses. They are made from a wide variety of materials including thermoplastic, elastomeric materials, neoprene, polyurethane and leather. They are secured by Velcro® tabs, with reinforcement for positioning or stability offered by metal or moulded thermoplastic components. The majority of brands are available in four or five sizes. The problems of fit may be compounded by the unusual shape of the thumb, in cases where arthritis has destroyed joint integrity. Individual moulding of components, as is possible with some brands (Rehband®), increases the potential to accurately fit the orthosis and therefore meet the desired objective.

Sillem et al.[11] compared a prefabricated neoprene hand-based thumb CMC orthosis to a thermoplastic hand based thumb MCP CMC immobilization orthosis. They found an equivalent effect on hand function, grip strength, and pinch strength, with the thermoplastic orthosis significantly better at reducing pain. The patients preferred the more flexible prefabricated orthosis. These findings are not dissimilar to those of Weiss et al.[15] While it is important to consider patient preference in deciding the type of orthosis, assessment findings and desired functional outcome should also influence intervention choice.

SUMMARY

The function of the hand is dependent upon a stable sensate thumb. Stability, essential for effective force transmission in the majority of grips and all pinches, can be achieved through orthoses incorporating joints of the thumb, and if necessary the wrist. Deficits in active and passive range of motion, particularly as they affect the web space can severely compromise the ability to position the thumb for opposition to the fingers. Addressing these deficits using orthotic intervention demands an understanding of the unique architecture of the thumb along with careful application of biomechanical principles in orthotic design and fabrication. Orthotic choice is based on what provides the optimal effect for which the patient is seeking intervention.

REFERENCES

1. Beasley J. Osteoarthritis and rheumatoid arthritis: Conservative therapeutic management. Journal of Hand Therapy. 2012;25(2): 163–172.

2. Colditz J. Anatomic considerations for splinting the thumb. In Hunter JM, Makin EJ, Callahan AD editors. Rehabilitation of the Hand: Surgery and Therapy. St Louis: Mosby; 1995. p 1161–1172.

3. Colditz JC. The Biomechanics of a thumb carpometacarpal immobilization splint: Design and fitting. Journal of Hand Therapy. 2000;13: 228–235.

4. Egan M, Brosseau L. Splinting for osteoarthritis of the carpometacarpal joint: a review of the evidence. American Journal of Occupational Therapy. 2007;61: 70–8.

5. Harvey L, de Jong I, Goehl G, Marwedel S. Twelve weeks of nightly stretch does not reduce thumb web-space contractures in people with a neurological condition:

a randomised controlled trial. Australian Journal of Physiotherapy. 2006;52: 251–258.

6. Leversedge FJ. Anatomy and pathomechanics of the thumb. Hand Clinics. 2008;24(3): 219–29.

7. Moulton MJ, Parentis MA, Kelly MJ, et al. Influence of metacarpophalangeal joint position on basal joint loading in the thumb. Journal of Bone and Joint Surgery. 2001;83A: 709–16.

8. Pellegrini VD Jr. Osteoarthritis of the trapeziometacarpal joint: the pathophysiology of articular cartilage degeneration. I. Anatomy and pathology of the aging joint. Journal of Hand Surgery. 1991;16A: 967–74.

9. Phelps PE, Weeks PM. Management of the thumb-index web space contracture. American Journal of Occupational Therapy. 1976;30: 543–550.

10. Rannou F, Dimet J, Boutron I, et al. Splint for base-of-thumb osteoarthritis: a randomized trial. Annals Internal Medicine. 2009;150: 661–9.

11. Sillem H, Backman CL, Miller WC, and Li LC. Comparison of two carpometacarpal stabilizing splints for individuals with thumb osteoarthritis. Journal of Hand Therapy. 2011;24(3): 216–25.

12. Steultjens EMJ, Bouter LLM, Dekker JJ, et al. Occupational therapy for rheumatoid arthritis. The Cochrane database of systematic reviews 2004;1:CD003114. 26

13. Towheed TE. Systematic review of therapies for osteoarthritis of the hand. Osteoarthritis Cartilage. 2005;13: 455–62.

14. Valdes K, Marik T. A systematic review of conservative interventions for osteoarthritis of the hand. Journal of Hand Therapy. 2010;23: 334–51.

15. Weiss S, LaStayo P, Mills A, Bramlet D. Splinting the degenerative basal joint: custom-made or prefabricated neoprene? Journal of Hand Therapy. 2004;17: 401–406.

16. Zhang W, Doherty M, Leeb BF, et al. EULAR evidence based recommendations for the management of hand osteoarthritis: report of a task force of the EULAR Standing Committee for International Clinical Studies Including Therapies (ESCISIT). Annals Rheumatic Disease. 2007;66: 377–88.

8

ORTHOTIC INTERVENTION AND CASTING IN THE PRESENCE OF NEUROLOGICAL DYSFUNCTION

INTRODUCTION

This chapter has been devoted to provision of orthoses for clients with neurological dysfunction. The need for a specific chapter arises in part from the fact that expertise in orthotic design and fabrication is the domain of the hand therapist who rarely treats clients with neurological dysfunction, while therapists who have experience and expertise in addressing issues related to hypertonicity and dyskinetic movement often do not have the same expertise in orthotic fabrication.

The objective of this chapter is to attempt to marry these domains of practice. Orthotic intervention for the client with neurological dysfunction is multifaceted and presents even the most competent therapist some of their greatest technical challenges.

Orthoses, braces and splints have been used for many years in neurological practice. As in other chapters of this book the term *orthosis* is used to describe all devices designed and fitted to the upper limb to achieve a specific purpose related to immobilization or mobilization of tissue, or facilitation of function (refer to Chapter One for further clarification).

Adults and children with cerebral palsy, stroke and traumatic brain injury do not present as a homogeneous sample. While the neurological injury is non progressive, the consequences of that injury over time are influenced by a myriad of factors such as age, growth, gravity, occupation, medical and therapeutic interventions. It is essential to consider these factors when implementing orthotic and casting interventions to manage muscle changes in the presence of neurological symptoms for the individual client.

LITERATURE REVIEW

Therapeutic management of the consequences of upper motor neurone symptoms in the upper limb has evolved over the past 50 years from biomechanical, neurophysiological, neurodevelopmental perspectives to those that emphasise neuroplasticity and motor control. Advances in knowledge pertaining to brain injury and plasticity, muscle histology and physiology, the nature of spasticity and hypertonicity are changing procedures and protocols and the way clinicians approach orthotic and casting interventions. This literature review explores knowledge related to orthotic and casting interventions in the presence of upper limb neurological dysfunction. The best available evidence is that which is least susceptible to bias, such as that provided by specific systematic reviews and randomized controlled clinical trials. However, conclusions drawn must be considered in the context of the life long nature of disability in this population and the research protocols used, particularly the intensity, duration and the type of intervention investigated. Research evidence gathered over weeks in certain phases of human development, recovery or rehabilitation, guide practice at these time frames. It is not realistic to generalise findings across the practice of adult and paediatric upper limb neurological rehabilitation. Therapists are urged to read study protocols in order to draw conclusions appropriate to guide practice for their client populations.

The introduction of Botulinum neurotoxin (BoNT – generic names Botox® or Dysport®) in the mid 1990's to manage upper limb hypertonicity in children and adults, has influenced the nature of clinical practice as it relates to orthotic and casting interventions. BoNT, an adjunct intervention rarely used in isolation to other therapies,[25] is considered in the context of the person's overall spasticity management. Its administration challenges therapists to determine the appropriateness of orthotic intervention for the upper limb while considering the aims of managing symptoms such as pain and contracture or improving function.[14] Ideally this reasoning occurs prior to the administration of BoNT. A reduction in hypertonicity of the upper limb musculature following injections provides a period of time when resistance in the muscles is reduced so that progressive mobilization with casts or orthoses can effectively impact joint and soft tissue contracture. Where improved functional movement is the goal of BoNT intervention an orthosis may be fabricated to position a joint/s in more mechanically efficient positions.

INDICATIONS FOR INTERVENTION

Traditionally the indications for orthotic intervention and casting have been considered to be modification of spasticity, prevention or modification of contracture, management of pain, maintenance of tissue integrity and to improve function and participation in activity.

MODIFICATION OF SPASTICITY

The muscle changes in the presence of hypertonicity are what sets this client population apart from other domains of hand therapy when considering orthotic and casting interventions. Hypertonicity is understood as two components. The first is the dynamic resistance of muscle to passive stretch caused by interaction of neural factors (exaggerated response to movement stimulus) and non-neural factors (active properties of muscle and connective tissue). The second is the static passive tendency of muscle to return to a resting position following stretch. Spasticity is the neural component of hypertonicity and is described by Lance[32] as a motor disorder characterized by a velocity-dependent increase in 'muscle tone' with exaggerated tendon jerks, resulting from hyper excitability of the stretch reflex. Muscle tone is the sensation of resistance that is encountered as a joint is passively moved

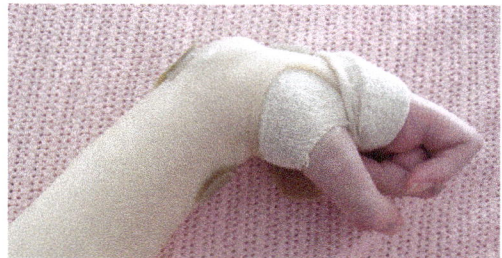

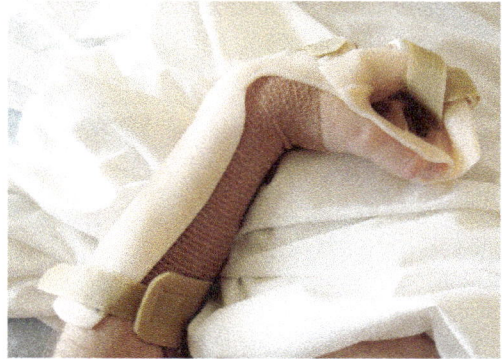

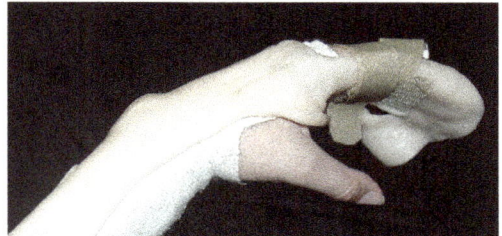

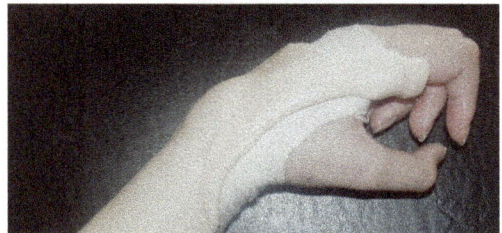

Figure 1: Long-term management of the consequences of hypertonicity is managed by a series of orthoses. Serial static principles were used to gain passive ROM in the wrist and finger flexors over a 3 year period. The client's capacity to actively isolate the index finger for a functional point only became evident once wrist and finger tendon unit lengths approached neutral. (Courtesy Terri Dival & Judith Wilton)

through a range of motion.[71] Hypertonia is linked with contracture, however the exaggerated reflexes of spasticity do not directly lead to contracture.[47] It is suggested that muscle contracture may actually potentiate the stretch reflex.

The historical premise that intermittent application of upper limb orthoses can impact spasticity has not been substantiated by research. Transient benefits can be related to the immobilization of the muscle, with no relation to type of orthosis. Immobilization of the wrist and fingers in neutral or extended positions, worn for periods ranging between 2-22 hours per day, over 4-8 weeks duration, have demonstrated no impact on spasticity.[34,35,36] No recent studies have investigated longer periods of orthotic intervention.

Interventions addressing hypertonicity in the elbow primarily focus on casting. The neurophysiological effects of casting on spasticity remain undefined. Childers et al.[7] found the level of motor neurone activity was decreased when a cast was applied. It is proposed that inhibition results from decreased sensory input from cutaneous and muscle receptors during the period of immobilization. The effects of neutral warmth and circumferential contact are also thought to contribute to modification of spasticity.[66]

CONTRACTURE PREVENTION OR MODIFICATION

In children with cerebral palsy atypical musculoskeletal development is a key component in development of contracture and deformity. Following acquired brain injury (ABI) contracture development is triggered by immobilization, disuse, muscle paralysis and weakness leading to loss of range of motion and over time potentially fixed contractures. Inability to use a joint actively over its full range of motion will lead to secondary changes in muscles and adaptation of connective tissues of the muscle tendon unit. The muscle changes may include atrophy as a result of protein degeneration, changes in fibre type and size, and sarcomere disorganisation.[21, 22] In addition the changes in the connective tissue within the muscle tendon unit and other tissues (skin, blood vessels, nerves, and myofascial tissues) are significant contributors to the development of contractures.[18]

Contracture, plus spasticity, contributes to increased resistance to passive stretch.[33, 47] In a longitudinal study of 27 subjects post stroke Ada and colleagues[1] identified the contributors to contracture were spasticity in the first four months and weakness in the subsequent 8 months. Pandyan[49] demonstrated wrist flexion contractures develop within 6–8 weeks post stroke in subjects who have no early functional upper limb recovery. Muscle strength was also identified as a significant predictor of elbow and wrist contractures by Kwah et al.[31] in a prospective study of 164 clients admitted to a stroke unit. While data did not identify which patients were most susceptible to contracture development 18% had developed an elbow contracture and 18% a wrist contracture at six months post stroke.

Pizzi et al.[50,51] confirmed an inverse correlation between passive ROM and time since stroke with contracture formation independent of pain and neglect.

As in other domains of hand therapy contractures are addressed by application of low load prolonged stress (gentle stretch) to the tissues at the end of their available range, for sufficient time to allow histological changes to occur in the tissues in response to the position imposed. For many years the neurological therapy literature supported use of orthotic interventions in submaximal passive range of motion (ROM) on the reasoning that full stretch at maximal range will increase hypertonicity, despite no evidence to support this premise. There is no evidence that placing spastic muscles on full stretch or maximal range will increase hypertonicity,[33] therefore to gain passive ROM principles applicable to mobilizing orthoses should be considered. Remodelling in tissues held in a lengthened position, for a period of hours over numerous days, ultimately depends on the ability of the cells to sense and transduce the mechanical force applied by the orthosis into biological action.

The term 'stretch' continues to be poorly defined in the neurological literature, particularly the description of therapy regimes that apply stretch to the upper limb via orthotic interventions (splints) and casting. The systematic review by Katalinic et al.[27] concluded stretch does not have clinically important effects. This conclusion is based on studies varying in intensity, duration and frequency of stretch intervention protocols for both

prevention and treatment of contractures, in upper and lower limb joints in adults and children. This highlights the need for further research refining the parameters of stretch interventions as applied over days, weeks and months for growing and mature musculoskeletal systems impacted by hypertonicity.

Gaining passive ROM is a common goal of intervention for this patient group, however there are few studies where orthotic mobilization principles were applied. Immobilization orthoses are fabricated at one wrist/hand angle, but in order to mobilize tissues they must be serially modified to hold tissues at the end of their passive ROM. The period of time allowed between modifications is dependent upon tissue response to the position prior to the orthosis being remoulded, in the new lengthened position. Harvey et al.[23] report on a study of serial static mobilizing orthoses applied to persons following acquired brain or spinal cord injury. Whilst the orthosis and protocol investigated failed to have an effect, results challenge therapists to explore the ways torque is applied via different orthoses and protocols. The authors' clinical experience would suggest use of serial static mobilizing orthoses worn over many years does result in gains in passive ROM (Figure 1). The effectiveness of orthoses to address contracture prevention and resolution in the long term has yet to be determined by quality clinical trials.

Differences in aetiology and age at onset are considerations for both short and long term interventions addressing passive ROM deficits in this client group. Adults have reached skeletal maturity whereas children continue to alter with respect to bone, muscle, and connective tissue growth and development. While it is accepted that the muscles of children with CP differ from normal age related muscles of children without spasticity[41,53] the time course of muscle development and how this might relate to the increasing muscle weakness and contracture is an area in need of further research.[3] Thus therapists in paediatric practice need to consider growth as a variable when determining appropriateness of interventions.

Serial casting has been used for many years to gain range of motion for clients with neurological dysfunction. Decisions to use casting are based largely on clinical experience as there is insufficient evidence to either support or refute the long-term effectiveness of upper limb casting for either adults or children with central nervous system (CNS) motor disorders.[2,20,37,41,44,64]

Clinical reasoning underpinning decisions to use casting have their genesis in biomechanical and to a lessor extent neurophysiological frames of practice. In a biomechanical rationale, casts apply low-load, long-duration stretch to address contracture. Biomechanical effects relate to changes in the length of muscle and connective tissues. Tardieu and Tardieu[63] propose that muscle contracture seen in persons with spasticity, is in part normal adaptation of muscle length in response to abnormal conditions. Histological changes in muscle, in response to being maintained in a shortened position, can be reversed by casting.[61] Adult muscle responds to stretching by adding new sarcomeres in series, thereby returning the sarcomeres to their optimum tension-generating length with no change in tendon length. The increase in passive ROM seen immediately post casting results from addition of sarcomeres to the muscle fibre, and lengthening of connective tissue elements.[60] In growing muscles, however, the initial increase in number of sarcomeres up to day five is followed by a decrease in sarcomere number, thereby decreasing muscle fibre length.[62] Muscle tendon length is maintained by lengthening of the tendon.[61,63] These findings suggest that extended casting protocols for young children should consider potential to increase tendon length rather than to influence muscle fibre length. It is stressed that cast lengthening of muscle contracture should be gradual, because a decrease in sarcomere number is greater than the decrease in length of muscle connective tissue.[63] Potential exists for muscle fibre breakdown from too fast or forceful stretching. Failure to retain range of motion following cessation of casting is due to accommodation of the muscle to the shorter length by the loss of sarcomeres and diminished tension in the connective tissues. Thus, the objective of casting intervention in the presence of contracture is to achieve and sustain the appropriate length of the muscle and associated connective tissues. Experience suggests that, in muscles with hypertonicity, shortening of muscle and connective tissues will recur unless stretch is maintained.[39,46,48,]

Much of the research on casting elbow and wrist flexion contractures in the presence of hypertonicity is undertaken in small case study designs. Two groups of studies are seen - those that apply a series of non removable circumferential casts worn for several weeks,[9,16,24,28,40,46,52,59] and those in which casts are bivalved and worn for several hours per day for many months.[10,38,58] Authors describe gains in range of motion following the application of a series of casts worn for 24 hours per day over 2-4 weeks; and maintenance of passive ROM in casts applied for 3-5 hours per day over many months.

Randomized control clinical trials are limited. In a study of the treatment of elbow flexion contractures in persons with ABI, Moseley et al.[46] compared the effectiveness of two weeks serial casting and a positioning programme of 1 hour stretch per day. The findings that serial casting resulted in greater gains in passive ROM compared to stretch are similar to an earlier study by Hill.[24] However, gains in passive ROM have not been shown to translate into improved functional use of the extremity.[24] Two randomized control trials conducted by Law and colleagues[38,39] investigated the effectiveness of intensive neurodevelopmental therapy (NDT) and casting in children with cerebral palsy. Neither casting nor intensity of NDT made a significant difference in hand function over no casting and regular occupational therapy. However, improvements in quality of movement after casting were greater in children 4 to 8 years old than in those under 4 years with authors suggesting differences were related to the age of the children. The increased quality of movement and increased wrist extension associated with cast use over six months was not evident 3 months after cast wear ceased.

The cast changing interval of 5-7 days appears in numerous studies, perhaps due to traditional practice and to convenience of the treatment setting[9] rather than evidence that this time frame leads to an optimal result. In adults with ABI in an inpatient rehabilitation setting Pohl and colleagues[52] found no difference in passive range of movement gains between groups who had casts changed every 5–7 days compared with 1–4 days. However they concluded a cast-changing interval of less than 5 days was superior to the 7 days cast-changing interval because it resulted in a shorter duration casting with fewer casts required, and a reduction of complication rates. In most studies the first cast is removed and immediately replaced with another cast at an increased angle within available range of movement with each successive cast incorporating gains in range of motion obtained from the previous cast.[16] Reasons for ceasing casting intervention relate to reaching normal ROM, achieving predetermined passive ROM goal, or exhausting the time interval or number of casts.

In nearly all studies casting is followed by another intervention designed to sustain gains in passive ROM achieved. Many involve immobilization orthoses and therapies to apply end range stretch. Numerous authors' concur with the findings of Pohl[52] that retention of gains in passive ROM post casting intervention can be achieved with customized orthoses for the wrist and elbow joints over 4 weeks.[9,69,70] Moseley and colleagues[46] found that positional stretch administered in either one 60-minute session or two 30-minute sessions per day, was ineffective with half of the gain lost within 24 hours and almost completely gone by four-weeks follow-up.

There is increasing evidence that casting joints at end range does have positive short-term effects on passive ROM. However much research is required to identify intensity, frequency and duration of casting intervention, address the impact of adjunct spasticity management therapies, and the effectiveness of follow-up interventions to maintain range of movement.[42]

INTERVENTION FOR LONG TERM MAINTENANCE OF INTEGRITY OF TISSUES

Post discharge from rehabilitation facilities, or following extended holiday periods, it is not uncommon to see regression in patients with neurological dysfunction. Pandyan et al.[49] demonstrated subjects most prone to wrist flexion contractures were those who showed no upper limb function within four weeks of their stroke. Strategies designed to prevent contractures should focus on this high-risk subgroup and begin early in rehabilitation. Pizzi et al.[51] studied persons 4 months post stroke and found an inverse correlation between passive wrist and elbow ROM and time since stroke. In the same sample improvements in passive range of wrist motion were recorded following 3 months wrist hand immobilization orthosis wear for 90 minutes per day. Benefits gained from rigorous therapy programmes may have

a longer duration if appropriate intervention is provided through orthoses or casts worn for specified periods during the day. It is suggested that interventions aimed at preventing contractures address joint movement and continue until functional recovery occurs.[49]

Where severe contracture and deformity leads to approximation of tissues, particularly in the elbow crease or the palm of the hand, intervention is essential to maintain extensibility and integrity of the skin tissues, prevent infection and wound formation, and enable cleaning and hygiene. Prevention of deformity and long-term maintenance are achieved by orthotic intervention. Sustaining effective intervention to address hypertonicity over a life span of cerebral palsy or following an ABI remains a challenge for therapists and clients.

INTERVENTION TO ADDRESS PAIN

Wrist pain may be a problem associated with malpositioning of paretic wrists and hands in the acute phases post stroke, and secondary to long term contracture in adult cerebral palsy clients or persons with ABI. Pain at the elbow and hand articulations has been found to correlate strongly with a reduction of the ROM of the wrist.[50] A wrist neutral functional realignment orthoses was shown to have positive effects on the prevention and development of hand pain in sub acute stroke patients.[4] Therapists concluded pain reduction could be associated with appropriate postural responses in the hand and wrist due to correct muscular and joint alignment or to protection offered during rehabilitation.

INTERVENTION FOR FUNCTION

The paucity of literature pertaining to the use of orthoses to facilitate functional use of the hand in the presence of neurological dysfunction is perhaps a reflection of the difficulties of research in this area rather than a window into the reality of practice. Requirements for functional hand use have greater implications for those persons with bilateral upper limb involvement.

Timing of orthotic application relates to the persons clinical goals. It is inappropriate to immobilize tissues limiting joint movement in early stages of rehabilitation following ABI when the emphasis is using neural plasticity to harness potential for recovery of muscle strength.[33] However once recovery has plateaued provision of an orthosis may assist specific functional tasks identified by the client, and or their carer. Assessment will determine the requirements of the orthosis, the design, and the materials. If the orthosis allows success in performance of functional objectives, repetition of the task or activity will afford opportunities to improve strength, range of motion, coordination and skill. Wearing a prefabricated wrist and hand immobilization orthosis at night, where the main aim was to reduce impairments such as spasticity or contracture, has been found to have no impact upon functional movement patterns evident during the day.[34,36]

Research findings from studies that investigated orthoses worn by children with cerebral palsy reveal trends toward more normal movement patterns and greater grasp skills.[5,13,26,43,55] The positive effect of hand orthoses in combination with adjunct therapies is generally evident for the duration of intervention, with diminishing effect over 2-3 months following cessation. There were differences in the sample populations, adjunct interventions and in gains associated with orthosis wear, but no significant relationship between orthosis type and change in hand function.

ELBOW/FOREARM INTERVENTIONS

Deficits in elbow and forearm motion and function in this client population present a challenge for therapists particularly as they impact upon the persons occupational tasks, posture and appearance; or ease of care for those in high dependency situations. Indications for interventions to address deficits in passive ROM as described in previous sections are applicable to the elbow. However where a variety of postures of the upper limb are required in the performance of functional tasks such as reach and hand orientation, rigid correction of deformity of the elbow and forearm is not always compatible with performance of daily tasks. For this reason options for functional intervention have focused on Lycra® and neoprene, particularly for children where the deficits in sensory input contribute to a modified motor output.

Research into the effectiveness of Lycra® arm sleeves using needle electromyography on normal subjects and persons with hemiplegia, indicated a change in muscle patterns consistent with the direction of application of the orthosis.[19,20] However, Gracies et al.[19] found no short-term benefit of Lycra® splints in adults with hemiplegia.

Elliott and colleagues[11,12] used a combination of sensitive 3D motion analysis with client centered assessments to assess the efficacy of Lycra® arm sleeve splints and goal directed training in children with CP. Wearing of Lycra® arm splints for three months, resulted in arm movements that were faster, more efficient, and required less secondary corrections. Whilst effects were only evident whilst splints were on, with only small improvements in range of pronation/supination, the Lycra® arm splints did make a quantifiable change to the attainment of movement goals of importance to the child.

The prefabricated neoprene orthosis designed to supinate the forearm has distal anchorage on the thumb and a serial static strap to rotate the forearm. It is secured at the distal end of the arm. Casey and Kratz[6] report success in facilitating supination with this type of orthosis in a single case study. The author's experience suggests this design is appropriate for clients who walk, who do not have a significant deformity of the wrist and who have functional extension of the arm.

THERAPIST'S CLINICAL REASONING

Studies that explored factors influencing therapist's clinical decision making in choice of intervention, for children and adults with upper limb performance dysfunction secondary to brain injury, reveal consistency across different settings and types of brain injury.[29,54] Factors essentially fall into two domains, those specific to the client such as neurological musculoskeletal upper limb performance dysfunction, severity, acuteness or chronicity of condition and associated sensory and cognitive performance components; and those related to environmental factors such as context of service provision, therapists experience and preferences. Experienced therapists consider the client and their families will have a significant impact on choice of interventions,[8] particularly those that require time and financial commitments. Once clinical decisions have been made therapists are encouraged to explain to the client and or their family, the rational behind the decision to commence an orthotic or casting programme. Kuipers and colleagues[30] in a study of the use of upper limb orthoses by persons with ABI found the clients' trust in, and agreement with therapists as to the goals of intervention, and the therapists' diligence in contacting clients for follow up, were influential factors on the clients' implementation of the program.

Orthotic interventions require clients to wear them in accordance with jointly agreed goals in order to be successful, with therapists having minimal direct control of intervention application. Casting is a more invasive intervention requiring modifications to several aspects of the clients daily activities therefore requires agreement prior to commencing intervention. However the therapist does retain some control over the intervention, as the client or family cannot easily remove it. These factors have a significant impact on the timing and effectiveness of intervention, but are not reported as considerations in orthotic/splinting and casting studies to date, making it difficult to apply evidence based results to the realities of clinical practice.

CONTRAINDICATIONS AND PRECAUTIONS TO ORTHOTIC AND CASTING INTERVENTION

Orthoses and casts applied to the upper limb of clients with neurological dysfunction have the potential to injure tissue. The consequences of injury from incorrect or poorly fabricated orthoses or casts, or inadequately planned protocols may be permanent. Therapists should be mindful of the potential harm associated with these interventions, and put in place appropriate strategies for initial surveillance and ongoing review.

The precautions relate to dissipation of pressure when fabricating orthoses for clients with neurological dysfunction. Appropriate resolution of forces created between the client and the orthosis, requires consideration of the dynamic aspects of hypertonicity and how it impacts upon all features of the

orthosis. Compromise of skin integrity and/or vascularity is a potential risk.

Casting is contraindicated when continued monitoring is not possible and in the presence of conditions such as significant oedema, impaired circulation, or heterotrophic ossification. Care is required where there are unhealed wounds. External padding of the cast may be necessary for persons with behavioural or cognitive problems to ensure they do not injure themselves, or others, with the cast.

SUMMARY

Numerous studies have addressed the issue of orthotic intervention and casting in the presence of hypertonicity. Patient characteristics differ between studies with regard to age, the underlying neurologic diagnosis and phase of recovery, severity of the problem/s associated with hypertonicity, the types of orthoses and casts used; the wearing schedules in terms of hours per day and total duration of orthotic intervention and the evaluation techniques used to determine the effectiveness of the intervention.

There is evidence of a change in clinical reasoning in relation to provision of orthotic and casting intervention, from that which specifically addresses hypertonicity and the consequences of deformity, to that which focuses on dysfunction and meeting the client's objectives in occupational performance. As there are a myriad of client centred factors that influence clinical reasoning and the diversity of reasons orthoses are prescribed, routine prescription based upon a standard protocol is not recommended. The task of finding practical orthotic solutions to complex and often technically difficult problems raised by clients continues to be the challenge for therapists in neurological practice.

Randomized clinical trials where hand orthoses are applied strictly according to requirements of a research protocol for short intervals of time, with efficacy determined at impairment levels, do not provide definitive answers on orthotic interventions for the individual client along the life long continuum of development, recovery or maintenance. Clearly our "best evidence" has many deficits and requires continued critical appraisal pointing to the need for continued research in this domain of practice. It also highlights the need for analysis and judicial use of information to underpin reasoning in clinical practice.

Where functional movement does not put the joint through a full range of motion, and daily passive range of movement or posturing does not adequately maintain range, orthotic intervention or casting may be indicated. These interventions address *peripheral* musculoskeletal responses to the central nervous system (CNS) dysfunction and therefore results are not permanent, as they do not influence the CNS.

Mobilizing orthoses, using serial static or serial progressive principles, are recommended to address deficits in range of motion where a low force is applied for long periods of time, as muscle spasticity and paresis remain potential contributors to contracture irrespective of tissue extensibility. Serial static orthoses are moulded in one position at the end range of the elastic limit of tissues with a period of time allowed for tissues to respond to the position prior to the orthosis being remoulded in the new lengthened position. The therapist undertakes incremental adjustments at intervals as gains are made in tissue extensibility and passive ROM. Refer to chapter 1 for more detailed information on nature of contracture and principles of application of mobilizing orthoses to address deficits in joint range of motion.

An orthosis is not unlike a prescribed medication in that each has adverse as well as positive effects. Prescription needs to be specific to the individual and made in consideration of other therapeutic, pharmacological, and surgical interventions. The time course of upper limb muscle contracture evolution and deterioration in persons with neurological dysfunction is used as a guide when to initiate interventions, with the optimal time to sustain interventions determined by recovery of active motion or potential long term complications.

ASSESSMENT TO DETERMINE APPROPRIATE ORTHOTIC / CASTING INTERVENTION

A comprehensive assessment is essential in determining if an orthosis, or casting, is an appropriate intervention for a client with neurological upper limb involvement. It should include observation of posture and movement patterns, passive and active range of motion as influenced by hypertonicity and discussion regarding the goals of the client and or carer.

POSTURE AND MOVEMENT CONSIDERATIONS

Describing the posture of the upper limb at rest, during walking or functional mobility and if possible purposeful use identifies muscle groups that may be overactive or weak and contribute to deformity. For example if a client's hand rests in greater than 45 degrees of wrist flexion this may be an indication of wrist or finger flexor spasticity, a lack of active wrist extension against gravity, or a combination of the two. Describing the posture will also provide information about approximation of skin surfaces, of particular interest the elbow crease, wrist crease, palm and the thumb. Postural observation will guide the clinician to the muscle groups that are contributing to the musculoskeletal problem and those that need closer biomechanical assessment.

Differences between unilateral or bilateral hand use, stresses associated with task performance, and retained primitive reflexes

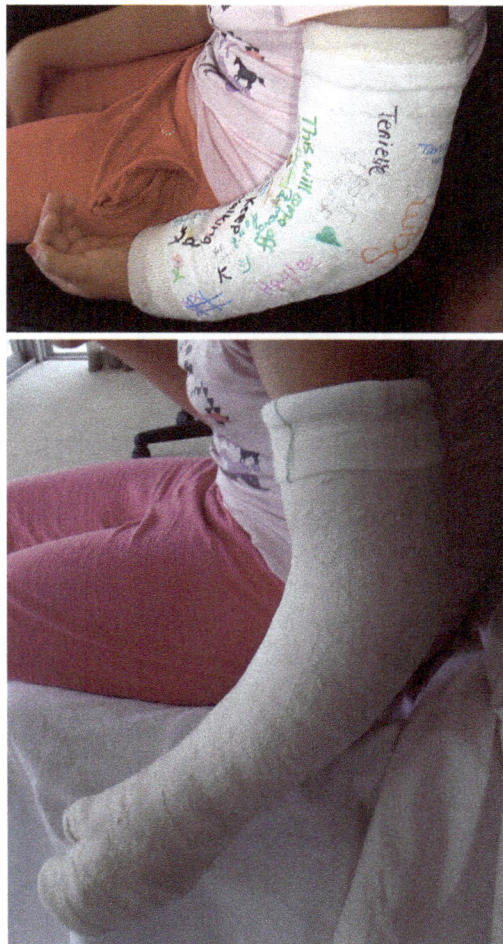

Figure 2: Serial Elbow Cast. Serial progressive casting undertaken in conjunction with Botox to effect passive extension deficit of the elbow in a child with an ABI.

that influence head and limb position, and the stability and mobility of the pelvis, trunk and shoulder girdle must also be considered as they often result in movement patterns different to those seen in clinical testing. As spasticity has its greatest impact upon intentional movement, observation of the limb during sleep may assist the therapist to determine if the problem is associated with contraction of muscles or contracture of connective tissue. Carer input may assist in this regard.

RANGE OF MOTION

Rapid passive range of motion opposing the action of the muscle group will elicit resistance if spasticity is present. Hypertonicity will be felt as a resistance to motion in any part of the range. The resistance felt may occur at the same point of initial catch on rapid passive movement. Assessment of passive range of motion will identify if there are any limitations at the end of the joint range or the presence of contracture. Limitations in active range of motion identify abhorrent movement patterns. Having a complete picture of range of motion will assist in determining the action of the orthosis and the forces required to balance and or restore movement for improved function or forces required to prevent shortening of musculature and joint structures.

CLIENT GOALS

The needs, goals and expectations of the client need to be assessed, as they are paramount to the success of orthotic intervention. If the client and carer do not appreciate the reason for the intervention then it will not be successful.[8,30] If the client does not have purposeful intent to use the limb, intervention focussed upon functional performance will not achieve any objective. Prevention of deformity for hygiene or pain relief then becomes the primary objective.

PATTERNS OF DEFORMITY AND INTERVENTION OPTIONS

The effects of neurological dysfunction on the hand and upper limb are unique to each individual, and tend to follow characteristic patterns of deformity. These are described as flexor or extensor patterns with shoulder retraction, depression, and internal rotation, elbow flexion, forearm pronation, wrist flexion, thumb and finger adduction and flexion. Alternatively the pattern may include shoulder retraction, depression, and internal rotation, elbow extension, forearm pronation, wrist extension, thumb and finger adduction and flexion. In clients with cerebral palsy scapular protraction and shoulder extension is also seen in association with the flexor pattern in the rest of the upper limb.

In the management of neurological dysfunction identification of the pattern of altered upper limb muscle function is of vital importance in defining the objectives for orthotic intervention.[54] The information included in this section will identify patterns of deformity and discuss various options for orthotic intervention. The patterns for orthoses are found in other chapters of this book.

ELBOW AND FOREARM

The predominate pattern of hypertonicity at the elbow is flexion and forearm pronation. This pattern will limit reach and orientation of the hand in functional performance, and alter postural symmetry that has an impact upon mobility. Severe flexion contractures of the elbow in dependant clients can limit the ease for carers to position or dress the client. The pattern of elbow extension, forearm pronation creates fewer problems for care, however severely impedes any potential to use two hands in functional tasks.

Regaining forearm supination ROM is challenging, particularly in the presence of pronation contracture and or pronator spasticity. If intervention is targeted at increasing passive range of motion or managing pain, casting and orthotic intervention is recommended. If intervention is targeted at improved active movement, particularly post BoNT then repetition of movement (active supination) is recommended within an activity based programme. If an orthosis with dynamic components is appropriate, then reasoning of the nature of the material, the purpose and timing of wear is an essential part of the clinical reasoning process.

Recommended Intervention

1. Serial Progressive Casting. In the presence of contracture, intervention should provide opportunities for the tissues to be held at end range, particularly when range cannot be maintained by active functional patterns of motion. Casting, over several weeks will maximize time tissues are held at end range, but is associated with the loss of limb function and normal deterioration associated with immobilization. When deciding to cast the elbow to address contracture, a realistic end range of motion is deter-

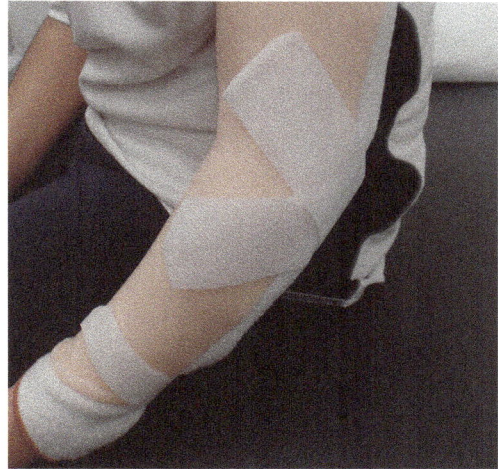

Figure 3: Anterior elbow immobilization orthosis used to sustain gains of casting. Remoulding to accommodate gains in ROM will change purpose of intervention to a serial static mobilizing orthosis.

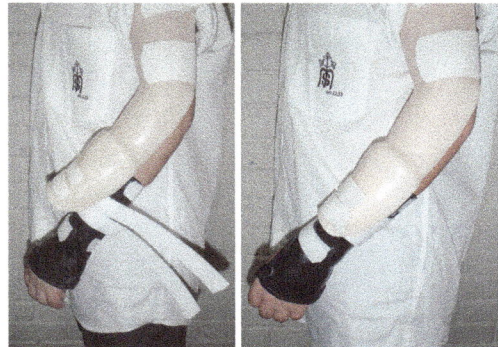

Figure 4: Forearm mobilization orthosis.

mined by the functional objective/s of the client, or the requirements of carers for passive motion in those persons dependent in personal care (Figure 2).

2. Anterior Elbow Immobilization Orthosis (Figure 3) is use to sustain gains of serial casting, or as a mobilizing orthosis to progressively gain passive ROM. The orthosis may be used in conjunction with other modalities such as BoNT or surgical releases.

3. Forearm mobilization orthosis (Figure 4). When the goal is to address passive ROM deficits serial progressive orthotic principles are applied. The orthosis consists of wrist and elbow components, with rotation straps winding around the forearm to sustain the end range position. The elbow component provides the stable base from which rotational force is applied to the forearm. The position of elbow immobilization is determined by elbow mobility and the need to address an end range position in this joint. Fabrication process is described in Chapter 4.

4. A custom made Lycra® arm orthosis is used for children in conjunction with interventions directed to attainment of movement goals specific to elbow and forearm. They have specific application for those clients with active movement and sensory impairment of proprioception and awareness.

5. The prefabricated forearm rotation neoprene orthoses provides a more gentle mobilizing force as it does not rigidly hold an end range position. Consisting of a thumb and hand component with strap that is spiraled up the forearm in the desired direction of rotation and secured to the arm. Good elbow extension is required to achieve appropriate rotation force. Caution is required when wrapping to ensure vascular supply to arm is not compromised.

6. Lycra® or 'soft splinting' should not be used to resolve deficits in passive range of motion or reduce contracture. For elderly clients with severe flexion contractures of the elbow foam rolls may be used to prevent approximation of tissues and skin breakdown in the elbow crease.

DEFORMITIES OF THE WRIST, FINGERS AND THUMB

The wrist and hand present a complex interaction of intrinsic and extrinsic musculature, in which hypertonicity dictates the predominant pattern of deformity, and ultimately the functional potential. In 1981, Zancolli and Zancolli[72] described a surgical classification of spastic hand deformities in the wrist and fingers, while House and colleagues[26] identified four patterns of deformity in the thumb. Building upon these classifications, Wilton[67, 68] developed a classification focused upon the functional deficits associated with paralysis and spasticity in the extrinsic and intrinsic musculature of the wrist, fingers and thumb. This Neurological Hand Deformity Classification (NHDC) was refined following a retrospective longitudinal case analysis of 115 video clips of 26 children with cerebral palsy performing upper limb gross and fine motor tasks, at multiple time points, during occupational therapy sessions between 1982 and 2012. The NHDC demonstrated excellent intra-observer and inter-observer reliability in describing the changes in hand deformity in children over time.[17]

In the NHDC, static and dynamic aspects of deformity are considered. The dynamic aspect requires consideration as to which muscles have a primarily role in the deformity or dysfunction evident. It is important to focus upon the wrist first and determine if the deformity arises from wrist, or finger, or both wrist and finger musculature. The classification of presenting hand deformity, and ability to record deformity progression, is the basis of clinical reasoning when determining appropriate intervention that may include orthoses and casts (Table 1).

It is recommended that classification is carried out through observation of the client's approach towards and attempted grasp and release of a daily functional item. Maintaining consistent and regular recording of the classification is essential to guide intervention and to monitor change over time. It is recommended that the movements during this task be visually recorded. The camera should be placed at a right angle to client on the opposite side to the limb being assessed. This will allow vision to determine the level of the wrist of flexion/extension, finger movement and thumb position.

FLEXION DEFORMITIES

F1 Wrist Flexion ≤ 20 degrees Thumb Adduction
Wrist and Finger Motion

Spasticity in flexor carpi ulnaris (FCU) means that approach to an object during function occurs with the wrist in 0-20 degrees of flexion. However, strength in the wrist extensor muscles can overcome the spasticity. There is no evidence of spasticity in the finger musculature.

Thumb Motion

In a large number of cases no deficit is seen in the thumb. The thumb deformity that is commonly associated with this wrist pattern is adduction of the thumb at the carpometacarpal (CMC) joint. Extension and abduction of the thumb are possible, but limited by a combination of contracture and contraction in the adductor pollicus muscle and first dorsal interosseus. Voluntary motion is still present in the thumb metacarpophalangeal (MCP) and interphalangeal (IP) joints.

Passive Range

Full passive ROM is available at all joints of the wrist and fingers. Contracture of the thumb index finger webspace will reduce ROM.

Functional Deficits

This pattern creates no impediments to function of the hand. Approach to objects for reach and grasp is generally in wrist flexion, with a tendency for hyperextension at the finger MCP and proximal interphalangeal (PIP) joints. Finger flexion is well controlled and is associated with wrist extension. Hyperextension, seen at the PIP joints, results from wrist flexion increasing the distance the extensor digitorum communis (EDC) tendons traverse before inserting on the proximal end of the middle phalanx. Less shortening of EDC is required to effect extension at the MCP and PIP joints. Transmission of force through the fingers, as required in typing, may be reduced if hyperextension of the PIP joints is associated with PIP joint laxity. MCP joint hyperextension

NEUROLOGICAL HAND DEFORMITY CLASSIFICATION

Type	F1. Wrist flexion ≤ 20°, thumb adduction	F2. Wrist flexion > 20°, active wrist & finger extension	F3. Wrist flexion > 20°, wrist extension powered by finger flexors and extensors
Associated thumb deformity	Not always present CMC Adduction	CMC adduction MCP extension IP hyperextension	CMC adduction MCP & IP vary
Associated finger patterns	Hyper extension of PIP joints	Hyper extension of PIP joints	Hyper extension of PIP joints
Primary location of spasticity	FCU AP	FDP & FDS AP, 1st DI	FCU, FCR, PL FDP & FDS AP
Muscles not effected by spasticity	Wrist extensors Extrinsic & intrinsic finger flexors & extensors	Wrist & thumb extensors Intrinsic finger musculature	Intrinsic finger musculature
Contracture	Thumb web space	FDP & FDS end range extension Thumb web space	FCU, FCR limiting end range wrist extension combined with loss of end range FDS & FDP. Thumb web space
Functional deficit	Nil Limited thumb abduction compromising thumb span to clear object for grasp	Palm orientation in grasp, wrist control during finger flexion Thumb disadvantaged effective opposition	Reach and grasp compromised by wrist extension powered by active finger extension or reversed tenodesis action

Table 1

F4. Wrist flexion > 20°, active finger flexion & extension, wrist extension absent	F5. Wrist flexion finger flexion, minimal active movement	E1. Wrist extension, finger movement powered by intrinsic muscle action	E2. Wrist extension, finger flexion, minimal active movement
CMC adduction MCP & IP vary	CMC adduction, MCP & IP flexion	CMC adduction MCP flexion IP neutral	CMC adduction, MCP & IP flexion
Hyper extension of PIP joints	Flexion of IP joints	MCP flexion IP extension	Flexion, adduction at MCP joints, flexion of IPs associated with wrist extension posture
FCU, FCR, PL FDP & FDS AP	Combined spasticity extrinsic & intrinsic musculature of the fingers and thumb	ECRL & ECRB, ECU contributes to ulnar deviation. Interossei, AP FPB	Combined spasticity extrinsic & intrinsic musculature of the fingers and thumb
Intrinsic finger musculature	Wrist musculature opposite to wrist position	FDP & FDS	Wrist flexor musculature opposite to wrist position
FCU, FCR, PL, FDP, FDS limiting end range extension. Thumb web space	Severe deformity in wrist, fingers & thumb muscles with deficits in volar skin & soft tissue	Intinsic finger flexors, thumb, palmar skin & fascial shortening. Hand hygiene critical.	Wrist extensors & dorsal wrist capsule. Palmar skin & fascial contracture potential severe deformity of wrist, fingers MCP joints & thumb.
Approach & grasp compromised by wrist position	No Function	Opening fingers & thumb for grasp disadvantaged by wrist extension - finger flexion/extension possible if wrist in neutral & thumb abducted.	No Function

213

frequently compensates for the deficit in thumb abduction when grasping objects as large as the palm of the hand.

Recommended Orthotic/Splinting intervention

Intervention should be directed to specific functional objectives.

1. No intervention is necessary for the wrist, as the gains from intervention would be outweighed by the loss of motion and sensation.

2. When the PIP joint deformity is associated with joint hypermobility, it may impact on functional performance. Small orthoses, manufactured to restrict PIP joint movement into hyperextension, can be useful for specific functional/vocational tasks that require pointing or keyboard access. (Refer to Figures 25 and 26, Chapter 6, page 167-168).

3. If the deficit in active thumb abduction does not significantly impede function, decreased passive range of movement of the webspace may be addressed by a CMC mobilization, hand based orthosis worn at night (Figure 11 and 12 Chapter 7, pages 184 and 186). Functional use of the hand is not compromised.

4. Where thumb function is limited by inability to abduct for effective opposition, the orthosis chosen should abduct and rotate the metacarpal without compromising grasp. Orthotic intervention options are:

    (a) Custom made thumb orthoses of either Lycra® or neoprene. The nature of these materials allows movement but can be bulky on small hands. Fabric based orthoses are inappropriate if the adduction pattern is very strong, or contracture of the webspace is significant.

    (b) Immobilization orthoses to address the CMC and MCP joints and control the metacarpal. The CMC/MCP immobilization orthosis incorporating a spiral design is recommended as it covers a relatively small area of the palm leaving the wrist and finger function unimpeded (Figure 4 and 6 Chapter 7, pages 178 and 181).

F2 Wrist Flexion > 20 Degrees, with Active Wrist and Finger Extension Wrist and Finger Motion

Spasticity is located in the wrist flexors FCU and flexor carpi radialis (FCR), and in the finger flexors, flexor digitorum profundus (FDP) and flexor digitorum superficialis (FDS). Strength in the wrist extensor muscles can overcome the resistance of spasticity in the wrist flexors as long as the fingers are flexed. Spasticity located in FDS and FDP muscles results in an inability to fully extend the fingers unless the wrist is flexed greater than 20°. Finger extension generally involves hyperextension of both the MCP and PIP joints due wrist flexion creating traction on the EDC tendons. Spasticity located in the intrinsic hand musculature may impact upon thumb and finger adduction.

Thumb Motion

On reach, the thumb may adopt a posture of adduction at the CMC joint, or CMC adduction with hyperextension of the MCP and IP joints. The thumb metacarpal is held in an adducted position by a combination of contracture and contraction in the adductor pollicus muscle and first dorsal interosseus. Action of extensor pollicus longus (EPL) and extensor pollicus brevis (EPB), acting across a hypermobile MCP joint, in the absence of flexor pollicus brevis (FPB) spasticity, creates the more distal deformity of IP hyperextension. Functionally this deformity develops as extensors work to bring the thumb away from the palm of the hand for grasp.

Passive Range

No deficits are evident in the wrist musculature. Shortening may be demonstrated in FDP and FDS at the end range of finger extension when the wrist is also extended. Contracture of the index thumb webspace is generally present.

Functional Deficits

When approaching objects for grasp, the fingers are hyper extended at the MCP joints. The palm is not orientated toward the object for grip. The fingers can be positioned over objects, a bar or handle, with increasing wrist extension evident as the fingers flex to grasp the object. With this pattern, the thumb is disadvantaged for effective opposition, particularly when associated with adduction at the CMC joint. Thus pulp-to-pulp pinch is generally unsuccessful unless the index finger is positioned in extension at the MCP and flexion at the PIP and DIP. To achieve thumb and finger opposition some clients will use a more lateral pinch with the middle finger accentuating the index finger position of hyperextension at the MCP and flexion of the IP joints.

Functional Requirements

These clients require greater control of wrist motion - in flexion so that the palm can be orientated towards the object on approach for grasp, and in extension, to give greater control to finger closure during grasp. Abduction of the thumb CMC joint and slight flexion of the MCP and IP joints increase the options for effective pinch.

Recommended Orthotic/Splinting intervention

Orthotic intervention for the wrist is not a primary consideration for these clients as wrist immobilization may reduce active control, weaken immobilized muscles, and compromise the ability to open hand for function. Therapy should focus on the development of active wrist control. Orthotic intervention should only be considered where clients require more effective control of their wrist position, promoting more efficient finger opening and closing to meet specific functional goals.

Orthotic considerations are:

1. Orthoses made from Lycra®, or other flexible fabric, allow movement of the wrist through mid range and therefore do not compromise finger function. Flexible boning or thermoplastic insert incorporated into the design can restrict maximal wrist flexion and extension allowing greater synergy between wrist and finger musculature (Figure 5). Orthoses may be custom made or prefabricated. Numerous circumferential designs are available from major hand therapy product suppliers. As the restriction of motion is dependant on the design of strapping, and the tension

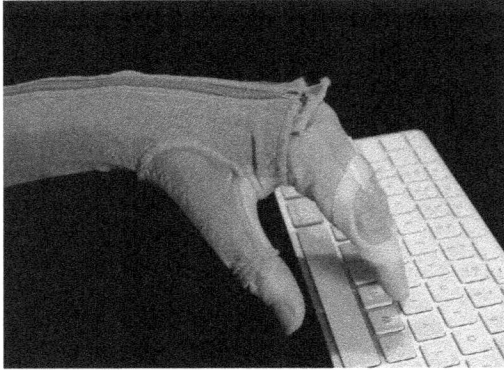

Figure 5: Lycra® Wrist Orthosis. The Lycra® wrist orthosis is combined with thermoplastic PIP extension restriction orthoses to overcome a pattern of deformity exacerbated when undertaking this demanding fine motor and cognitive task.

required to secure the orthosis, therapists must choose the product with these biomechanical considerations in mind.

2. Correction of the wrist position, and reduction of the distance over which the EDC tendons traverse at the wrist, will resolve much of the hyperextension deformity at the PIP joint. Orthoses to restrict the hyperextension (see Figure 5) are only necessary if the joints 'lock' in hyperextension thus restricting coordinated flexion, or if the hyper mobility of the joints compromise function.

F3 Wrist Flexion > 20 degrees. Finger Flexors and Extensors Power Wrist Extensor Motion

Wrist and finger motion
Spasticity is located in FCU, FCR, FDP and FDS. Wrist extensor motion may result from the action of EDC, or from reverse tenodesis action powered by active flexion of the fingers during grasp. Hyperextension of the PIP joints may be present.

Thumb Motion
The predominant posture of the thumb with this wrist pattern is adduction at the CMC joint and hyperextension of the MCP joint. As described in the previous classification, this deformity is a combination of contracture and contraction of intrinsic muscles acting on the CMC joint and extrinsic extensors acting across the MCP joint.

Passive Range
Deficits in extensibility are evident in the extrinsic wrist and finger flexor musculature resulting in deficits at the end of passive extension range. Spasticity located in FDS and FDP is evident on passive extension of the wrist as the IP joints will flex. On passive extension of the fingers the wrist will flex.

Functional Requirements
These clients require greater extension of the wrist to enable the fingers to effectively grasp objects towards the palm of the hand. Positioning of the thumb so that it can oppose the index finger will also increase options for effective grasp and pinch.

Recommended Orthotic/Splinting intervention
The objective of intervention may be to improve hand function, to prevent further contracture, or to address pain in the wrist. The associated deformity in the thumb will determine limitations seen in the webspace and range of motion.

Options for intervention are:
1. Function specific wrist immobilization orthoses may be required for school age children and adults. Determining the

wrist position that allows finger flexion and extension movement is critical. Orthoses considered are similar to those identified for F2 Classification, however are generally positioned in greater degrees of wrist flexion.

2. Orthotic intervention to address loss of passive ROM should only be considered if there is evidence of contracture in FCU, FCR, FDP and FDS. The wrist hand orthosis (mobilization), dorsal volar design, (Figure 6) can be used to address contracture during non-functional periods of the day, or at night..

3. Serial casting can be used to address contracture in the wrist flexors and extrinsic finger flexors. However, potential to further weaken wrist extensor musculature from sustained immobilization must be considered.

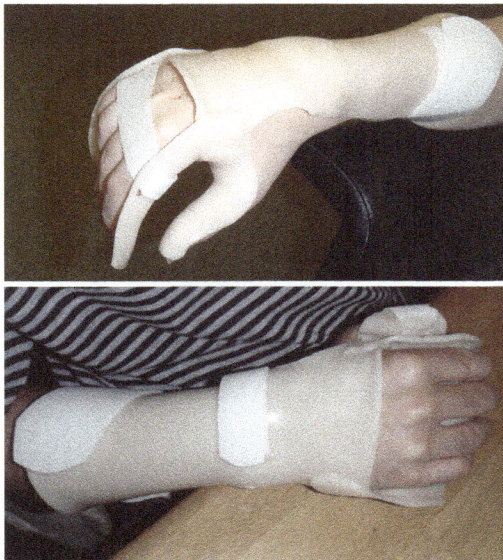

Figure 6: Wrist Hand Orthosis Mobilization. This orthosis can address wrist, finger and thumb position at end range to address contracture. Radial and palmar views (a and b).

F4 Wrist Flexion > 20 Degrees, Active Finger Flexion And Extension, No Active Wrist Extension,

Wrist and finger motion

Spasticity is located in FCU, FCR, Palmaris Longus (PL), FDP and FDS. Strength in the ECRL and ECRB muscles is insufficient to overcome spasticity in the wrist flexors and the effects of gravity. Wrist movement in direction of extension may result from the action of EDC, with the wrist remaining in its flexion range. Mid range flexion of the fingers is possible, however the position of wrist flexion disadvantages the finger flexors as maximum muscle shortening is achieved before end joint range is reached. During approach to an object active finger flexion enables grasp. Extension of the wrist is not independent of finger flexion motion. Hyperextension of the PIP joints is present.

Thumb Motion

The predominant posture of the thumb with this wrist pattern is adduction at the CMC joint and hyperextension of the MCP joint. As described in the previous classification, this deformity is a combination of contracture and contraction of intrinsic muscles acting on the CMC joint and extrinsic extensors acting across the MCP joint.

Passive Range

Significant deficits in extensibility are evident in the extrinsic wrist and finger flexor musculature resulting in passive ROM deficits in extension. Reduced extensibility may also be present in EDC, limiting full passive finger flexion. Spasticity located in FDS and FDP is evident on passive extension of the wrist. It is also evident on passive extension of the PIP and DIP joints, as the wrist will move into flexion if the wrist is not immobilized.

Functional Requirements

These clients require greater extension of the wrist to enable the fingers to grasp objects towards the palm of the hand. Positioning of the thumb so that it is moved out from in the palm and can oppose the index finger may increase options for effective grasp and pinch.

Recommended Intervention

The objective of intervention may be to improve hand function, to prevent further wrist contracture for ease of management, or to address pain in the wrist. With the predominance of hypertonicity in the wrist flexor musculature the fingers cannot be tightly fisted and therefore there is rarely a risk of breakdown of skin in the palm of the hand. The associated deformity in the thumb will determine limitations seen in the webspace and range of motion.

Options for intervention are:

1. Orthotic intervention to address passive ROM deficits in wrist and finger musculature can be worn at night if spasticity is not evident during sleep. The wrist hand immobilization orthosis (dorsal volar design) is recommended (Figure 6).

2. Serial casting can be used to address contracture in the wrist flexors and extrinsic finger flexors. Casting is more effective than orthotic intervention to improve the passive extension ROM as it maximizes the time tissues are held at end range. With greater length in the flexor muscles the wrist can approach a more neutral position and thus improve the biomechanical advantage to extrinsic finger flexor and extensor musculature during grasp. Gains from casting must be maintained with an ongoing orthotic programme.

3. Wrist immobilization orthoses are used to gain a better wrist position whilst not compromising the ability to extend the fingers during reach and approach for functional tasks. The pattern of spasticity in FDS and FDP will determine the angle to which the wrist can be extended while still allowing finger extension. To accommodate this an orthosis may be fabricated with the client's wrist in flexion. Orthoses that address this deformity require rigid materials to hold the position. A wrist immobilization orthosis with dorsal forearm and palmar components is recommended (Figure 7). Good contour and avoiding pressure on the dorsal aspect of the wrist and across palmar surface is essential as it is challenging to immobilize the wrist while accommodating flexion forces. The use of adhesive backed silicone gels can be advantageous in addressing pressure issues.

4. Orthotic options for the wrist should also incorporate components to address the thumb deformity. Abduction of the CMC joint, stabilization of the MCP joint in a few degrees of flexion, and prevention of hyperextension of the IP joint will position the thumb for effective opposition. To achieve this combination rigid components are used. Where a wrist

immobilization orthosis is not an option, as it would compromise finger function, orthoses designed to specifically address the thumb deformity can improve hand function. Thumb CMC/MCP immobilization design is recommended as it provides the necessary control to position joints.

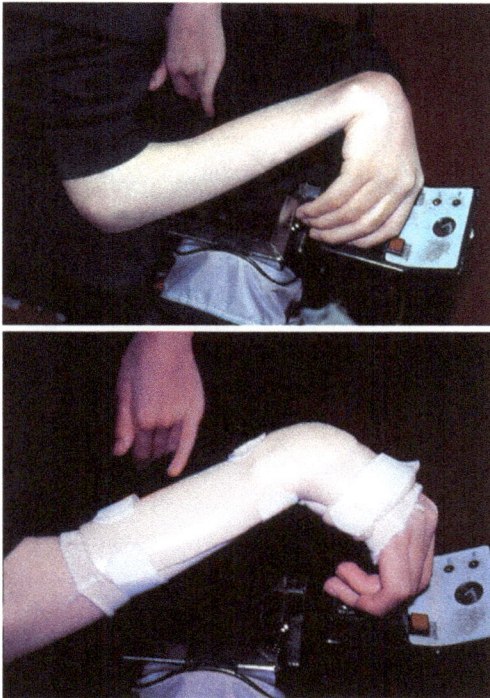

Figure 7: Severe flexion deformity of the wrist is exacerbated by functional use of the hand a. Immobilizing the wrist in maximum passive extension with a Dorsal Wrist Immobilization Orthosis increases options for finger and thumb function b. Gel inserted prior to fabrication of the splint modifies contour over the dorsum of the wrist. A customized lining 'sock' is worn under the orthosis.

F5 Totally Fisted Hand With Wrist Flexion

Wrist and finger motion

Hypertonicity and contracture in the wrist flexor musculature determines the position of the wrist. Combined with hypertonicity in the extrinsic and intrinsic flexor musculature of the fingers and thumb, the potential exists for a severe deformity. No active wrist motion is evident. Fingers are generally flexed at all joints with minimal active motion.

Thumb Motion

Severe adduction contracture of the thumb is always present. The posture of the rest of the thumb may vary depending upon the contribution of other thumb muscles. Where FPL is involved the thumb is flexed across the palm and is trapped under the flexed fingers by a combination of contracture and contraction. Another common posture involves adduction of the metacarpal and flexion at the MCP joint against the radial side of the flexed index and middle fingers. Ulnar rotation often results from the sustained force applied to the fingers. Secondary connective tissue contracture compounds the problem.

Passive Range

Significant deficits in end range motion result from contracture in muscles, skin and connective tissues across joints, web spaces and palm. Contracture is not always equal across the four fingers with the most severe deformity commonly in the ring finger. Constant approximation of tissues can lead to problems with skin integrity, nail care and hygiene.

Recommended Intervention

The critical issue in this type of hand deformity is to maintain range of motion so as to prevent fixed contractures, maceration, infection, and breakdown of the skin on the palm and thumb. The objective is to stop approximation of the skin, to allow some air to circulate and tissues to dry. Orthotic intervention must be sustained and reviewed on a regular basis.

A spacer between the palm and fingers is required. Prefabricated palm protectors and custom made soft rolls can be compressed so they only create an interface between tissue layers. If placed between the fingertips and the palm hyperextension of DIP joint will be exacerbated. Ideally spacers should be placed proximal to the distal phalanx to create gentle pressure on the proximal and middle phalanges, and not the distal phalanx. Incorporation of thermoplastic materials on the

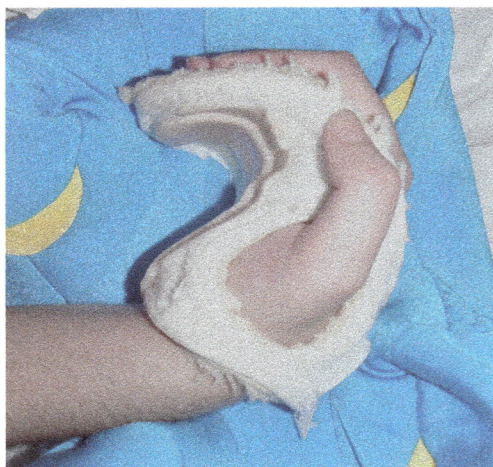

Figure 8: Reinforced soft palmar protector. Bonding thermoplastic material to create a roll on the palmar surface prevents strong flexion of fingers hyperextending DIP joints.

under surface of palm protectors is used to achieve better contour along volar surface of the proximal and middle phalanges as evident in Figure 8. Thermoplastic materials that become 'sticky' when dry heated (e.g. Orfit®) can be adhered directly to the palmar surface of the palm protector. Using serial static mobilizing principles, reheating the whole protector in hot water, allows the degree of finger extension to be gradually modified as changes in tissue extensibility occur. In acute phases post ABI where very high hypertonicity is evident this may be a safe intervention to prevent palmar maceration.

EXTENSION DEFORMITIES

E1 Wrist Extension With Finger and Thumb Flexion At The MCP Joints

Wrist and finger motion

Spasticity is primarily located in the wrist extensor muscles ECRL, ECRB, ECU and in the hand intrinsic muscles. Hypertonicity in ECRL and ECRB influences both active and passive wrist range of motion. The wrist posture is extension. The strength of the wrist flexors is able to overcome the resistance in the wrist extensors allowing active wrist flexion motion to neutral and therefore capacity to extend the fingers in approach to objects.

Hypertonicity in the hand intrinsic muscles in combination with an extended wrist promotes flexion and adduction at the MCP joints of both the fingers and thumb. With flexion of the MCP joints the intrinsic pull on the lateral bands of the extensor mechanism is facilitated across the dorsal aspect of PIP joint and PIP joint hyperextension deformities may result. Contraction and contracture in the intrinsic finger musculature, combined with shortening in the EDC muscle tendon unit, limits motion into MCP extension, MCP abduction, and composite flexion at MCP, PIP, and DIP joints when the wrist is in neutral. Potential to move out of the pattern of finger MCP flexion adduction and IP extension is greater when the wrist is held in neutral.

Thumb Motion

The thumb metacarpal is held in an adducted position by contraction in the adductor pollicus muscle and first dorsal interossei. The MCP joint is held in flexion by spasticity in the FPB that does transmit some of its force to the IP joint, thus maintaining it in extension. When contracture is evident in FPL wrist extension will increase IP flexion. Contracture of the skin and connective tissue across the flexor surface of the MCP joint is common.

Passive Range

Deficits in range of motion may be evident with loss of extensibility often present in the skin, palmar fascia, intrinsic finger musculature, wrist extensors and EDC as seen by difficulty in achieving an intrinsic minus finger position, or full passive flexion of the fingers with the wrist approaching neutral. With progression of this deformity contracture of the thumb is common as it is trapped under the flexed fingers. Sustained pressure of fingers flexed against the palm of the hand

can also result in hyperextension deformities of the DIP joints. Deficits are seen in extensibility of the skin and connective tissue over the dorsum of the wrist, the palm, and the webspace of the thumb and fingers.

Functional Requirements

These clients require the wrist to be positioned in a more neutral position to orientate the hand to approach objects and increase efficiency of the FDP and FDS fingers. In addition, the thumb must be extended out of the palm of the hand if any grasp is to be effective.

Recommended Orthotic/Splinting intervention

This pattern of deformity requires constant monitoring as it can lead to significant contractures of the thumb and finger MCP joints and ultimately a breakdown of skin in the thumb webspace and the palm of the hand. Hygiene is often a concern. The objective of intervention may be to improve hand function, to prevent further wrist contracture for ease of management, or to prevent risk of maceration of skin in the palm of the hand. Critical analysis of contracting forces, and the deficits in passive ROM, considering passive insufficiency of extrinsic and intrinsic finger musculature, will determine joint positions in both immobilization and mobilization orthoses.

Orthotic intervention options are:

1. Wrist immobilization orthoses made of thermoplastic materials are used to sustain a neutral wrist position. Designs must incorporate components on both

volar and dorsal surfaces of the hand to achieve effective immobilization. The volar component incorporates the thumb in abduction and extension (Figure 9). This orthosis can be used to address the wrist contracture whilst also facilitating functional use of the fingers.

2. Mobilizing serial static principles underlying application of wrist hand orthoses to address ECRL and ECRB contracture. The critical issue in addressing this contracture is to address end range positions, which are contrary to most hand therapy practice. The wrist should be immobilized in the direction of flexion, the MCP joints that are contracted in flexion need to be extended and abducted, and the PIP joints that have limited flexion due to limited finger extensor tendon extensibility need to be flexed. Making this orthosis in two separate parts – dorsal wrist forearm component to maintain wrist in neutral, and palmar finger component to extend MCP joints and flex PIP and DIP joints – facilitates ease of application (Figure 10).

3. Serial casting the wrist into flexion is an option should range of motion deteriorate despite orthotic intervention.

The authors highly recommend therapists monitor clients with this deformity over the long term as prevention of significant contracture in the intrinsic musculature and palmer fascia is a far easier intervention than attempting to correct deformity once it becomes fixed.

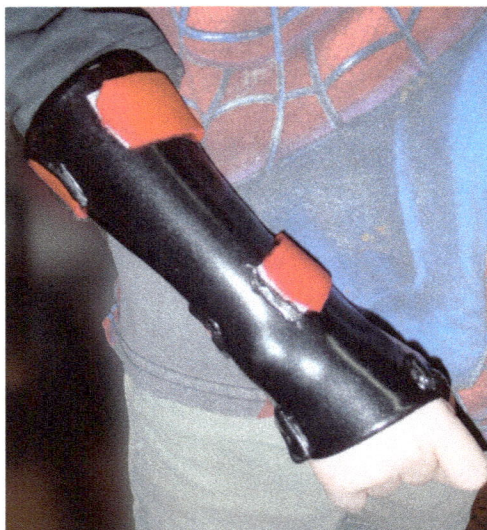

Figure 9: Wrist immobilization orthosis in neutral to facilitate function in the fingers and thumb.

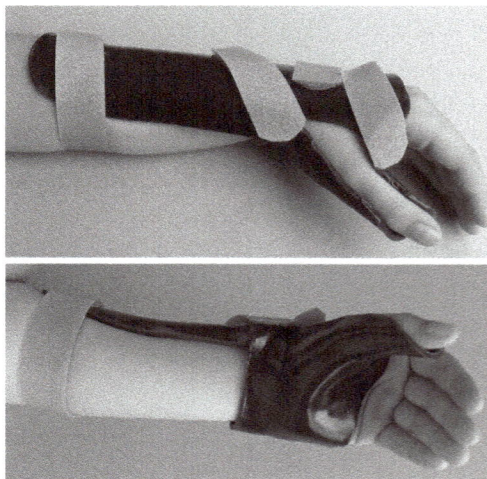

Figure 10: Wrist Immobilization Orthosis Two Piece Option. The nature of forces generated in this deformity requires reciprocal parallel forces to be applied to hold the wrist in neutral to flexion. The wrist is immobilized between dorsal and volar components secured with Velcro®. Extending the palmar component can effectively control the fingers.

E2 Totally Fisted Hand With Wrist Extension

Wrist and finger motion

The degree of hypertonicity in the wrist extensor musculature will determine the position of the wrist. Combined with hypertonicity in the extrinsic and intrinsic flexor musculature of the fingers and thumb, the potential exists for a severe deformity and compromise of palmar skin integrity. Minimal active motion is evident. Fingers are generally strongly flexed and adducted at the MCP joints with minimal active motion in PIP joints.

Thumb Motion

Severe contractures of the thumb are always present. Minimal CMC abduction is possible due to combined Adductor Pollicus, first dorsal interosseus and soft tissue contracture. FPB has a major impact on flexion of the MCP joint with the thumb flexed across the palm, flexed or extended at the IP joint, and trapped under the flexed fingers by a combination of contracture and contraction.

Passive Range

Significant deficits in end range wrist motion result from contracture in wrist extensor muscles and connective tissue. Hypertonicity and contracture of intrinsic finger muscles can result in volar movement of the proximal phalanx at the MCP joints and loss of finger and thumb palmar fascia and skin. Constant approximation of tissues can lead to problems with skin integrity, nail care and hygiene.

Recommended Intervention

The critical issue in this type of hand deformity is to maintain range of motion so as to limit potential for fixed contractures, maceration, infection, and breakdown of the skin on the palm and thumb. The objective is to stop approximation of the skin, to allow some air to circulate and tissues to dry. Orthotic intervention must be sustained and reviewed on a regular basis. Type of intervention is likely to be determined by the patient's age and capacity of their tissues to tolerate the force.

Options for intervention are:

1. Protection of palmar skin is best achieved by positioning the wrist in flexion that increases potential length in extrinsic finger flexors so some extension is possible.
2. Customised palmar protectors and custom made soft rolls (as described for F5 deformity above) are recommended.

PROCEDURES

Incorporation of upper limb orthoses into therapy programmes for clients with neurological conditions presents therapists with some unique challenges not experienced in other areas of practice. Clients cannot always position their limbs, or sustain a position that is ideal for the therapist when fabricating an orthosis. Spasticity will often increase due to anxiety or excitement associated with the fabrication procedure, on movement of the limb as the client attempts to assist, and in response to the tactile and temperature stimulus of the procedure. The therapist must not only control the thermoplastic material, but also control the limb. Therefore, it is recommended the fabrication procedure be broken down into smaller components, and material that has a memory is used. Attention should also be given to the environment in order to reduce any factors that may increase hypertonicity during orthotic fabrication.

A thorough understanding of biomechanical principles, as outlined in Chapter 2, is critical in the design of orthoses for this client group. The forces applied by the hand to the orthosis, and its various components, are significant. Thus reactive forces generated by the orthosis are equally great. Prior to designing an orthosis it is essential to analyse the normal forces generated by the hand, in addition to those generated by the spastic muscles. Considering the force application as a series of reciprocal parallel forces that address each joint in sequence will enable therapists to determine how to use forces to stabilize as well as mobilize joints. From this information it is possible to determine the direction, location and intensity of forces that will be created at the orthosis-hand interface when the orthosis is achieving its objective. Minimization of pressure is essential and is achieved by the strategic use of 'fat like' gels or high-density foam padding and thick 'hand socks'.

Many of the thermoplastic orthoses used to immobilize or restrict joint function are described in the chapters on orthotic fabrication for the elbow, wrist, fingers and thumb.

Orthoses may immobilize joints, or mobilize joints if reviewed and remoulded at intervals appropriate to contracted tissue response. This section outlines some procedures that make it easier to fabricate orthoses for the client with neurological dysfunction.

Wrist Hand Orthosis Pattern

An orthosis that incorporates both dorsal volar components (Figure 6) is recommended to address contracture and spasticity in both the wrist and fingers. This design is superior to the volar designs (Figure 5 in Chapter 5, page 116) because

- It uses an effective lever system to apply extension force to the wrist and fingers
- The pressure, resulting from force applied to position the wrist and counteract the force of the spastic muscles, is widely distributed across the dorsum of the wrist and the volar surface of the hand by well contoured thermoplastic material
- It allows greater control over the wrist and hand so that one therapist can fabricate it
- It can be easily adjusted to accommodate increased extension of the wrist and fingers
- It can be applied independently by the client using one hand.

There are generally three issues to address when fabricating orthoses in the presence of hypertonicity - the wrist, the fingers, and the thumb. Prior to fabrication, determine the angles at which joints are to be immobilized and the padding and linings to be incorporated. Then determine the best position of the limb for fabrication of the orthosis using the position of proximal and distal joints to decrease the effects of spasticity in the muscles traversing the joint to be addressed. Experiment with various limb postures to achieve the best position for the client and therapist. Initially therapists may require an additional person to position the limb with the second applying the material. Three millimetre non-perforated Orfit® or Aquaplast® materials are used for this orthosis. Dense stockinette or woollen socks are used as a lining. They can be easily washed and replaced and are preferable to lining materials that are adhered to the orthosis. Allowance is made for the density of the lining material.

Procedure To Take A Pattern

Mark the following points referring to Figure 11.

1. The length of the orthosis from wrist to proximal end is two-thirds the length of the forearm. This roughly equates to the length of the hand. Measure length using a tape and mark with a small dot.

2. Position the wrist at an angle close to the angle to the finished orthosis. Allow the fingers and thumb to remain flexed. Lie pattern material over the dorsum of the hand and mark the points as illustrated in Figure 11a.

    1-2   Medial and lateral aspects of the hand just proximal to the heads of the finger metacarpals.

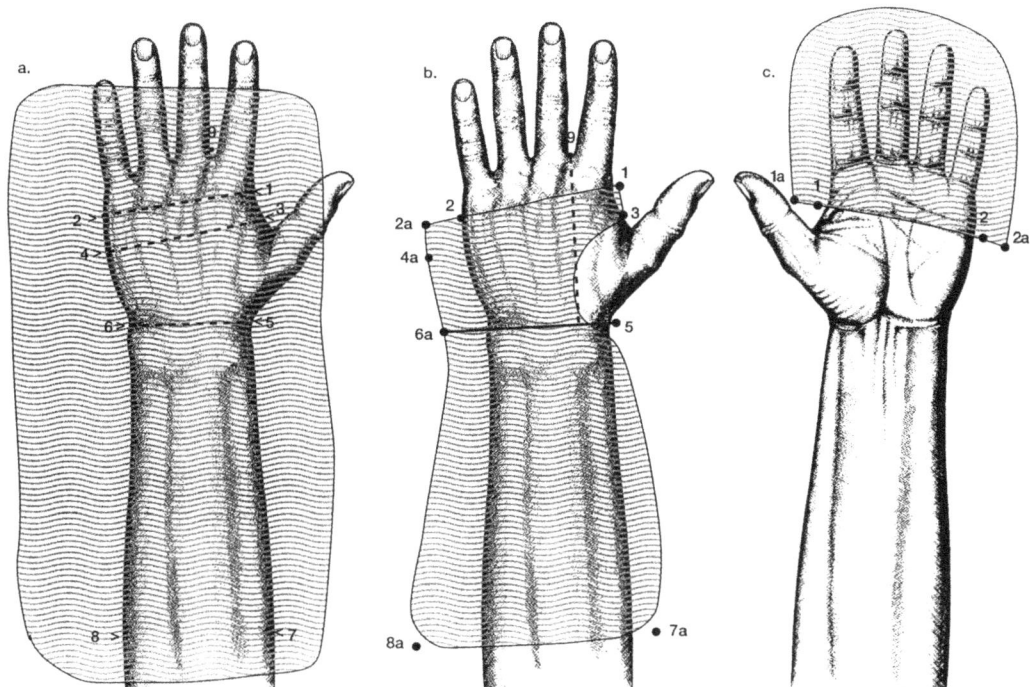

Figure 11: Pattern Wrist Hand Orthosis -Dorsal Volar Design.

3-4 Medial and lateral aspects of the hand at the thumb web level.

5-6 Medial and lateral aspects of the wrist at mid-carpal level.

7-8 Medial and lateral aspects of the forearm at the length previously determined.

9 Index and middle finger web.

The width of the orthosis should be half the circumference at the forearm and wrist. This can be determined by wrapping the pattern material around and marking the desired width at the forearm and wrist. These width points are indicated on the diagram as 2a, 4a etc.

The volar finger component extends from the heads of metacarpals to the tips of the fingers. Flex the client's wrist to take the pattern. This will disadvantage the finger flexor muscles when contracting actively or in association with tone. Mark the medial and lateral aspects of the hand just proximal to the heads of the finger metacarpals as illustrated in Figure 11c. Add 1-1.5 cm to the length and width (radial and ulnar) of the finger component.

To shape the pattern:

1. Join points 1 and 2 (MCP line).
2. Join points 3-4 (thumb line).
3. Join points 5-6 (wrist line).
4. Draw a vertical line from point 9 to intersect the wrist line.
5. Starting at point 2a, draw a line around the forearm through points 4a, 6a, and 8a curve sharply around to 7a then up to 5. The curve through 7a should be shallow to ensure this aspect of the orthosis does not impede elbow flexion.

6. The line between 5 and 3 touches the vertical line 9 allowing clearance for the thumb.
7. Points 1 and 3 are joined.
8. Cut the two pattern pieces out. When fitted to the hand, the proximal edge of the palmar component is aligned to the thumb line of the dorsal component. Check for fit on the patient, prior to transferring it to the thermoplastic material.

The thumb position can have a significant influence upon the tone in the fingers and rest of the hand. An extra piece of thermoplastic material is cut out. The length of thumb, and the width of the thumb at the IP and MCP joint levels determine the dimensions. For children under six the thumb and the finger component can be combined in one piece of material.

Fabrication Procedure

Moulding the orthosis follows the same sequence as taking a pattern:

1. Pad out any bony prominences on the dorsum of the wrist. If the wrist will be in greater than 40° of flexion, pressure will be exerted across the carpal region. 'Stiff' exercise putty is used to shape an inverse mould space for the adhesive backed high-density padding or gel. Mould a piece, no thicker than 3mm over the area requiring protection. If the wrist is in a more neutral or extended position the padding is only required over the ulnar head and radial styloid. Intimate contouring of thermoplastic material in the vicinity of the wrist is essential.

2. Place heated material over the dorsum

of the wrist and hand. Position the wrist while letting the fingers and thumb flex.

3. Prior to removing from the hand, mark the location of the distal edge of the orthosis across dorsum of the MCP joints. Remove it from the hand. Gently remove exercise putty maintaining its shape. Used as a pattern to cut gel (or high density foam) to the shape ensuring adhesive backed surface will adhere to the inside of the orthosis. Chamfer edge of gel to ensure smooth transition between gel and thermoplastic material. Reheat, smooth and flare the edges, proximal, distal and around the thumb.

4. Place the cooled forearm component on the dorsum of the hand, ensuring it is aligned to the marker. Allow the wrist to flex till relaxation is evident in the fingers while maintaining contact of the dorsal component with the back of the hand. The heated finger component is accurately positioned under the MCP joints and adhered to the forearm component on both radial and ulnar sides. Intimate moulding of the transverse palmar arch is crucial if this orthosis is to be comfortable.

5. Remould the finger component distal to the MCP joints to the predetermined angle of finger extension. This stage can be done without applying the orthosis to the client. Maintain transverse and longitudinal arches.

6. In adult clients, where the circumference around the MCP heads is greater than the circumference just proximal to MCP joints, an opening may be required on one side of the orthosis. Therefore, just before

the material is completely cool, unstick the bond on the ulnar aspect of hand. The relative position of these two pieces of material is maintained by a Velcro® strap.

7. Apply straps at the proximal end of the orthosis, and at the wrist if the original pattern of tone was wrist extension. Finger straps applied to the proximal phalanx should have good contour.

8. Apply orthosis and determine strapping required for the fingers and forearm. Secure these straps before applying thumb component.

9. The thumb component is adhered to the palmar surface of the finger component. It is important that the thumb piece is of sufficient width to mould intimately around the MCP joint to achieve a positional force on the metacarpal in the desired position of abduction or extension of the thumb. The bond between these two pieces of material must be very smooth.

10. If necessary a strap, is applied to secure the thumb in the orthosis.

Casting Procedure

Prior to initiating a casting programme for clients not within a hospital setting, commitment of carers to the programme is essential. The impact of the cast on posture and functional tasks such as showering, mobility, and dressing must be considered, and any problems resolved prior to initiating casting. It is also essential that the therapist and client are available for follow up for the duration of the programme. Holiday periods and summer months should be avoided. It is also suggested casts are not applied on Fridays unless weekend surveillance is possible.

Two persons are required. The person holding the limb is responsible for determining the angle the joint is to be cast whilst the other applies the cast. Prior to casting the angle at which each joint is to be immobilized must be determined. Fixing this angle by taping the goniometer provides an easy reference during the process.

Fabrication Procedure

Stockinette, cast padding, thin wool felt, and plaster are required to manufacture this cast. Instructions are given for procedures for both the elbow and wrist components.

1. Measure stockinette the length of cast plus allowance for turning over plaster at proximal and distal ends (width of 7 cm for most adults and 5 cm for small adults and children). For casts traversing the hand cut a small hole for the thumb. If elbow is to be cast at greater than 45° flexion, slit the stockinette at the anterior elbow crease horizontally from one condyle to the other. Overlap the proximal and distal portions.

2. Wool felt strips, 3 cm in width, are applied to protect ends of plaster and bony prominences relevant to each cast:
   - The circumference of the arm/forearm proximal end
   - The posterior two-thirds of the elbow across the humeral condyles
   - Longitudinally down posterior aspect of arm, over olecranon, and down shaft of the ulna
   - The circumference of wrist just proximal to the ulna head
   - The circumference over the finger MCP joints.
   - Two strips are required to protect the thumb. The first piece is the length from the index finger PIP to the proximal wrist crease. Cut an oval hole in the middle and place over the thumb at the level of the MCP joint. Proximal end may be tucked under wrist felt. The second piece, the length from the index PIP joint across the webspace to the IP joint of the thumb, is threaded through the hole of the first. Tuck end under finger MCP felt.

3. Tape wool felt strips in place over the stockinette.

4. Apply cast padding in a circumferential manner: three to four rolls of 7 cm padding are required depending upon the size of the limb. Start at proximal end placing edge of padding so that it overlaps half the width of the felt. Wrap it around twice before proceeding distally, overlapping the previous layer by half, end by wrapping twice overlapping half the felt at distal end. Additional padding is applied for
   - elbow casts in a figure eight around the elbow twice overlapping the olecranon by 2 cm
   - wrist and hand casts in a radial direction across the volar surface of the wrist. Unwrap

a portion about 30 cm long and split in half. One portion is wrapped around the hand while the other is spiralled around the thumb. An additional piece is then added for the fingers.

5. Return to the proximal edge of the padding and apply a single wrap proximal to distal. Repeat so there are three layers in total. The padding should feel even throughout the length of the arm. Bulking or puckering of padding may be smoothed out.

6. Apply plaster using exactly the same procedure as the padding. Begin at the proximal end 1.5 cm distal to the edge of padding. Place small tucks in plaster as necessary. At end of each roll, moisten hands and smooth plaster in the direction wrap was applied. Repeat for a total of three layers.

8. When plastering through the webspace, pinch the plaster so that it lies in the trough formed by the padding. If fingers are not included in cast do not plaster over the distal palmar crease to allow full movement of the MCP joints.

9. After completing the second plaster layer, mould well to ensure conformity. Form the transverse palmar arch by applying gentle pressure with fingers on the volar surface, and the palm of hand on the dorsal surface. Hold for 2-3 minutes until plaster has set slightly before applying a third layer.

10. Finish the cast by turning the padding, felt and excess stockinette over the proximal and distal edges of the plaster and secure with a small strip of plaster bandage. Felt strips through the thumb webspace can be trimmed and then tucked in before securing stockinette with a small strip of plaster bandage.

11. Check to ensure two fingers can fit snugly in at each end of the cast. The cast will take 24-48 hours to dry so should be placed upon a soft surface and pressure avoided.

Post casting the size, colour, and temperature of the hand, and the capillary refill of nail beds should be monitored. Staff and family members should be instructed how to monitor the cast and procedures to follow should emergency removal of cast be necessary.

Casts may be worn for 4-10 days in a series over 3-4 weeks. Casts are removed by soaking in water, or with a plaster saw. On removal of the cast, the limb is re-evaluated, washed, gently mobilized and then recast, if appropriate. To bivalve the last cast saw the cast in half and carefully cut through the padding and lining. The stockinette is removed and a thin strip of felt taped over the edges of the plaster. New stockinette, and Velcro® straps are secured in place with thin strips of plaster. When applying a bivalved cast, it is important that the limb is positioned accurately in the cast to ensure no problems arise from pressure.

WEARING SCHEDULE

The literature on upper limb orthotic and casting interventions shows great variability in wearing schedules in hours per day as well as total duration in days, months and even years. Interventions to address functional goals have obvious application schedules, while interventions that address prevention of muscle and connective tissue contracture in persons with CNS dysfunction may require a life long commitment. Interventions using mobilizing principles to address deficits in passive ROM require regular review and modification until ROM goals have been achieved. Then maintenance protocols should be implemented.

Studies by McPherson et al.[44] and Rose and Shah[56] give indications to positive short-term outcomes. Tardieu and Tardieu[63] suggest sustained stretch should last for 6 hours daily to prevent deformities in spastic muscles, while studies by Sheenan et al.[57] and Lannin et al.[34, 36] suggest 10 -12 hours per day over periods less than 5 weeks have minimal clinically significant effect. High quality studies over many months and even years are required.

Immediately following initial orthotic or cast application surveillance for at least one hour is required to ensure no problems arise. Patients, parents or carers assume respon-

sibility for the intervention at this time. If there are no issues the time of application is increased gradually to the maximum recommended. Issues of concern regarding casts should be addressed immediately, with orthotic wear ceased until adjustments can be made.

Wearing Recommendations

1. Orthoses designed to address functional objectives should be worn during functional times only and never worn during periods of rest or sleep.
2. In the presence of spasticity with associated contracture, evidence suggests a period of orthosis wearing of six hours per day is necessary to maintain extensibility of tissues in the long term. Orthoses should not compromise potential to use the affected hand.
4. Orthoses designed to address range of motion deficits may be worn at night when their impact upon functional performance is minimal. In addition, this affords extended periods during which tissues can be maintained at end range. ROM gained by serial casting must be sustained by bivalve casts or orthoses until the risk of potential contracture is diminished or active motion is sufficient to maintain joint motion.
5. Orthoses that have a preventative objective, whether that is to protect skin integrity or maintain length of tissue, need to be worn for as long as the risk exists. A lifetime of orthotic intervention is often a possibility.

CONCLUSION

The efficacy of orthoses and casting for clients with upper limb hypertonicity has been investigated in numerous studies and examined in a number of systematic reviews.[2, 27, 35, 37, 45, 64, 65] The conclusion from these findings is that there is insufficient evidence to establish or disprove the effectiveness of these interventions for upper limb hypertonicity in adults and children with congenital and acquired CNS dysfunction. It is suggested that the scarcity of high-level research evidence is not surprising as evaluating the efficacy of upper limb interventions requires great attention in the research design to the variability of CNS motor disorder presentation and the desired individual clinical outcomes.[33]

When attempting to make sense of the recommendations pertaining to use of orthotic interventions for persons with neurological dysfunction, therapists must consider the purpose of the intervention as one would in other domains of hand therapy. A 'hand orthosis' is not a panacea for hand dysfunction with significant differences between orthoses that immobilize compared to those that mobilize tissues. Hand orthoses worn during sleep will not improve function during the day, orthoses that immobilize joints are more likely to contribute to loss of range of motion than increase it, orthoses worn intermittently for a 4 week interval are unlikely to prevent loss of range of motion in joints over many months and years when the primary cause of contracture formation has not been resolved.

Information contained in this chapter reflects the authors many years of clinical experience in addressing upper limb neurological dysfunction combined with a considered analysis of the literature. It provides a framework for clinical reasoning based upon the clients presentation, peripheral musculoskeletal problems associated with hypertonicity and spasticity, understanding of the common patterns of deformity, options for intervention using a variety of designs and materials, and practical suggestions in design and fabrication, to assist those therapists prepared to undertake this challenging yet rewarding area of orthotic intervention.

References

1. Ada L, O'Dwyer N, O'Neill E. Relation between spasticity, weakness and contracture of the elbow flexors and upper limb activity after stroke: an observational study. Disability and Rehabilitation. 2006;28: 891–897.

2. Autti-Ramo ISJ, Anttila H, Malmivaara A, Makela M. Effectiveness of upper and lower limb casting and orthoses in children with cerebral palsy: an overview of review articles. American Journal Physical Medicine and Rehabilitation. 2006;85: 89–103.

3. Barrett R, Lichtwark G. Gross muscle morphology and structure in spastic cerebral palsy: a systematic review. Developmental Medicine and Child Neurology. 2010;52(9): 794–804.

4. Bürge E, Kupper D, Finckh A et al. Neutral functional realignment splint prevents hand pain in patients with subacute stroke: a randomized trial. Archives of Physical Medicine and Rehabilitation. 2008;89(10): 1857–1862.

5. Burtner PA, Poole JL, Torres T et al. Effect of wrist hand splints on grip, pinch, manual dexterity, and

muscle activation in children with spastic hemiplegia: a preliminary study. Journal Hand Therapy. 2008;21: 36–42.

6. Casey CA, Kratz EJ. Soft tissue splinting with neoprene: The thumb abduction supinator splint. American Journal of Occupational Therapy. 1988;42: 395–398.

7. Childers MK, Biswas SS, Petroski G, Merveille O. Inhibitory casting decreases a vibratory inhibition index of the H-reflex in the spastic upper limb. Archives Physical Medicine Rehabilitation. 1999;80:714–716.

8. Copley J, Turpin M, Brosnan J, Nelson A. Understanding and negotiating: Reasoning processes used by an occupational therapist to individualize intervention decisions for people with upper limb hypertonicity. Disability and Rehabilitation. 2007; 1–13.

9. Copley J, Watson-Will A, Dent K. Upper limb casting for clients with cerebral palsy: a clinical report. Australian Occupational Therapy Journal. 1996; 43: 39–50.

10. Cruickshank DA, O'Neill DA. Upper extremity inhibitive casting in a boy with spastic quadriplegia. American Journal of Occupational Therapy. 1990;44: 552–555.

11. Elliott CM, Reid SL, Alderson J, et al. Lycra arm splints in conjunction with goal-directed training can improve movement in children with cerebral palsy. NeuroRehabilitation. 28(1), 47–54.

12. Elliott CM, Reid SL, Hamer P, et al. Lycra(*) arm splints improve movement fluency in children with cerebral palsy. Gait and Posture. 2011;33(2): 214–9.

13. Exner CE, Bonder BR. Comparative effects of three hand splints on bilateral hand use, grasp, and arm-hand posture in hemiplegic children: A pilot study. Occupational Therapy Journal of Research. 1983;3:75–92.

14. Fehlings D, Novak I, Berweck S, et al. Botulinum toxin assessment, intervention and follow-up for paediatric upper limb hypertonicity: international consensus statement. European Journal of Neurology. 2010;17 (Suppl. 2): 38–56

15. Flett PJ. Rehabilitation of spasticity and related problems in childhood cerebral palsy. Journal of Paediatrics and Child Health. 2003;39: 6–14.

16. Freehafer NA. Flexion and supination deformities of the elbow in tetraplegia. Paraplegia. 1977/78;3: 221–225.

17. Georgiades M, Elliott C, Wilton J et al. Description of the progression of hand deformity in children with cerebral palsy. Perth; Edith Cowan University.

18. Gorter J, Becher J, Oosterom I, et al. 'To stretch or not to stretch in children with cerebral palsy.' Developmental Medicine and Child Neurology. 2007;49: 10.

19. Gracies JM, Fitzpatrick R, Wilson L, et al. Lycra® garments designed for patients with upper limb spasticity: mechanical effects in normal subjects. Archives of Physical Medicine and Rehabilitation. 1997;78(10):1066–71

20. Gracies JM. Pathophysiology of impairment in patients with spasticity and use of stretch as a treatment of spastic hypertonia. Physical Medicine Rehabilitation Clinics North America. 2001;12: 747–68.

21. Gracies JM. Pathophysiology of spastic paresis. I: Paresis and soft tissue changes. Muscle Nerve 2005;31:535–551.

22. Gracies JM. Pathophysiology of spastic paresis. II: Emergence of muscle overactivity. Muscle Nerve. 2005;31:552–571

23. Harvey L, De Jong I, Goehl G, Mardwedel S. Twelve weeks of nightly stretch does not reduce thumb webspace contractures in people with a neurological condition: a randomised controlled trial. Australian Journal of Physiotherapy. 2006;52(4): 251–8.

24. Hill J. The effects of casting on upper extremity motor disorders after brain injury. America Journal of Occupational Therapy. 1994;48: 219–24.

25. Hoare BJ, Wallen MA, Imms C, et al. Botulinum toxin A as an adjunct to treatment in the management of the upper limb in children with spastic cerebral palsy

(UPDATE). Cochrane Database Systematic Reviews. 2010: CD003469.

26. House JH, Gwathmey FW and Fidler MO. A dynamic approach to the thumb in palm deformity in cerebral palsy. Journal of Bone and Joint Surgery. 1981;63A: 216–225.

27. Katalinic OM, Harvey LA, Herbert RD, et al. Stretch for the treatment and prevention of contractures. The Cochrane Collaboration. 2010 Published by John Wiley and Sons, Ltd.

28. King T. Plaster splinting as a means of reducing elbow flexor spasticity: A case study. American Journal of Occupational Therapy. 1982;36: 671–673.

29. Kuipers K, McKenna K, Carlson G. Factors influencing occupational therapists' clinical decision making for clients with upper limb performance dysfunction following brain injury. British Journal of Occupational Therapy. 2006;69: 106–114.

30. Kuipers K, Rassafiania M, Ashburnera J, et al. Do clients with acquired brain injury use the splints prescribed by occupational therapists? A descriptive study. NeuroRehabilitation. 2009;24: 365–375.

31. Kwah LK, Harvey LA, Diong JHL, Herbert RD. Half of the adults who present to hospital with stroke develop at least one contracture within six months: an observational study. Journal of Physiotherapy. 2012;28: 41–47.

32. Lance JW. What is spasticity? Lancet. 1990;335(1): 606.

33. Lannin NA, Ada L. Neurorehabilitation splinting: Theory and principles of clinical use. NeuroRehabilitation. 2011;28: 21–28.

34. Lannin NA, Cusick A, McCluskey A, Herbert RD. Effects of splinting on wrist contracture after stroke: A randomized controlled trial. Stroke. 2007;38: 111–116.

35. Lannin NA, Herbert RD. Is hand splinting effective for adults following stroke? A systematic review and methodologic critique of published research. Clinical Rehabilitation. 2003;17(8):807–16.

36. Lannin NA, Horsley SA, Herbert R, McCluskey A, Cusick A. Splinting the hand in the functional position after brain impairment: a randomized, controlled trial. Archives of Physical Medicine and Rehabilitation. 2003;84: 297–302.

37. Lannin N, Cusick A. A systematic review of upper extremity casting for children and adults with central nervous system motor disorders. Clinical Rehabilitation. 2007;21: 963–976.

38. Law M, Cadman D, Rosenbaum P, et al. Neurodevelopmental therapy and upper-extremity inhibitive casting for children with cerebral palsy. Developmental Medicine and Child Neurology. 1991;33: 379–387.

39. Law M, Russell D, Pollock N, et al. A comparison of intensive neurodevelopmental therapy plus casting and a regular occupational therapy program for children with cerebral palsy. Developmental Medicine and Child Neurology. 1997;39: 664–70.

40. Lehmkuhl LD, Thoi LL, Baize C, et al. Multimodal treatment of joint contractures in patients with severe brain injury: cast, effectiveness and integration of therapies in the application of serial/inhibitive casts. Journal Head Trauma Rehabilitation. 1990;5: 23–42.

41. Lieber RL, Steinman S, Barash IA, Chambers H. Structural and functional change in spastic skeletal muscle. Muscle and Nerve. 2004;29:615–27.

42. Lockhart J, Margallo K, Russell D. Serial casting in the upper extremity of children with cerebral palsy: A Review of the literature. CanChild Centre for Childhood Disability Research. Canada. 2010. p. 1987–1990.

43. Louwers A, Meester-Delver A, Folmer K, et al. Immediate effect of a wrist and thumb brace on bimanual activities in children with hemiplegic cerebral palsy. Developmental Medicine and Child Neurology. 2011;53(4): 321–6.

44. McPherson JJ, Kriemeyer D, Alderks M, et al. A comparison of dorsal and volar resting splints in the reduction of hypertonus. American Journal of Occupational

Therapy. 1982;36: 664–670.

45. Mortenson PA, Eng JJ. The use of casts in the management of joint mobility and hypertonia following brain injury in adults: a systematic review. Physical Therapy. 2003; 83: 648–53.

46. Moseley A, Hassett L, Leung J, et al. Serial casting versus positioning for the treatment of elbow contractures in adults with traumatic brain injury: a randomized controlled trial. Clinical Rehabilitation. 2008;22(5): 406–17.

47. O'Dwyer NJ, Ada L, Neilson PD. Spasticity and muscle contracture following stroke. Brain. 1996;119: 1737–49.

48. O'Dwyer NJ, Neilson PD, Nash J. Mechanism of muscle growth related to muscle contracture in cerebral palsy (review). Developmental Medicine and Child Neurology. 1989;31: 543–7.

49. Pandyan AD, Cameron M, Powell J, et al. Contractures in the post-stroke wrist: a pilot study of its time course of development and its association with upper limb recovery. Clinical Rehabilitation. 2003;17(1): 88–95.

50. Pizzi A, Carlucci G, Falsini C, et al. Evaluation of upper-limb spasticity after stroke: a clinical and neuro-physiologic study. Archives of Physical Medicine and Rehabilitation. 2005;86:410–5.

51. Pizzi A, Carlucci G, Falsini C, et al. Application of a volar static splint in poststroke spasticity of the upper limb. Archives of Physical Medicine and Rehabilitation. 2005;86: 1855–9.

52. Pohl M, Rückreim S, Mehrholz J, et al. Effectiveness of serial casting in patients with severe cerebral spasticity: a comparison study. Archives of Physical Medicine and Rehabilitation. 2002;83:784–90.

53. Pontén E, Gantelius S, Lieber RL. Intraoperative muscle measurements reveal a relationship between contracture formation and muscle remodelling. Muscle and Nerve. 2007;36(1):47–54.

54. Rassafiani M, Ziviani J, Rodger S, Dalgleish, L. Occupational therapists' decision-making in the management of clients with upper limb hypertonicity. Scandinavian Journal of Occupational Therapy. 2008;15(2): 105–15.

55. Reid DT, Sochaniwskyj A. Influences of a hand positioning device on upper extremity control of children with cerebral palsy. International Journal of Rehabilitation Research. 1992;15:15–29.

56. Rose V, Shah S. A comparative study on the immediate effects of hand orthoses on reduction of hypertonus. Australian Occupational Therapy Journal 1987;34: 59–64.

57. Sheenan JL, Winzeler-Mercy U, Mundie MH. A randomized controlled pilot study to obtain the best estimate of the size of the effect of a thermoplastic resting splint on spasticity in the stroke-affected wrist and fingers. Clinical Rehabilitation. 2006;20: 1032–1037.

58. Smith LH, Harris SR. Upper extremity inhibitive casting for the child with cerebral palsy. Physical and Occupational Therapy in Paediatrics. 1985;5: 71–79.

59. Steer V. Upper limb serial casting of individuals with cerebral palsy-a preliminary report. Australian Journal of Occupational Therapy. 1989;36: 69–77.

60. Tabary JC, Tabary C, Tardieu C et al. Physiological and structural changes in the cat's soleus muscle due to immobilization at different lengths by plaster casts. Journal of Physiology. 1972;224: 231–244.

61. Tardieu C, Huet de la Tour E, Bret MD, Tardieu G. Muscle hypoextensibility in children with cerebral palsy: I. Clinical and experimental observations. Archives of Physical Medicine and Rehabilitation. 1982;63:97–102.

62. Tardieu C, Tabary J, Tabary C, Huet DeLa Tour E. Comparison of the sarcomere number adaptation in young and adult animals. Influence of tendon adaptation. Journal of Physiology. 1977;73:1045–55.

63. Tardieu Y, Tardieu C. Cerebral palsy. Mechanical evaluation and conservative correction of limb joint contracture. Clinical Orthopaedics and Related Research. 1987;219: 63–69.

64. Teplicky R, Law M, Russell D. The effectiveness of casts, orthoses, and splints for children with neurological disorders. Infants Young Children. 2002; 15: 42–50.

65. Tyson S, Kent R. The effect of upper limb orthotics after stroke: A systematic review. NeuroRehabilitation. 2011;28: 29–36

66. Wallen M, O'Flaherrty S. The use of the soft splint in the management of spasticity of the upper limb. Australian Journal of Occupational Therapy. 1991;38: 227–231.

67. Wilton JC. Casting, splinting, and physical and occupational therapy of hand deformity and dysfunction in cerebral palsy. [corrected] [published erratum appears in Hand Clinics 2004; 20: 227]. Hand Clinics. 2003;19: 573–584.

68. Wilton JC. Hand splinting: principles of design and fabrication. London: WB Saunders, 1997: 168–97.

69. Yasukawa A. Case report – upper extremity casting: adjunct treatment for a child with cerebral palsy hemiplegia. American Journal of Occupational Therapy. 1990;44: 840–46.

70. Yasukawa A, Malas BS, Gaebler-Spira DJ. Efficacy for maintenance of elbow range of motion of two types of orthotic devices: a case series. Journal Prosthetics Orthotics. 2003;15: 72–77

71. Young RR. Spasticity: a review. Neurology. 199;444: 512–520

72. Zancolli EA, Zancolli ER. Surgical management of the hemiplegic spastic hand in cerebral palsy. Surgical Clinics of North America. 1981;61: 395–406.

APPENDIX

Abbreviation Key

ABI	acquired brain injury		FCR	flexor carpi radialis
ADL	activities of daily living		FCU	flexor carpi ulnaris
AHTA	Australian Hand Therapy Association		FDP	flexor digitorum profundus
AP	adductor pollicus		FDS	flexor digitorum superficialis
APB	abductor pollicus brevis		FPB	flexor pollicus brevis
APL	abductor pollicus longus		FPL	flexor pollicus longus
AROM	active range of motion		HTTP	high temperature thermoplastics
ASHT	American Society of Hand Therapists		IP	interphalangeal
BoNT	Botulinum neurotoxin		ISO	International Organization for Standardization
CP	cerebral palsy		LTTP	low temperature thermoplastics
CMC	carpometacarpal		MCP	metacarpophalangeal
CNS	Central nervous system		NDT	neurodevelopmental therapy
DIP	distal interphalangeal		NHDC	Neurological Hand Deformity Classification
DI	dorsal interossei		PIP	proximal interphalangeal
DRU	distal radioulnar		PL	palmaris longus
ECRB	extensor carpi radialis brevis		PROM	passive range of motion
ECRL	extensor carpi radialis longus		PRU	proximal radioulnar
ECU	extensor carpi ulnaris		ROM	range of motion
EDC	extensor digitorum communis		TAC	torque angle curve
EPB	extensor pollicus brevis		TERT	total end range time
EPL	extensor pollicus longus		TFCC	triangular fibrocartilage complex
ERT	end range time		TROM	torque range of motion

Orthosis Splint

Articular
impacting on joint motion

Non Articular
impact soft tissue not joints,
anatomic segment

Immobilization
Prevent
movement at
joints.
Static

Mobilization
Gain specific
passive / active
ROM.
Serial static
Serial Progressive
Dynamic

Restriction
Pathology
specific
movement
control.

**Torque
Transmission**
neural
pathology.

UL Joint to Which Intervention Directed
shoulder, elbow, forearm, wrist, finger and thumb joints

Basis of Orthosis
Describes inclusion of proximal or distal joints

Finger

Thumb

Hand

Wrist &
Hand

Wrist &
Forearm

Forearm &
Elbow

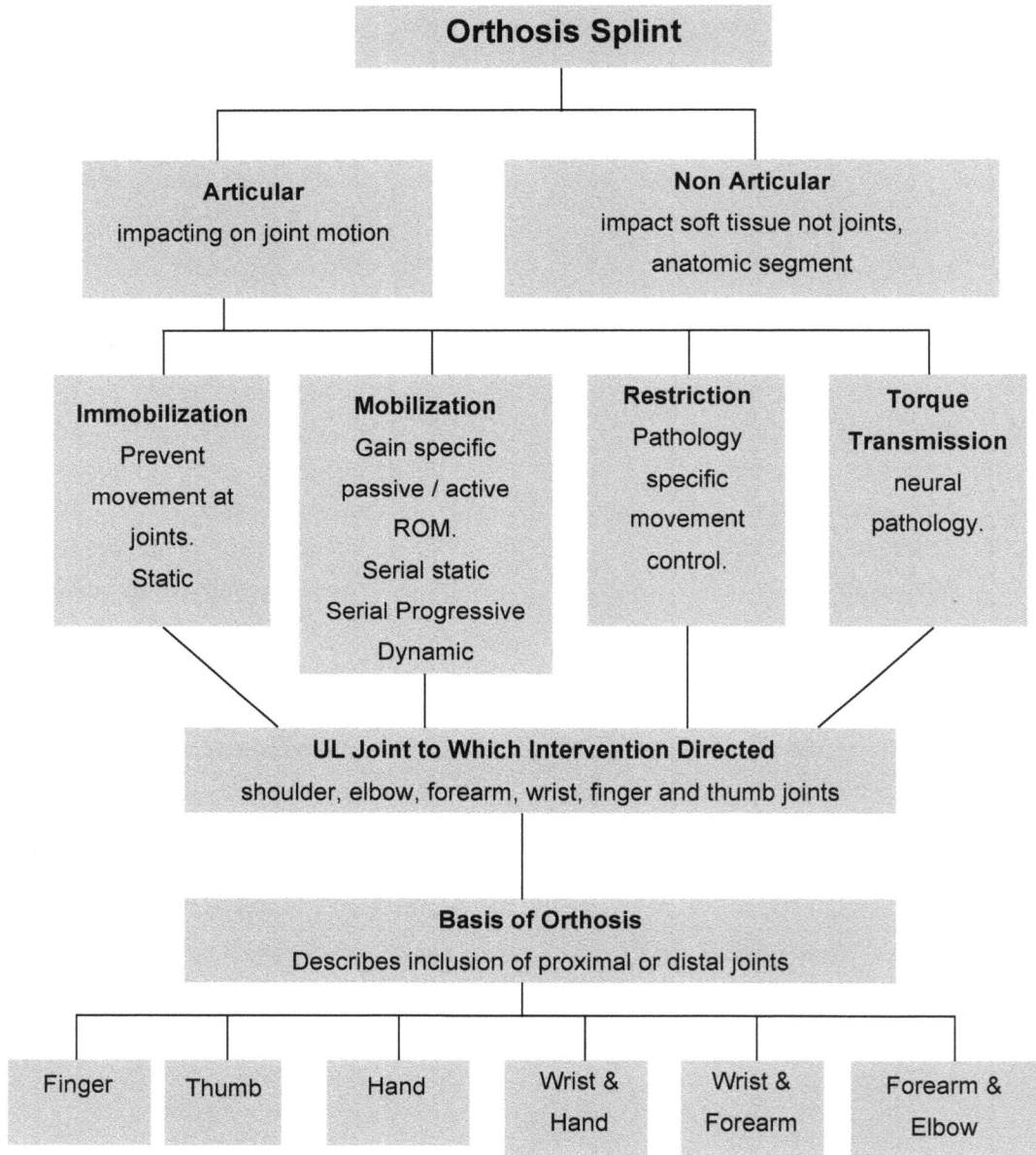

The full AHTA Splint/Orthosis Schedule is available via the Australian Hand Therapy Association website. Members may access via the Library Resources. Non members may request a copy via 'Help' link.   www.ahta.com.au

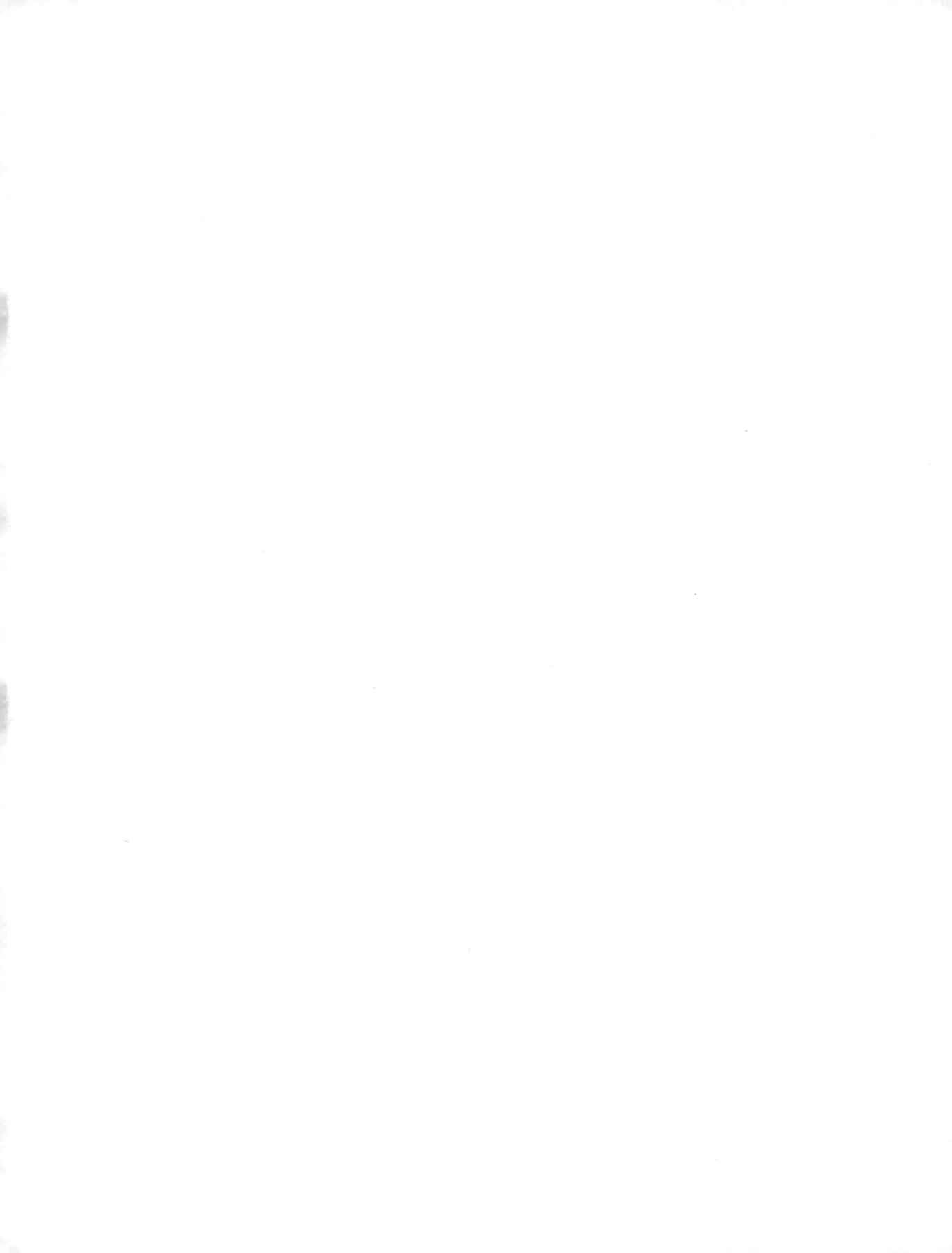

www.ingramcontent.com/pod-product-compliance
Lightning Source LLC
Chambersburg PA
CBHW050105220326
41598CB00043B/7392